AN INTRODUCTION TO
NEUROSURGERY

BRYAN JENNETT M.D. F.R.C.S.

Professor of Neurosurgery
The Institute of Neurological Sciences, Glasgow
and The University of Glasgow

Foreword by

CHARLES WELLS C.B.E. S.Pk. LL.D. F.R.C.S.
Professor Emeritus of Surgery, University of Liverpool

Third Edition

WILLIAM HEINEMANN MEDICAL BOOKS LIMITED
LONDON

First published 1964
Second edition 1970
Reprinted 1973
Third edition 1977
Reprinted 1978

© by Bryan Jennett, 1977

ISBN 0 433 17302 5

Text set in 10/11 pt Monotype Times New Roman, printed by letterpress,
and bound in Great Britain at The Pitman Press, Bath

Foreword

"There is a rare and enviable quality and clarity in Mr Jennett's prose."   Lord Cohen of Birkenhead

These words are taken from the introduction to another important work by the same author, published only two years ago. In his foreword Lord Cohen also remarks that "he (Mr Jennett) has been singularly successful in finding apt quotations for his . . . headings." I am sure that I could have found for my own heading no fitter words than Lord Cohen's to express my admiration for the way in which this present work is written.

The 1962 monograph is described in the foreword as a "study in depth" of three hundred and eighty-one patients suffering from epilepsy following a blunt head injury. What is remarkable is that the same quality and clarity should distinguish, as it most certainly does, so different a contribution as this, which is a study in breadth. The author is never superficial but, by the avoidance of repetition, by a nice choice of words and by a strict economy in their use, he surveys, indeed he explains, possibly for the first time in this small compass, the whole field of neurosurgery. What is even more remarkable is that he contrives this in a positive and unequivocal fashion, never too dogmatic and never departing from the logic of his argument. The reader is informed by the author briefly, clearly, precisely and is left in no doubt about his meaning.

Few surgeons today can avoid the trend towards specialisation but none can afford to ignore his grounding in the general discipline of surgery itself, and none can afford to ignore the changing concepts of neurophysiology or their impact upon neurosurgery. The one touches his daily work: the other may face him as an urgent challenge at any moment. Many who are conscious of these responsibilities will read this book with pleasure and consult it with profit.

I join Lord Cohen with pride in claiming some part in the early days of Mr Jennett's medical and surgical education in Liverpool, but his rare gift of communication is his alone.

Charles Wells

Kuala Lumpur
March, 1964

Preface to the First Edition

The pioneering days are over. Neurosurgery is an accepted part of medical practice, more widely available than ever before and expanding rapidly.

Yet as recently as 1961 a *Lancet* Editorial* referred to the delay in the diagnosis and treatment of conditions requiring neurosurgery in these words: "Even now, thirty five years after modern neurosurgical methods were instituted in this country, the neurosurgical specialty may still lack the full confidence of the public or the profession. Or is the neurosurgeon right when he says that early symptoms and signs are not known as well as they might be . . .?"

Part of the responsibility for this must lie with the specialty for not having made itself more intelligible and more accessible. As a result there is insufficient general awareness of what can and cannot be done, and of what is regarded as urgent and why. Neurosurgery is still often regarded as mysterious and difficult, and in any event of very limited value to most patients; consequently it is too often turned to only as the last resort.

This book endeavours to dispel the mystery, and to encourage the increasing numbers who are becoming involved with neurosurgery in one role or another to understand its principles. Clearly such a book should not try to be comprehensive. Selected topics are treated at relative length rather than more topics sketchily; operative details are included only for those urgent procedures which may require to be done as emergencies in general surgical units, and to illustrate principles of approach. For those who wish to know more suggestions for further reading are made; these references have been chosen for their authority and scope, for their inclusion of adequate reference to previous literature and for their ready availability.

The neurosurgeon's work has expanded in the last decade to include the surgical treatment of subarachnoid hæmorrhage, the treatment of movement disorders by stereotaxic surgery, and an increased share in the surgery of trauma. Brain tumours no longer take up most of his attention. Rapid advances in neuroradiology, and the development of other diagnostic aids, has brought about changes in the diagnostic approach to intracranial conditions.

The implications of these developments has not yet been widely recognised. Neurosurgery in Britain is the child of traditional neurology but its relationship to the wider fields of modern surgery and radiology is gradually becoming as important. A carefully taken and detailed history of the patient's illness will always be paramount in diagnosing

* *Lancet*, 1961, ii, 917, "Time in the Machine."

disorders of the nervous system. But many of the clinical signs and syndromes, traditionally elicited with such skill and care, are proving to be less reliable localising features with the development of a more dynamic concept of the disorganisation of the nervous system caused by disease.

It may be more important initially for the surgeon to know in which compartment of the skull the disease is situated, rather than which precise aspect of nervous function is most affected. The appropriate investigation can then be initiated and there will be no delay if urgent surgery is needed. Consideration has always to be given to the urgency and priority that diagnostic and therapeutic measures should command; life-saving treatment cannot always be delayed until investigations are complete and the exact anatomical and pathological diagnosis is beyond doubt. Instead of the traditional exposition of the anatomy and examination of the nervous system there is therefore a discussion of the symptoms and signs of mass lesions in which the emphasis is on localisation within the main compartments of the skull.

It is impossible to acknowledge, even if it were possible to remember or recognise, all the influences and help which are drawn on in writing a book. My friend Robert Tym, as well as writing the last two chapters, read and re-read the text as did my wife, Dr Sheila Jennett. They both knew the kind of book I wished to write and did their best to keep me to my intentions and I am grateful to them for their diligence and perseverance in trying to bring me to order. Dr John Evanson read most of the chapters from the viewpoint of a physician, and Mr Michael Lee those on spinal conditions from an orthopædic standpoint; each made constructive suggestions.

The illustrations are the work of Dr Robert Ollerenshaw and Mr R. Neave in Manchester, and Mr Gabriel Donald and Mr Hugh Gray in Glasgow; Dr Roger Whittaker composed the arterial tree for Fig. 15 from a study of many normal angiograms. I am grateful to Mr Richard Johnson and Dr Reginald Reid in Manchester and to Mr J. Sloan Robertson and Dr Leslie Steven in Glasgow for allowing the reproduction of radiographs taken in their departments. Permission to reproduce illustrations was kindly given as follows: *Acta Radiologica* Fig. 5a, *The British Journal of Radiology* Fig. 18, Butterworths Fig. 5b, *The Journal of the Faculty of Radiologists* Fig. 20, The Controller, H.M. Stationery Office (from *Medical Research Council War Memorandum No. 7—Aids to the Investigation of Peripheral Nerve Injuries*) Fig. 50b and c. The authors are acknowledged in the legends.

Mr Owen R. Evans and Miss Ninetta Martyn of Heinemann's have shown courtesy and patience in meeting the various demands and crises which they must by now have come to expect from authors.

GLASGOW   W. B. J.
March, 1964

Preface to the Second Edition

In the six years since the first edition there have been significant technical developments affecting methods of investigation and treatment, and most changes in the text apply to these areas. Investigation by radioactive isotopes has developed rapidly and the section on brain scanning has been expanded to include other radio-isotope techniques. Better understanding of the effects of anæsthesia on intracranial pressure has called for major rewriting in Chapter 7. The section on the endocrine effects of pituitary tumours and the tests available has been re-arranged and expanded. Many small alterations have been made in the head injury chapters to take account of improved understanding of various aspects both of pathology and of management. Chapter 11 (previously 13) has been largely rewritten because so much has recently been published about both hæmorrhagic and ischæmic vascular lesions; the same goes for hydrocephalus and spina bifida, and the opportunity has been taken to include some other cranial and spinal deformities in these chapters.

The last part deals with lesion-making in the nervous system, a field in which the widespread adoption of stereotaxic techniques is opening up new possibilities. One chapter deals with the principles of stereotaxis and lesion-making, and there follow modifications of the original material on pain, movement disorders and hypophysectomy, together with a new section dealing with surgery for epilepsy and psycho-surgery.

As an introduction this book aims to provide a framework within which more detailed and up-to-date information can be accommodated. With this in mind some reorganisation of the chapters into different parts has been undertaken. The first part now deals with intracranial space-occupying lesions in general, rather than with tumours in particular, and the first chapter has been expanded to take account of the more dynamic aspects of the physiopathology of expanding intracranial lesions. The sections of the previous Chapters 1 and 2 which dealt with mental symptoms have been combined to form a separate new chapter. At the end of the chapter on neuroradiology a scheme outlining the strategy of investigation has been included, as a summary of Chapters 5 and 6. The pathology and clinical aspects of intracranial tumours are now brought together in a single chapter (9) and the nomenclature of neuro-ectodermal tumours has been adjusted, under the guidance of Professor Hume Adams, to conform with current thinking among British neuropathologists. All drug dosages have been converted to the metric system and temperatures to Centigrade. The American names of drugs mentioned are given on page 356.

An introductory book is no place to quote statistics from personal clinical series, but in response to specific suggestions three sets of figures have been given: the incidence of different intracranial tumours in a series of over 1,600 collected in the Glasgow Institute; some data of use in predicting the risk of late traumatic epilepsy, based on my own studies; and some very approximate figures about the results of conservative and surgical treatment of intracranial aneurysms, based on recent reports. The plea for more references has been met by almost 200 new items under "Further Reading" at the end of each chapter, but no references are included in the text in order to make this as easy as possible to read.

W.B.J.

The University
Glasgow
January, 1970

Preface to the Third Edition

The years since the last edition have seen some changes of emphasis in attitude in certain areas of neurosurgery. There have been three international symposia devoted wholly to intracranial pressure in the last 5 years, and these are reflected in the re-writing of the chapter (1) on the physiopathology of intracranial pressure. Better understanding of altered states of consciousness and the assessment of coma have necessitated re-writing the chapter on mental disorders associated with intracranial organic pathology; this now includes a discussion of brain death and related unresponsive states.

The development of EMI scanning (computerised axial tomography) has transformed the investigation of intracranial disease—for those fortunate to have access to this new machine. The chapters (5, 6) on preliminary investigations and contrast radiology have been restructured with this development in mind, but alternative methods will obviously remain important, both for circumstances in which EMI scanning is unavailable, as well as for conditions for which it is inappropriate or provides incomplete information. The important topic of head injury has received a good deal of study in the last few years, and the rethinking of some aspects of this problem are mainly reflected in a restructured chapter 12, which now includes classifications of severity of injury and of outcome after brain damage. Several of the topics previously dealt with under post-operative care and complications (chapter 8) have been transferred to chapter 13, which deals with the management of head injury; after all an operation can be regarded as a planned and controlled head injury. The chapters on tumours (9) and on vascular lesions (11) include comments on newer methods of treatment, chiefly chemotherapy and microsurgery respectively.

Stereotaxis is much less frequently done than previously and this is reflected in shortening the text on this and re-distributing the material which was formally in Chapter 21. The reference lists have been considerably expanded and up-dated.

More than twenty new illustrations are included. I acknowledge permission as follows: fig. 1 is from "Clinical Neurosurgery", published in 1975 by Williams & Wilkins; fig. 5a is from *Nursing Times*, fig. 5b from the *Journal of the Royal College of Physicians*; figs. 7, 61 and 77 are from "Scientific Foundations of Surgery" (Heinemann); figs. 20, 52, 54 and 56 are from "Operative Surgery", Volume 14 (Butterworth); fig. 58 is from *The Lancet*; fig. 59 is from "Epilepsy after Non-missile Head Injuries" (Heinemann); fig. 71 is from Lewin's "The Management of Head Injuries" (Bailliere, Tindall).

I am grateful to Mr. Graham Teasdale for his advice about many of the chapters which have been revised; Dr. Leslie Steven has kindly provided EMI scan prints. My secretaries Sally Brown and Margaret Smith have miraculously transformed scribbled manuscripts into acceptable typescript. As usual Miss Ninetta Martyn of Heinemann's has been patient and helpful.

B.J.

THE UNIVERSITY
  GLASGOW
January, 1977

Contents

List of Illustrations

"Life is the art of drawing sufficient conclusions from insufficient premises."

SAMUEL BUTLER
Notebooks, 1912

I: Intracranial Space-Occupying Lesions

Introduction

Tumour surgery once made up the bulk of the neurosurgeon's work. Although this is no longer so the diagnosis and management of patients suspected of harbouring various intracranial space-occupying lesions illustrate most basic techniques of diagnosis and management.

Local masses commonly disclose their whereabouts by interfering with the function of the neighbouring part of the brain and producing focal signs. How they do so is uncertain, but possible mechanisms are displacement or distortion of nervous structures and alterations in local blood flow due to occlusion of arteries or veins, with the development of areas of ischæmia or congestion.

But the effects of local intracranial masses extend much further than the immediately adjacent brain. They are space-occupying lesions within the cranium, the only body cavity which is wholly rigid and inelastic. Consequently raised intracranial pressure develops and eventually compression of the brain as a whole becomes a feature of most tumours, as of other intracranial masses such as abscess and hæmatoma. Because tumours usually grow gradually it is easier to study the evolution of the various phases of brain compression in patients with tumours than in those with more rapidly developing mass lesions, in whom the clinical course is often telescoped into a few days or even hours. The processes involved are the same, however. What follows about tumours applies to other lesions; they may be indistinguishable but can often be recognised because of their clinical context, such as the association of hæmatoma with recent head injury or of abscess with chronic ear disease.

Brain compression is important because it frequently dominates the clinical picture and threatens the patient's life, and the methods of investigation and treatment employed may have to be modified on this account. The features of raised pressure, which are the same wherever and whatever the mass may be, are discussed in the first chapter. The next discusses mental disorders, which may or may not reflect localised lesions.

The remaining chapters deal with symptomatology, diagnosis and treatment in the order in which the clinician normally works. That is to

1

say they consider in turn the questions: where is the mass in the skull? (Chapter 3), are there serious brain shifts? (Chapter 4), are clinical impressions confirmed by investigations? (Chapters 5 and 6), what is to be done about it? (Chapter 7), and what may happen after operation? (Chapter 8). The clinical characteristics and management of the commoner pathological types of intracranial mass lesion are discussed in the three chapters of Part II.

CHAPTER 1

Raised Intracranial Pressure

Physiopathology
> Blood volume
> CSF volume and circulation
> Brain volume
> The mass itself
> Effect of pressure on function

Clinical
> Headache
> Papillœdema
> Vomiting

Physiopathology

Changes in intracranial pressure (ICP) reflect changes in the volume of the intracranial contents, which are made up of brain, cerebrospinal fluid and blood (fig. 1). Although each of these may change in volume the rapidity with which each can alter varies greatly—brain and CSF volume changing much less rapidly than intracranial blood volume. Fluctuations in blood volume occur frequently in patients already suffering from more slowly developing space-taking lesions which affect the brain or ventricle size, and the effects of these may thus be aggravated or mitigated; moreover blood volume changes can readily be influenced by clinical manoeuvres, which give them additional importance.

Intracranial blood volume

Cerebral arterioles dilate rapidly if $PaCO_2$ rises above or PaO_2 falls below normal, and as a result ICP rises (fig. 2). Changes in blood gases are usually due to respiratory inadequacy, itself the result of hypoventilation or of pulmonary insufficiency. Hypoventilation may be due to respiratory depression from drugs or from some cerebral condition; sometimes it is due to respiratory obstruction from the aspiration of vomit, from swallowing the tongue or from glottic closure during the onset of an epileptic fit. Any element of respiratory obstruction will cause an additional rise in ICP by passive venous engorgement, because

3

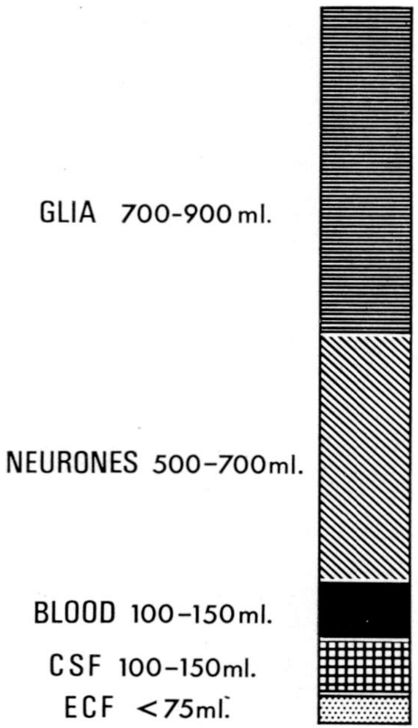

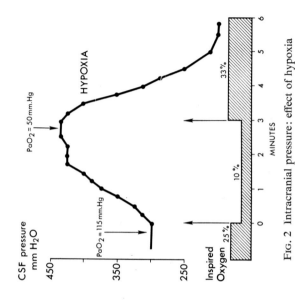

Fig. 2 Intracranial pressure: effect of hypoxia

Response is vasodilatation with increased intra-cranial blood volume; increasing inspired CO_2 percentage has a similar effect. (Record from anaesthetised, curarised dog maintained by mech-anical ventilator.)

Fig. 1 Intracranial contents, by volume

Only the blood volume can be rapidly altered. Note the small volume of extracellular fluid (ECF).

the intracranial venous sinuses are in direct contact with the superior vena cava, no valves intervening; any increase in central venous pressure is therefore immediately transmitted to the intracranial cavity. Patients who are unconscious are liable to one or more of these events, as are any patients suffering from acute brain damage (whether traumatic or not). An epileptic fit may aggravate the situation, as may the administration of pre-medication or of analgesic drugs. These factors, alone or in combination, may precipitate a crisis in a patient whose capacity to compensate for temporary rises in intracranial blood volume is already impaired (see page 7).

CSF volume and circulation

CSF is mainly secreted from the choroid plexuses in the lateral ventricles and passes by way of the foramen of Monro (interventricular

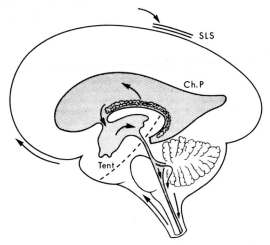

FIG. 3 CSF pathways
Most CSF follows path shown from lateral ventricle choroid plexus to fourth ventricle and then via cisterna ambiens to supratentorial subarachnoid space; some exchange with blood probably occurs throughout the system. (S.L.S. = superior longitudinal sinus; Ch. P. = choroid plexus; Tent = tentorial hiatus.)

foramen) into the third ventricle, down the aqueduct of Sylvius (iter) to the fourth ventricle; from there it escapes into the cisterna magna through the median foramen of Magendie and the lateral foramina of Luschka (fig. 3). Some fluid then passes into the spinal subarachnoid space but probably most passes up through the cisterna ambiens, a narrow space between the mid brain and the edge of the tentorial hiatus (fig. 9), to gain the subarachnoid space over the surface of the cerebral hemispheres, from which it is absorbed into the sagittal sinus by way of the arachnoid villi. A certain amount of CSF is produced and absorbed all along this route but most is produced in the lateral ventricle and most is absorbed by the sagittal sinus. Obstructive hydrocephalus can develop due to a space-occupying lesion encroaching on a part of this system, and in this way a small tumour may have a profound effect on intracranial pressure. The narrower part of this system blocks most readily, leading to dilatation of whatever cavities are above the obstruction. If this block is of the foramen of Monro, one or both lateral ventricles dilate; if of the iter the third ventricle is also involved and if at the outlet from the fourth ventricle then that ventricle will also dilate (fig. 24). Patients with obstructive hydrocephalus can develop very high intracranial pressures which may persist over long periods, although possibly the pressure fluctuates during this time; it is such patients who commonly develop secondary changes in the skull related to the raised pressure (page 54, and fig. 13).

Brain volume

Brain oedema is still incompletely understood, but most agree that two main types can be distinguished, although they may co-exist. *Vasogenic œdema* is characterised by an increase in extracellular fluid, largely due to increased permeability of the endothelium of brain capillaries. This is the type of oedema that is commonly associated with tumour, abscess, contusion, haemorrhage or infarct. It is often focal and may therefore contribute to brain shift and herniation. *Cytotoxic œdema* is associated with swollen cells, glia or neurones, due to the accumulation of intracellular water and sodium. The common cause is hypoxia, particularly due to cardiac arrest; this effect is therefore often seen throughout the brain.

The mass itself

The accumulation of additional intracranial material, be it tumour, pus or blood, must eventually raise pressure but first causes displacement of some normal intracranial contents. The extent of the changes produced will depend mostly on the size of the lesion but somewhat on the speed of development, and on the extent to which the pathological process destroys brain, rather than expanding it with pathological tissue. These factors, and the amount of cerebral œdema or swelling induced by the lesion, largely account for the wide discrepancy found in the effects produced both clinically and pathologically by what may at first seem similar masses in terms of size and site.

Volume/pressure relationships

Another factor which influences the effect which alterations in the volume of various intracranial contents have on ICP is the elastance or stiffness of the brain (inverse of compliance). This depends in part on the extent to which normal compensatory processes have been exhausted. At first CSF and blood are displayed from the intracranial cavity into the more distensible spinal canal, and brain then takes up the sub-arachnoid space vacated by CSF. Brain shifts may also develop, with the formation of internal herniae and the development of the characteristic clinical effects related to these (page 51). Once these compensatory mechanisms are exhausted then the slightest additional increase in blood volume, as due to temporary cerebral vasodilatation, can produce a marked rise in intracranial pressure, and this may precipitate a clinical crisis. This is because each quantum of additional volume causes a much greater effect on pressure when compensatory reserves are no longer available (fig. 4). Intracranial elastance is not,

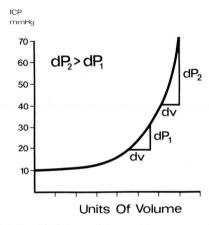

FIG. 4 Relationship between intracranial pressure and volume of space-occupying lesion

At first compensation is possible, but once these mechanisms are exhausted a small increase in volume causes a large increase in pressure. Compensation takes a finite time, and although the graph is relatively independent of the time scale over days, weeks or months, a really sudden increase in volume might produce an immediate rise in pressure, even when the total volume is quite small.

however, dependent only on the existing volume of intracranial contents and their proportional disposition. Certain other factors, which are to some extent under clinical control, have been found to affect elastance to a greater or lesser degree than they affect intracranial pressure directly see page 8).

Elastance is measured at the bedside by observing the effect on ICP of the injection into or aspiration from the ventricle of 1 ml. of fluid; a change of pressure of more than 3 mmHg. indicates increased elastance (or tightness).

Compensatory mechanisms at first maintain a normal pressure in the face of added volume (fig. 4). Blood and CSF are displaced from the intracranial cavity into the more distensible spinal canal, and brain takes up subarachnoid space vacated by CSF. According to the size of the mass brain shifts next develop as parts of the brain are extruded from areas of highest pressure to less compressed areas, forming the internal hernias recognised by pathologists, and producing the characteristic clinical effects related to them (page 51). As these compensatory mechanisms became extended the tightness or elastance of the brain (= inverse of compliance) increases. This can be measured by the increase in ICP resulting from a unit change in volume (fig. 4). The elastance of the brain is affected by many factors other than the actual level of the ICP:

Increased elastance	Decreased elastance
Hypercapnia (any degree)	Hypocapnia (any degree)
Hypoxia ($PaO_2 <$ 50 mmHg)	Hyperoxia (PaO_2 1000–1500 mmHg)
REM sleep	Hypothermia
Volatile anaesthetic agents	Barbiturates
Nitrous oxide	Neuroleptanalgesia
	Increased intrathoracic pressure

This quality of the brain is of considerable clinical significance, because on the elastance of the brain at any time will depend the effect of any event which increases intracranial volume—such as oedema, or temporary vasodilation (due to various causes such as blood gas changes, respiratory obstruction, or epileptic fits, *inter alia*). If elastance is high such an agent may precipitate a clinical crisis. When ICP measurements are available the elastance may be tested by observing the volume-pressure response—the change in pressure which immediately follows a 1 ml. change in intracranial volume (by intra-ventricular aspiration or injection): normally the change is less than 3 mmHg.

Measurement of ICP

Increasing use is now made of direct measurement of ICP, and this has emphasised what was already suspected—that clinical signs of raised pressure are very unreliable. The measurements have also indicated that the level of pressure is often variable, particularly when it is raised; therefore single observations (e.g. during ventricular tapping or at lumbar puncture) can be misleading. Recent symposia have reviewed the various technical methods available; no general agreement has been reached as to the most suitable for clinical work. An intraventricular catheter allows calibration for absolute values and makes it possible to measure the pressure-volume response, and to reduce pressure by aspiration. If the ventricles are very small it may be difficult to keep the recording going, but in that event a subdual recording can be made. There is a small but definite risk of infection and that is why some centres favour an extradural or subdural sensor, although calibration is not possible and access to the ventricle is denied. Measurements of ICP can be of use in diagnosis by establishing whether or not pressure is increased; for example in patients with hydrocepahlus or suspected papilloedema, and in patients with post-traumatic and post-operative deterioration. They make it possible to monitor treatment which can be changed if it is not effective in lowering pressure. And it may be of use in prognosis, in that high pressure which fails to respond to treatment indicates an inrecoverable situation.

EFFECT OF RAISED INTRACRANIAL PRESSURE ON FUNCTION

The effect on function of raised intracranial pressure alone is difficult to study because in clinical practice, there is almost always the effect of the primary pathological process which is itself directly influencing brain function locally; in addition there are the effects of brain shifts on areas of brain remote from the primary mass. What is known clinically is that some patients with a high intracranial pressure may be alert and sometimes quite free of symptoms, as in the condition of pseudo tumour

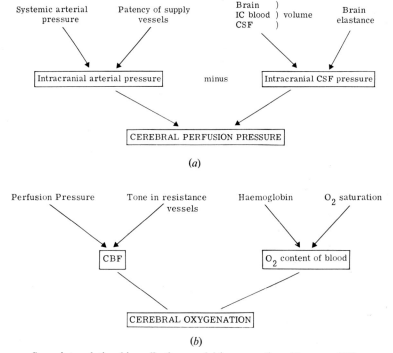

Some interrelationships affecting cerebral oxygenation, (*See page* 100).

(page 50). Others are in serious trouble, being drowsy and disorientated; immediate improvement may follow treatment which deals only with the intracranial pressure, such as aspirating CSF from the ventricle It would appear that pressure alone, with no local mass capable of producing brain shifts, produces few symptoms, at least until a certain critical level of pressure is reached. That critical level is when the perfusion pressure is so reduced that cerebral blood flow falls so that cerebral oxygenation and other metabolic requirements are no longer adequately met. Mean perfusion pressure is the mean arterial pressure minus the intracranial pressure and is normally about 100 mmHg; animal experiments suggest that when this falls below c.40 mmHg cerebral hypoxia may develop, but no data is avalable for man. The importance of considering intracranial pressure in conjunction with mean arterial pressure is obvious and is a factor of great importance in considering anaesthesia for neurosurgical patients (page 97). One effect of a rapidly rising intracranial pressure, as occurs for example with extradural hæmatoma, is to raise the arterial blood pressure and in such circumstances intracranial pressure may reach very high levels without any appreciable change in perfusion pressure; it is the brain shift induced by such a lesion which is the vital factor, until the pressure outstrips compensatory mechanisms, when the brain as a whole will suffer. Other inter-relationships which affect and are affected by intracranial pressure are discussed on p. 103.

Clinical

Two-thirds of patients with space-occupying lesions suffer from the classical triad of headache, papillœdema and vomiting and most of the remainder have at least two of these complaints. Many also show mental disorder of some kind, from drowsiness to coma, from mild personality change to profound dementia.

None of these features is peculiar to raised pressure; indeed with the exception of papillœdema there are many commoner causes of each of them alone. It is their occurrence together which raises the suspicion of raised intracranial pressure, although the evidence for a causal relationship between high pressure and the classical symptoms is very incomplete and there is no consistent correlation between the height of the pressure and the severity of the symptoms. The complexities of this relationship have been discussed but pending a more exact explanation these features are conventionally ascribed to raised intracranial pressure, and are spoken of as the "general" symptoms and signs of intracranial tumour, in contrast to localizing features.

Headache

MECHANISM OF PRODUCTION

Most structures in the head are insensitive to pain, and neurosurgeons used to operate almost exclusively under local anæsthesia knowing that the bony skull and the brain itself could be handled painlessly. Distension or traction affecting the arteries of the scalp and at the base of the brain, or the venous sinuses and their main tributaries, gives rise to ill-localised pain. More localised pain results from stretching or distortion of certain areas of the dura mater and of the trunks of the fifth, ninth and tenth cranial nerves. Headache can also originate in spasm of the large muscles at the base of the skull, and this may occur alone or as an added reflex activity when one of the other painful mechanisms is in play. Whatever the origin the final common path for pain is limited to the trigeminal, glossopharyngeal and vagus nerves together with the posterior roots of the first three cervical segments.

CHARACTERISTICS OF PRESSURE HEADACHE

The patient commonly wakes with a headache which disperses within an hour or so. It may disappear for days or even weeks, and sometimes after months of regular morning headache there may be a complete remission although the pressure is unrelieved. Pressure headaches are frequently not of very great intensity, being described as throbbing or bursting, aggravated by coughing, sneezing, stooping down or exertion, and may be relieved by aspirin or codeine tablets or by going to bed for a few days.

The distribution of the headache seldom gives any useful clue to the site of the tumour. Not only is the headache often felt at a situation remote from its production, but the site of production may be remote from the tumour. Most pressure headaches are felt bilaterally in the frontal or occipital regions. However, headache which is initially or exclusively occipital, radiating down the neck, is likely to be due to a mass in the posterior fossa: tumours in the cerebello-pontine angle often cause persistent aching in these areas.

Severe internal hydrocephalus may produce a syndrome of intense episodic headache associated with acute rises of pressure, which may be precipitated by neck or head movements. These so-called *hydrocephalic attacks* can be alarming; the patient may cry out with pain, consciousness may be clouded, pulse and respiration become irregular and occasionally death supervenes. These attacks warn of dangerously high pressure requiring prompt relief.

SOME OTHER CAUSES OF HEADACHE

1. **Hypertension.** Although there may be a specific vascular component to hypertensive headaches they are largely due to raised pressure and may therefore be indistinguishable from those due to tumour. Occurring in the morning, and sometimes accompanied by vomiting, they are frequently more severe than tumour headaches. Episodes of hypertensive encephalopathy can closely resemble hydrocephalic attacks. The relief of hypertensive headaches when the blood pressure is

lowered by drugs is not a reliable diagnostic test, for a similar improvement can be expected in tumour cases due to the lowering of intracranial tension secondary to the drop in arterial pressure. The remarkable efficacy of splanchnicectomy in relieving hypertensive headache, even when the blood pressure is not greatly altered, has never been satisfactorily explained.

2. **Migraine.** These severe episodic headaches usually begin in the teens, tend to run in families and are sometimes accompanied by focal neurological disorders such as visual phenomena (fortification spectra, hemianopia or blindness), paræsthesiæ or weakness on one side of the body, and dysphasia; numbness round the lips on both sides is another common complaint. The headache is often a hemicrania, altering from side to side in different attacks, and lasting for several hours to a day or so. It seldom returns within a fortnight; more commonly attacks recur monthly or even sporadically over the years. Some patients recognise specific precipitating factors such as menstruation, the week-end, or emotional stress. Vomiting is common and alarming prostration can occur. Ergot preparations, if given at the outset, may abort an attack.

3. **Anxiety states and neurosis.** Headache is one of the commonest of psychosomatic symptoms, but when of this origin tends to have certain characteristics. Unremitting over weeks, months or years, with even an hour's relief denied, it is often said to be *worse* at times, but never *better*; the sensation is of pressing, burning or "like a tight band round the head," and it is uninfluenced by analgesics.

4. **E.N.T., eye and dental disease.** Sinusitis, glaucoma and toothache all give rise to pain in the trigeminal distribution, but there is often radiation or referral to the head; secondary muscle spasm can also cause headache, as it does with cervical spondylosis.

5. **Meningism.** Irritation of the basal meninges, whether by blood from subarachnoid hæmorrhage, or by pus in meningitis, gives rise to severe pain in the head and neck associated often with great restlessness and noisiness.

6. **Temporal arteritis.** The elderly patients to whom this condition is confined complain less of headache than of localised pain or tenderness in the scalp, and the affected artery may be palpated. The pain can be very severe and unremitting until the artery is divided surgically or cortisone is given. A third develop visual symptoms, sudden blindness or field defects.

7. **Lumbar puncture headache—low pressure state.** Traction and distortion of structures at the base of the brain, similar to that which occurs with *raised* pressure, may be responsible for the headache sometimes complained of after drainage of CSF by lumbar puncture. This often appears to be aggravated by sitting up, and may be relieved by a high fluid intake; low CSF pressure may therefore be one factor but it cannot be the only one because headache is so variable after lumbar puncture, some patients denying any discomfort whatever.

Papillœdema

Anatomically the optic nerve is an extension of the brain, complete with meningeal coverings and subarachnoid space. Intracranial tension is thereby transmitted to a site where its effects may be directly observed, although two factors limit the reliability of such observations. One is the time needed for papillœdema to develop, probably some days of abnormally high intracranial pressure (although large blot or splash hæmorrhages may occur at the time of a severe subarachnoid hæmorrhage). The other is that even long-standing raised pressure may fail to be reflected in the optic fundus if the subarachnoid extension is cut off from the general subarachnoid space, either on account of individual structural anomalies or because a tumour is obliterating the space around one optic nerve.

MECHANISM OF PRODUCTION

As intracranial pressure rises CSF is forced out along the subarachnoid sheath of the optic nerve, and this pressure is exerted on the central vein of the retina where it crosses the subarachnoid space. Œdema of the nerve head develops and the retinal veins are engorged.

Unilateral swelling may result from an orbital lesion affecting one optic nerve but can also occur with generalised pressure if the intracranial mass is so situated that it compresses one nerve, blocking the subarachnoid space around it. This leads to primary optic atrophy on that side, and the occurrence of papillœdema in one eye and optic atrophy in the other constitutes the Foster Kennedy syndrome.

Papillœdema seldom develops in infants, except following sagittal sinus thrombosis, because the skull bones can separate and the sutures spread; the fontanelle tension is the best guide to pressure at this age. The elderly less often have papillœdema as a sign of intracranial tumour because the somewhat atrophied brain, with large subarachnoid spaces and dilated ventricles, leaves more room than is usually available for an expanding lesion. Raised pressure develops late, and a tumour may readily be confused with a vascular lesion, in that there are focal signs without pressure.

APPEARANCE

The essential component is swelling of the nerve head, and this may be measured in dioptres by comparing the lenses required to bring the disc and then the peripheral retina into focus. This manœuvre requires experience, and even skilled observers often come to conflicting conclusions about the degree of swelling. It is more useful to build up a qualitative assessment based on a number of factors.

The earliest change is filling of the optic cup, the depression in the nerve head from which the vessels emerge and where the nerve fibres seen end-on normally form a stippled patch known as the lamina cribrosa. Then the medial half of the disc becomes pink and its edges indistinct. Eventually no normal disc remains visible and the vessels climb out over the heaped-up pink swelling which has replaced it. The veins appear engorged at an early stage and later flame-shaped hæmor-rhages may develop, often alongside vessels. In severer degrees small circular "blob" hæmorrhages and exudate appear.

Papillœdema eventually subsides either because of a natural resolu-tion of the process responsible for it, or following surgical relief of pressure. Depending on the severity and duration of the swelling the disc may be restored to normal appearance and the nerve to full function, or *consecutive optic atrophy* may develop. Once started, atrophy often progresses even though the pressure has been relieved, and the patient is left blind; the pale discs remain permanently blurred at the edges. Fear of this sequel puts urgency into the treatment of patients with a high degree of papillœdema even when this is asymptomatic and when there is not any immediate danger from brain stem com-pression.

SYMPTOMS

Most patients are unaware of papillœdema and are surprised by the seriousness with which their other complaints are taken after their fundi have been examined. Eventually vision is affected, and a number of brain tumours are first detected by opticians who examine the fundi before prescribing glasses. The visual fields show enlargement of the blind spot and later peripheral constriction of the field. Children are curiously reluctant to complain of deteriorating vision, especially children under about 9 years of age, and not uncommonly papillœdema is discovered which has progressed almost to blindness without any other feature of raised pressure having become obvious.

Intermittent loss of vision is more common than steady deterioration. These episodes are termed *amblyopic attacks* (syn. obscurations of vision, amaurosis fugax) and consist of brief periods of partial or complete blindness, lasting usually less than a minute, occurring many times a day, often for several months. There may be complete blacking-out of vision, or only blurring, or greying with loss of colour perception. Episodes are precipitated by sudden rising from the horizontal or sitting position, and are particularly common on getting up from bed first thing in the morning; stooping is another trigger. Postural alterations in local blood supply probably account for these attacks. They occur only with severe papillœdema, usually after some weeks or months of head-ache. This symptom, which is often misinterpreted as a form of epilepsy, vertigo, dizziness or fainting, is important to recognise because it indi-cates that sight is in peril and relief of pressure is urgently needed whatever the underlying cause.

Bilateral Fundal Changes

1. **Arterial hypertension** may produce papillœdema which is indistinguishable from that due to an intracranial mass. Nonetheless the abnormalities of the retinal vessels, silver wiring and tortuosity, may indicate a hypertensive retinopathy, as well as an excess of hæmorrhages and exudates in relation to the degree of swelling of the nerve head. But there is no certain way of distinguishing the two conditions.

2. **Pseudopapillœdema** can be diagnosed with confidence only if an unchanging fundal picture is observed on repeated examinations over many months in a patient with no other signs of raised pressure. This is a congenital anomaly of the fundus, the disc being blurred and appearing swollen, but the retinal vessels are not engorged and there are no hæmorrhages; vision is unaffected.

3. **Metabolic disorders.** Prolonged carbon dioxide retention in advanced emphysema, may be associated with venous congestion in the fundus and eventually frank swelling.

Unilateral fundal changes

1. **Retrobulbar neuritis** is the condition most often mistaken for papillœdema, and the distinction is vital because the immediate management and the ultimate prognosis are so different. In most instances this is an incident in a demyelinating disorder, and though recovery is usually complete and rapid there remains the likelihood of further episodes of disseminated sclerosis. Normally only one eye is affected, though the second eye may later become involved. Visual acuity is affected early and severely, the patient presenting with loss of vision in one eye. This proves to be due to a paracentral scotoma—a patch of blindness affecting central vision so that reading is impossible though objects may be seen in the periphery of the visual field; as soon as an object is looked at it disappears because it then comes in the region of central vision. The globe is often painful to move, and tender on palpation. The marked swelling of the disc may be indistinguishable from papillœdema, but hæmorrhages are very rare and exudates unknown.

2. **Orbital tumour** by compressing or invading the optic nerve may lead to local congestion, and the tumour itself may appear in the fundus. There will usually be proptosis, failure of vision and sometimes limitation of eye movement.

3. **Thrombosis of central retinal vein** is sudden in onset with loss of vision, as in retrobulbar neuritis, but the fundal changes are quite different with hæmorrhages spreading widely to the peripheral retina, which is œdematous, and severe engorgement of veins. Cavernous sinus thrombosis and carotico-cavernous fistula may give a similar but less acute and dramatic appearance.

Vomiting

This may be a sign of increased pressure but also occurs as a focal manifestation of lesions in the fourth ventricle. Such lesions almost always bring about raised pressure due to obstruction to CSF flow and it may not be easy to determine which mechanism is operative at any one time.

Vomiting **due to pressure** usually occurs before breakfast, frequently as an accompaniment of morning headache. Although referred to as projectile this is seldom a striking feature; certainly it can occur without much nausea and so without warning. Children with tumours more frequently vomit than adults and often without any complaint of headache. This may be related to the great frequency in children of posterior fossa tumours which produce both raised intracranial pressure and local pressure on the medulla. Five-sixths of gliomas below the tent have vomiting compared with less than half those above the tent.

Vomiting **due to a local lesion** in the fourth ventricle is more likely to appear long before headache, and may be a daily occurrence for many months before signs of pressure or neurological disorder lead to the correct diagnosis.

The two commonest causes of morning vomiting are pregnancy and migraine, the latter usually recognisable by the episodic nature of the attacks and other features such as hemicrania and visual disorders.

FURTHER READING

Behrman, S. (1966). Pathology of papilloedema. *Brain*, **89**, 1–14.
Cutter, R W. P., Page, L., Galicich, J. and Watters, G. V. (1968). Formation and absorption of CSF in man. *Brain*, **91**, 707–720.
Ethelberg, S. and Jenson, V. A. (1952). Obscurations and further time-related paroxysmal disorders in intracranial tumour. *Archives of Neurology and Psychiatry* (*Chicago*), **68**, 130–149.
Fox, J. L. (1964). Development of recent thoughts on intracranial pressure and the blood-brain barrier. *Journal of Neurosurgery*, **21**, 909–967.
Jennett, W. B., Barker, J., Fitch, W. and McDowall, D. G. (1969). Effect of anæsthesia on intracranial pressure in patients with space-occupying lesions. *Lancet*, **i**, 61–64.
Langfitt, T. W., Weinstein, J. D., Kassell, N. F. and Simeone, F. A. (1964). Transmissions of increased intracranial pressure 1. within the craniospinal axis. *Journal of Neurosurgery*, **21**, 989–997.
Langfitt, T. W., Weinstein, J. D., Kassell, N. F. and Gagliardi, L. J. (1964). Transmission of increased intracranial pressure 2. within the supra-tentorial space. *Journal of Neurosurgery*, **21**, 998–1005.
McDowall, D. G. (1970). Cerebral circulation. *International Anaesthesiology Clinics*, Vol. 7. Little, Brown, Boston.
Miller, J. D. (1975). Volume and pressure in the craniospinal axis. *Clinical Neurosurgery*, **22**, 76–105.
Symposium (1973). Brain oedema—pathophysiology and therapy. In: *Advances in Neurosurgery* 1. Eds. Schurmann, Brock, Roulen and Voth, Springer, Berlin.

International Symposia on Intracranial Pressure

Brock, M., Dietz, H. (1972). Intracranial Pressure. *I Experimental and Clinical Aspects*. Springer, Berlin.

Lundberg, N., Ponten, U. and Brock, M. (1975). *Intracranial Pressure II*. Springer-Verlag, Berlin.

Beks, J. W. F., Bosch, D. A and Brock, M. (1976). *Intracranial Pressure III* Springer-Verlag, Berlin.

CHAPTER 2

Mental Disorders with Intracranial Lesions

Syndromes associated with impaired consciousness

Syndromes in alert patients

> Non-localising
> Localising

Pseudodementia

Other causes of organic dementia

Brain lesions are often expected to produce some mental symptoms and acute brain damage (whether due to trauma, haemorrhage or infection) usually does cause impaired alertness of some degree. Changes associated with slowly developing lesions, such as intracranial tumour, are often unobtrusive and noticed only by the patient's close relatives or friends. The doctor may learn of such subtle changes only if he directly questions the relatives: despite improved understanding and more realistic attitudes to mental illness, there is still a stigma which seals the lips of those who suffer, and those who witness, symptoms which are believed to mean a failing mind. When such conditions eventually cause raised ICP and brain shift then impaired alertness will often obscure more subtle features of mental abnormality. It is useful therefore to separate the two main types of mental disorder which can be recognised in association with organic brain disease—those associated with impaired consciousness, and those occurring in patients whose conscious state is not depressed, but in whom the content of consciousness is abnormal.

Syndromes associated with impaired consciousness

Impaired responsiveness is an expression of dysfunction of the brain as a whole—and it has been said that coma indicates brain failure, as uraemia bespeaks renal failure. The agents responsible may be reversible, such as depressant drugs, metabolic disorder and acute but transitory lesions, like mild concussion or meningitis. Structural damage causing prolonged disturbance of responsiveness may do so either by affecting the brain stem reticular formation and its upward projections; or by extensive bilateral involvement of the cerebral cortex. In either event the cerebral cortex as a whole is inactive to a greater or lesser degree.

Assessment of Coma

In gauging deterioration or improvement during the acute stage of many conditions the degree and duration of coma or altered consciousness usually overshadows all other clinical features in importance. It is therefore of considerable practical value to be able to record changing states of altered consciousness reliably. It was for this purpose that the **Glasgow Coma Scale** was introduced, and has subsequently been widely adopted. Observer-error trials have shown it to be reliable in the hands of non-specialist medical and nursing staff, including those for whom English is not their first language. The scale is a simple descriptive one, which avoid defining series of composite levels; it therefore takes account of the fact that different types of response may vary independently. It avoids making an arbitrary division between consciousness and unconsciousness, because altered consciousness is in fact a continuum. The three behavioural responses recorded relate to motor activity, verbal performance and eye opening (fig. 5).

If commands cannot be obeyed **motor activity** is reported as the response to a standard painful stimulus—pressure on the nailbed with a pencil. The response is recorded as *localising* if the other hand comes over to the site of the stimulus; as *flexor* if the elbow flexes, as *extensor* if it extends. This avoids the use of the terms decerebrate and decorticate, with the anatomical implications which these carry. The response of the upper limbs is usually the most reliable but the lower limbs should also be tested. It is the response of the best limb which is indicative of the conscious level; if one limb (or side) is clearly worse than the other this is evidence of focal damage in the nervous system.

In the **verbal** sphere *orientation* implies awareness of self and environment—the patient known where he is, why he is there and also the year, the season and the month. *Confused conversation* covers varying degrees of disorientation and confusion in a patient able to respond to questions in a conversational manner. *Inappropriate speech* indicates intelligible articulation limited to exclamatory or random words, usually shouting and swearing, with no sustained conversational exchange. *Incomprehensible speech* refers to moaning and groaning without recognisable words. Too much emphasis has probably been placed on the failure to speak in previous assessments of conscious level—there are many reasons why patients may not speak, including

INSTITUTE OF NEUROLOGICAL SCIENCES, GLASGOW
OBSERVATION CHART

NAME

RECORD No.

DATE

TIME

C O M	Eyes open	Spontaneously
A S C	Best verbal response	To speech
		To pain
		None

A S C	Best verbal response	Orientated
		Confused
		Inappropriate Words
		Incomprehensible Sounds
		None

Eyes closed by swelling = C

Endotracheal tube or tracheostomy = T

A L E	Best motor response	Obey commands
		Localise pain
		Flexion to pain
		Extension to pain
		None

Usually record the best arm response

Pupil scale (m.m.)
1
2
3
4
5
6
7
8

Blood pressure and Pulse rate
240
230
220
210
200
190
180
170
160
150
140
130
120
110
100
90
80
70
60
50
40
30
Respiration 20
10

Temperature °C
40
39
38
37
36
35
34
33
32
31
30

PUPILS	right	Size
		Reaction
	left	Size
		Reaction

+ reacts
− no reaction
c, eye closed

L I M B	A R M S	Normal power
		Mild weakness
		Severe weakness
		Spastic flexion
		Extension
		No response
M O V E M E N T	L E G S	Normal power
		Mild weakness
		Severe weakness
		Extension
		No response

Record right (R) and left (L) separately if there is a difference between the two sides.

(a) Observation chart

F<small>IG</small>. 5

INSTITUTE OF NEUROLOGICAL SCIENCES, GLASGOW
OBSERVATION CHART

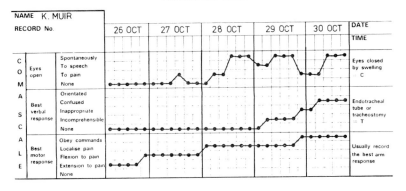

(b)   Coma scale

FIG. 5 (*continued*)

dysphasia, tracheostomy and inability to converse in a particular language.

Eye opening indicates whether the arousal mechanisms in the brain stem are active and, as will be described below, it is possible to have an aroused patient who is not aware and whose cerebral cortex is not functioning. *Eye opening to speech* is a response to any verbal approach, spoken or shouted and not necessarily the command to open eyes; eye opening to *response to pain* should depend on a stimulus in the limbs, because facial stimulation may cause reflex eye closure as part of a grimace. An advantage of this scale is that a measure of conscious state may be obtained even if one of the elements of the scale cannot be tested (e.g. the patient has a tracheostomy or the eyes are too swollen to open after local injury).

Coma has been defined in a number of studies as a patient who will neither obey commands, nor give better than an incomprehensible verbal response, nor will open the eyes, even to pain. The use of the Glasgow Scale makes it unnecessary to define terms such as light or deep coma, or stupor. When the latter is used it usually refers to a patient who will, in terms of the Glasgow scale, make at least a brief verbal response, albeit confused, but who is asleep or very drowsy until actively roused; it seems likely that most such patients would obey commands and would open their eyes, at least to painful stimuli.

At the lower end of the scale of unresponsiveness is the condition of **brain death**—now increasingly recognised as of importance in order to avoid undue prolongation of life-support measures for patients who cannot survive following massive brain damage. This has usually been due to primary intracranial damage (commonly trauma or haemorrhage) or resuscitation after a cardiac arrest.

Brain death is a product of our time, a result of efficient and widely available resuscitation procedures, which result in many patients with cardiac or respiratory arrest being intubated and ventilated as a routine primary measure. Once this has been done the patient may still be apnoeic but with good heart action and the question then is whether the continued apnoea is due to a reversible cause, such as depressant or relaxant drugs, or compression of the brain stem by a removable intracranial mass. In the neurosurgical ward this may be an intracranial haematoma, either traumatic or post-operative, or it may be another mass lesion such as an abscess or tumour. The urgency is to diagnose and deal with these conditions. Once these have been excluded or dealt with, and the patient still remains apnoeic, the question of brain death arises for the first time.

The need to exclude the possible influence of depressant drugs and muscle relaxants cannot be too strongly emphasised, because these can produce a suspension of brain stem activity indistinguishable from that due to brain death. They can become a problem in the case of the patient found unconscious in the street with no clear history of some intracranial ictus; and in patients suffering cardiac arrest in hospital, particularly in the operating theatre, when drugs will usually have been administered recently. Hypothermia should also be excluded because this again can produce brain stem inactivity and a clinical picture indistinguishable from brain death. Given these provisos, which in effect means that the patient's condition is undoubtedly due to structural brain damage—usually head injury or intracranial haemorrhage, the criteria of brain death can be applied. These have been the subject of much discussion in recent years and details still vary from one country or one institution to another. However, a consensus is emerging that the diagnosis should rest on clinical criteria and that investigations such as EEG, cerebral angiography and the like are necessary.

It must be established that the patient is apnoeic, by discontinuing the ventilator and watching for the return of spontaneous respiration as the PCO_2 builds up well above the threshold stimulus (40 mmHg). Providing the PCO_2 is above 36 mmHg. when the ventilator is disconnected an adequate CO_2 level will be achieved within 3 or 4 minutes. During this time oxygen should be supplied by a tracheal catheter at 6 litres per minute. If the PCO_2 cannot be measured, or if there is reason to believe that it is low due to prior hyperventilation, an adequate CO_2 level may be ensured by having the patient breathe 5% CO_2 in oxygen for 5 minutes prior to discontinuing ventilation.

It should then be established that other brain stem reflexes are all absent—that there is no pupil reaction (the size is irrelevant): that there is no facial or corneal reflex response to local stimulation; that the oculovestibular reflexes are absent (i.e. no eye movement during or following slow injection of 20 ml. of ice cold water into each external auditory meatus, clear access to the drum having been established on both sides). Spinal cord function may be preserved for some time after brain death, and reflex movement of the limbs may therefore persist; this may give rise to misunderstanding unless explained to all the staff, including the nurses.

Codes of practice for diagnosing brain death commonly require that criteria be shown to persist for certain periods of time. Two examinations, 30 minutes apart, when done approximately 6 hours after the initial ictus, should be adequate; the 6 hour delay gives time for the diagnosis to be established and remediable causes of the condition excluded; but in the case of cardiac arrest in a patient already in hospital this would be an unnecessarily long time to wait in most instances.

Other unresponsive states

Given the rigorous application of the criteria set out above there is no reason why any other states should be confused with brain death. However, there are other states which may cause difficulty for inexperienced staff and it is well to be quite clear about these

1. Apnoea associated with consciousness

Respiratory paralysis and inability to move may result from polyneuritis, poliomyelitis or myasthaenia gravis and such patients may survive for long periods if artificial ventilation is maintained; rarely this condition may result from a brain stem stroke. These patients have some brain stem reflexes preserved but eye movements and eyelid blinking are possible, and the patients may learn to communicate by a code using this residual voluntary movement. This tragic state has been described as the 'locked-in' syndrome.

2. Persistent vegetative state

This describes the survivor of acute brain damage who is breathing spontaneously but who remains unresponsive and speechless, with no psychologically meaningful response, because the cerebral cortex is functionally inactive. This may result from neocortical necrosis following cardiac arrest, or because the cortex has become disconnected from the brain stem arousal centres by extensive white matter damage, usually due to head injury. Brain stem and subcortical systems are still functioning, at least partially, and the patient has sleep/wake rhythms; when his eyes are open he may 'look' or even follow visual or auditory stimuli, and this frequently leads relatives to conclude that consciousness is returning. By the same token relatives may interpret postural or grasp reflexes as voluntary movements or responses to commands. There may be some incomprehensible vocalisation, but no recognisable words are ever uttered. This state can usually be suspected a week or two after the ictus, once the brain stem arousal system recovers from the initial lesion. The eyes then open, and the patient is awake—but the failure to show evidence of awareness or to speak, with only primitive responses, indicates that survival may be in the vegetative state. It has been loosely described as persisting or prolonged coma, but this is inappropriate in view of the fact that the patient is in fact aroused and awake, although not aware.

3. Akinetic mutism

This describes patients who are clearly functioning at a much higher level than those in a vegetative state but who will not speak. Their motor responses are commonly normal, without the spasticity of all four limbs with only reflex postural movements seen in the vegetative state. Such patients will make psychologically meaningful responses of some kind and will often speak a little, sometimes only in a whisper. It is a relative state of akinesia, in that some movement can usually be provoked. Patients have been known to remember events around them during this state, which has therefore been described as a state of receptivity *without* reactivity.

NON-LOCALISING SYNDROMES IN ALERT PATIENTS

Organic dementia

This usually affects all three aspects of normal mental function, although one may be more severely impaired than the others; these are intellect, memory and personality.

Intellectual function is concerned with problem solving, that is dealing with novel situations. Although formal tests may indicate marked limitation of ability in this field the patient may well be able to conduct himself appropriately both at work and at home if his life is largely routine and presents few new situations from day to day. If, however, his occupation is less stereotyped deficiencies at work may be the means whereby his illness first comes to light.

Poor memory is a common complaint, and because it is socially acceptable may be the cliché whereby a patient expresses a wide range of limitations in his mental capacity. Testing may reveal the defect to be primarily in his intellectual or language function, rather than of memory itself. Impairment of recent memory is, however, a common feature of organic dementia, whilst distant (childhood) memories remain intact. When memory is predominantly and severely affected a focal lesion may be suspected (*vide infra*).

Personality can be regarded as comprising drive, affect and social restraint or social judgement. Lack of drive, or apathy, is quite the commonest feature and is often first noticed in a falling off in interest in leisure activities. A man may continue to perform quite exacting work under the stimulus of bread-winning and protected by long established routine, yet come home exhausted, sink in a chair and dream away the evening. This change in personality (if such it is!) may lead to recommendations to take a holiday, to pull himself together or take vitamin pills. Eventually more serious lapses appear, many of which can be traced to failing recent memory: appointments are forgotten, articles mislaid, shopping expeditions left half completed. Carelessness in personal appearance combined with falling standards at work lead to dismissal, and the patient takes to sitting for long periods looking into space, accessible yet making little spontaneous attempt to keep in contact with his surroundings.

The severity of organic dementia seems often to be related to age, and the form it takes may reflect the basic personality of the individual. Insight may be retained, or be lost early on, but in either event memory for distant events, even those of childhood, is well preserved. When certain aspects of personality are predominantly affected there will be suspicion of a local lesion in the frontal lobes (*vide infra*).

Cerebral irritation or traumatic delirium

This is a state of restless, disorganised behaviour commonly seen during the recovery of consciousness after head injury, but occasionally seen after other disorders. It may be looked on as a kind of mental dystonia in which a normal afferent input evokes a disinhibited and uncontrolled response—it could be looked on also as a state of misdirected alertness rather than impaired alertness. There may be motor restlessness, attempts to get out of bed, and even to attack attendants; a lot of shouting and swearing is common and yet this may be interspersed with periods of apparent lucidity and appropriate response.

LOCALISING

Frontal lobe—behavioural disorders

In spite of the reputed function of this part of the brain in controlling higher mental activity and the consistent effect produced by psychosurgery in this region, mental syndromes due to local disturbances are quite unusual. They are nothing like as common as those due to diffuse pathology such as have been described above. Moreover a fairly extensive frontal lobectomy can be performed without any obvious impairment of mental functioning, but as soon as there is bilateral frontal damage symptoms do become manifest. The most obvious syndrome produced is that commonly referred to as "Witzelsucht syndrome", the nearest English translation being "pathological joking". The essential component is a lack of social restraint, the contribution of which to normal behaviour is clearly appreciated only when it is defective. There is incomplete awareness of the subtleties of social appropriateness; the patient may make tactless remarks and joke in unlikely situations yet the superficial impression is of unusual liveliness and genuinely quick wit. The clue to this being more than natural exuberance lies in mis-judgements of manners, an overstepping of good taste which is difficult to describe but easy to recognise. The euphoria of these patients, which is both enjoyable and contagious, usually precludes their having insight into their condition. When frontal lesions affect primarily the corpus callosum the effect is of a very profound dementia occurring as the primary clinical event.

Dominant temporal lobe
"Dysphasia (language disorders)"—see p. 36.

Non-dominant parietal lobe
"Spatial Disorders"—see p. 38.

Limbic system—memory disorders
All available evidence points to the limbic system as vital for active memorising. A memory record of immediate recent experience is essential for orientation and for the execution of planned, purposeful activity; a crippling dementia results if this record breaks down. Memory involves the perception and temporary storage of experience, followed after some delay by permanent registration; subsequent recall may be deferred indefinitely. Organic lesions usually affect only the permanent registration of new memories, without interfering with the recall of established memory, even those of childhood. The evidence for the implication of the limbic system is fourfold:

1. **Temporal lobe epilepsy** frequently consists of fragmentary memories and feelings of *déjà vu*, whilst automatisms are always associated with amnesia for the period of the attack.
2. **Temporal lobe stimulation** during operations under local anæsthesia provokes memories; moreover active memorisation is suspended during such stimulation.
3. **Pathological lesions** affecting the mammillary bodies consistently cause defective memorising as an isolated feature.
4. **Surgical excision** of the temporal lobe, if carried out bilaterally causes severe impairment of recent memory.

However, the two commonest conditions affecting recent memory in surgical practice—head injury and slowly developing space-occupying lesions—are associated with diffuse brain damage. The same is true for the memory failure of senility, of presenile dementia and of arterio-sclerotic dementia. In all of these conditions the memory defect affects only recent events.

Certain other abnormalities of nervous activity may be interpreted by the patient or his relatives as a failure of memory, but these should be clearly recognisable:

1. **Language disorders** may be described as "forgetting" names or words.

2. **Agnosia** affecting extrapersonal space may lead to a patient failing to recognise familiar surroundings and to say he has "forgotten" his way about.

3. **Apraxia** involves an ideomotor defect which the patient can usually describe, but he may say he has "forgotten" how to perform an action.

4. **Psychopathological amnesia** is distinguished by its sudden onset and its totality; not only recent events are forgotten but the patient can recall nothing about himself, his family or his past.

CONDITIONS MISTAKENLY INTERPRETED AS MENTAL DYSFUNCTION

Temporal lobe epilepsy can take the form of automatisms during which complicated and purposive, yet entirely inappropriate, activities are carried out for which the patient has no subsequent memory. The clue to the nature of such behaviour is the tendency for it to be stereotyped from one attack to another, and the invariable amnesia for events occurring during the episode. Some temporal lobe seizures consist entirely of subjective mental experiences which when described may suggest a functional disorder of the mind.

Disorders of language function are not always recognised immediately for what they are and profound dementia may be suspected when it is only the lines of communication which are affected. Nominal dysphasia, showing itself in the "forgetting" of names, is often regarded as due to a failing memory, whilst the faltering and inappropriate words slowly forced out by the patient with severe expressive dysphasia are easily taken as evidence of an equally disorganised mind. When the receptive side of language function is also affected, the appearance is even more suggestive of dementia. For here is a man who appears not to be able or willing to co-operate even in simple physical tests—in fact he cannot understand what he is being told to do, does not know what question is being asked; and the more verbal explanation offered the less likely is he to grasp what is wanted. Other evidence of left hemisphere dysfunction, hemiparesis or hemianopia, often accompanies dysphasia.

Topographical disorientation, a manifestation of dysfunction of the right parietal lobe, consists in an inability to recognise even familiar surroundings (p. 32). A man may be unable to pick out his own front door when he returns from the office, be unable to find the bathroom in his own house. The nature of this disorder may be suspected from its association with other signs of right hemisphere dysfunction such as hemianopia, and tests involving the drawing of maps and plans or the copying of designs may bring out the defect quite clearly. If these additional signs are not elicited primary dementia may be suspected, and the psychiatrist is liable to be called before the surgeon.

SOME OTHER CAUSES OF ORGANIC DEMENTIA

Cerebral atrophy in its pure form consists of progressive dementia occurring usually in men in their fifties and associated with marked dilation of the ventricular system. There are no signs of pressure, and the hydrocephalus is secondary to atrophy of the brain; an air encephalogram often shows an excess of air on the surface of the brain where the subarachnoid space is unnaturally large over the shrunken gyri.

Presenile dementia, associated with the names of Pick and Alzheimer, occurs in the forties and is rapidly progressive. There are many organic signs, such as dysphasia and hemiplegia, but no signs of raised pressure.

Cerebral arteriosclerosis betrays itself by small vascular accidents and by the appearance of sclerotic vessels in the retina. The onset of dementia is usually much slower with tumour than in the conditions just mentioned. There may be characteristic neurological syndromes such as Parkinsonism or pseudobulbar palsy, and epilepsy is common. Generalised arteriosclerosis is usually evident.

Psychosis. A tumour rarely produces symptoms which closely resemble primary psychiatric disorders, although if insight is retained for long with the organic dementia syndrome the awareness of failing mental powers may give rise to secondary depression. But mania, endogenous melancholia, schizophrenic withdrawal, violent behaviour, persecution, obsessions and hallucinations are rarely encountered. Nevertheless most neurosurgeons know patients who have had courses of electroconvulsive therapy in an attempt to disperse symptoms which were basically due to brain tumour or chronic subdural hæmatoma.

It is not possible from the nature of the mental symptoms to distinguish these organic conditions from dementia due to a space-occupying lesion; absence of pressure is not a reliable criterion because tumours may grow for long periods without evidence of raised intracranial pressure. For this reason patients developing dementia which is thought to be organic are usually investigated to exclude a mass, a very important step to take before accepting the uniformly gloomy prognosis associated with each of the other conditions described.

FURTHER READING

Cramond, W. A. (1968). Organic psychosis. *British Medical Journal*, **2,** 497–500.

Jennett, B. and Plum, F. (1972). Persistent vegetative state after brain damage. *Lancet*, **i,** 734–737.

Olin, H. S. and Weisman, A. D. (1964). Psychiatric misdiagnosis in early neurological disease. *Journal of the American Medical Association*, **189,** 533–538.

Plum, F. and Posner, J. B. (1972). *Diagnosis of Stupor and Coma.* 2nd edition. Davis, Philadelphia.

Teasdale, G. and Jennett, B. (1974). Assessment of coma and impaired consciousness. A practical scale. *Lancet*, **ii,** 81–84.

Williams, S. E., Bell, D. S. and Gye, R. S. (1974). Neurosurgical disease encountered in a psychiatric service. *Journal of Neurology, Neurosurgery and Psychiatry*, **37,** 112–116.

In: Scientific Foundations of Neurology (1972). Eds. Critchley, O'Leary and Jennett Heinemann, London.

Critchley, M. *Communication: recognition of its minimal impairment.* pp. 221–227.
Humphrey, M. E. *Personality.* pp. 211–216.
Newcombe, Freda. *Memory.* pp. 205–211.
Oldfield, R. C. *Intelligence,* pp. 201–205.
Plum, F. *Organic disturbances of consciousness.* pp. 193–201.

CHAPTER 3

Localising Symptoms and Signs

Limitations of localisation

Anatomical classification of intracranial masses

Supratentorial localising features
Epilepsy
Dysphasia (disorders of language function)
Parietal spatial disorders
Hemianopia
Hemiplegia

Infratentorial

Trans-tentorial

Limitations of localisation

Effective and expeditious relief of brain compression depends on the surgeon's ability to recognise the site of the primary expanding lesion. There is no equivalent in neurosurgery of exploratory laparotomy, no means of opening the skull and passing a hand round the brain from lobe to lobe looking for lesions. Accurate localisation rests on the interpretation of focal dysfunction in the nervous system and on the results of radiological and other studies.

Faith in the tendency of lesions to run true to physiopathological form, by producing only those disorders which would be anatomically anticipated, has been undermined by a better understanding of the organisational complexity of the nervous system and the subtleties of brain compression.

As stimulation and ablation studies in human subjects accumulate it has become apparent that concepts of localisation of function in the brain have hitherto been too rigid. Owing to the complexity of neuronal connections lesions in a single site may produce a wide range of phenomena in different individuals, whilst the same clinical syndrome can result from lesions in a variety of sites. The added effects of shifts and of pressure, and the part played by speed of development and spread of œdema, are difficult to allow for. "Always" and "never" are words seldom appropriate in describing the symptomatology of brain tumours; action must never be delayed until the completion of some syndrome, or relief denied a patient because of some apparent anomaly in the clinical picture.

However, the development of modern radiological techniques has added a new dimension to diagnosis in the nervous system. As a

Anatomical classification of intracranial tumours

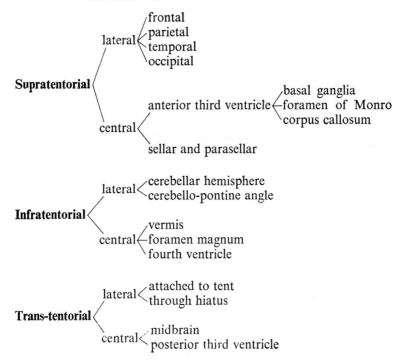

Supratentorial
  lateral
    frontal
    parietal
    temporal
    occipital
  central
    anterior third ventricle
      basal ganglia
      foramen of Monro
      corpus callosum
    sellar and parasellar

Infratentorial
  lateral
    cerebellar hemisphere
    cerebello-pontine angle
  central
    vermis
    foramen magnum
    fourth ventricle

Trans-tentorial
  lateral
    attached to tent
    through hiatus
  central
    midbrain
    posterior third ventricle

result the surgical neurologist now looks to the examination of the nervous system for a different order of accuracy in localisation than was expected when he had to rely solely on clinical assessment to indicate where he should operate.

But neuroradiological investigations are not diagnostic slot machine; choice must be made between different techniques in respect of safety and the likelihood of their yielding the required information. Both for planning radiological and other studies, and for devising appropriate surgical measures when the situation is too urgent to wait for X-rays or when investigations have failed to pin-point the tumour, the surgeon needs to know first and foremost which compartment of the skull is most likely to harbour the lesion.

The tentorium is the most important divider in the cranium (fig. 9)

Lesions above and below this structure produce distinctive syndromes call for different methods of investigation and carry their own perils. The chief concern is whether a mass is more likely to be above the tentorium or below, mainly central or lateral, and on the right side or the left. When dealing with rapidly advancing brain compression it is frequently difficult enough to localise a mass even within these crude limits, but it is vital to concentrate efforts on trying to do so.

Tumours which grow through the tentorium *laterally* may produce features typical of disorder in *both* the main cranial compartments. By contrast *centrally* situated tumours, in the posterior part of third ventricle or midbrain may cause only internal hydrocephalus and midbrain signs, without any evidence of tumour *either above or below* the tentorium.

The clinical features characteristic of each location will now be described, but the possibility of large masses remaining neurologically silent and producing signs only of pressure must not be forgotten.

Laterally placed supratentorial tumours

Epilepsy

Fits have already occurred in up to half the patients admitted with supratentorial tumours, and in 80% of those with more than two years history. In half the cases with epilepsy this was the initial symptom of the illness. Epilepsy is as likely to occur whether the tumour is extracerebral or intracerebral, but is three times more likely to complicate a fronto-parietal than an occipital tumour.

The variety of episodes now recognised as epileptic is enormous yet there is still a tendency to restrict the term to convulsions accompanied by tongue biting and incontinence of urine. No generally accepted classification of fits exists but it is most useful to distinguish between non-focal and focal seizures, accepting as focal any attack which suggests at any stage in its development, activity confined to one area of the cerebral cortex, no matter how widely it subsequently spreads. Many patients suffer from more than one type of attack, but if any is focal this is of localising significance.

TYPES OF ATTACK

In **non-focal** fits loss of consciousness is the primary event. Convulsions usually follow, affecting all four limbs though one side may be more active than the other. Occasionally there is little or no convulsive activity, the patient falling unconscious and remaining limp throughout the attack. A focal fit which spreads until all the limbs are involved may mistakenly be regarded as non-focal if it is not observed from the beginning. With careful observation fewer and fewer attacks are regarded as non-focal. Petit mal is another form of non-focal epilepsy, but is rarely if ever due to a space-occupying lesion; the term is usually confined to very frequent and brief attacks in children, associated with a specific EEG pattern (3 per second spike-and-wave).

Focal epilepsy takes many forms, best classified by the part of the brain which the paroxysm apparently first involves:

1. **Pre-central gyrus** (motor strip) activity leads to twitching of one side of the body, which begins in one area and may remain localised or spread until the whole limb, the whole side of the body or all four limbs are involved. This is Jacksonian or focal motor epilepsy; the clue to localisation is the first part to move, usually thumb, foot or face which have large cortical areas of representation. The part initially affected may be paralysed for a period of minutes or hours after the fit has finished (Todd's palsy); this may be valuable localising evidence when the onset of the seizure has not been witnessed.

2. The **speech centre** in the left temporal lobe may be the focus of activity, recognised by sudden dysphasia, either an inability to speak or to understand the speech of others. Spread will usually be first to the face.

3. The **frontal eye-field** causes the head and eyes to turn towards the opposite side; consciousness is almost always lost before any spread of activity to the limbs.

4. The **post-central gyrus** gives sensory epilepsy, feelings of numbness, tingling or a sensation of movement in a limb (or part of it) which may be followed by twitching in the same distribution.

5. The **visual cortex** in the occipital lobe causes hallucinations of light and colours, not recognisable as objects or people, in the opposite visual field to the lesion.

6. **Temporal lobe epilepsy** is now regarded as the explanation of many phenomena previously unexplained or ascribed to other causes. It is the commonest form of focal epilepsy although frequently less dramatic and obvious than the focal motor form. All types of attack include an *altered state of consciousness* but additional features enable three main kinds of seizure to be recognised.

(i) **Momentary absences** are pure lapses of consciousness during which contact is lost with the surroundings, the flow of speech broken, the thread of conversation lost. The patient does not fall and the episode may pass unnoticed by onlookers or may be mistaken for petit mal.

(ii) **Psychic phenomena** are experienced by the patient, often with little outward change in behaviour. Olfactory hallucination, invariably unpleasant and usually unrecognisable, associated with a feeling of unreality or detachment from the surroundings constitute an uncinate fit. Other sensations commonly reported are inexplicable fear, *déjà vu*—as though the situation and happenings occurring in reality around the patient had been lived through before, alterations or distortions of size and distance, and impressions of dissociation of body from soul. Some of these are transitorily experienced by normal people in the moments before falling asleep and when dozing after waking. If direct questions about these kind of phenomena are not asked the patient seldom volunteers an account of them, fearing ridicule or the suspicion of mental illness.

(iii) **Automatisms** comprise complex and perfectly executed activities, essentially purposeless, for the duration of which the patient is subsequently amnesic. Often an attack consists of only simple automatic activity, usually stereotyped, such as closing a door, crossing a room, clapping hands, or uttering some stock phrase. But sometimes he may travel across a city to a place never visited before, driving his car or using public transport and seemingly in full possession of his faculties. He then suddenly regains full consciousness and is perplexed by his whereabouts and is at a loss to explain how he got there.

IS IT EPILEPSY?

Unless an attack has been witnessed by an expert it may be impossible to decide its nature. In favour of epilepsy are altered consciousness with subsequent amnesia for the incident, cyanosis and frothing at the mouth, temporary bilateral pupillary dilatation, a bitten tongue or lip, incontinence of urine, injuries sustained during an attack, or Todd's palsy during recovery. None of these need accompany an epileptic attack, but if they do the presumption of epilepsy is high. Episodic disorders other than epilepsy may lead to confusion, particularly as they also may be associated with brain tumours; to recognise epilepsy proper is to localise the lesion as almost certainly supratentorial.

(i) **Opisthotonus** occurs in brief attacks usually when the brain stem is compressed acutely, such as by a foraminal cone (p. 50). Arching of the neck and lower spine backwards is often accompanied by decerebrate rigidity of all four limbs (extensor or tonic spasms).

(ii) **Decerebrate attacks** (extensor spasms) are due to compression at a rather higher level, in the midbrain, and more often result from tentorial coning (p. 45). Increased extensor tone causes straightening of the affected limbs with pronation of the forearm and plantar-flexion of the foot. Often the limbs of only one side are affected, and sensory stimuli may set off a spasm which may be associated with respiratory overactivity (rather than the apnœa of epilepsy), and possibly by pupillary changes.

(iii) **Chalastic fits** are a contrasting type of disorder because they are characterised by limpness and atony. They occur when pressure is dangerously high from tumours in either compartment of the skull, but particularly with tumours near the third ventricle. The knees suddenly give way and the patient falls to the ground without loss of consciousness, hence the term "drop epilepsy" is sometimes used.

(iv) **Hydrocephalic attacks** (p. 10).

(v) **Amblyopic attacks** (p. 14) though sometimes reported as black-outs are purely visual phenomena.

(vi) **Hysterical fugues** closely resemble epileptic automatisms and the distinction will depend on the setting and background of the incident. If epileptic the patient often suffers also from some attacks of a different nature which are more readily recognisable as epileptic.

(vii) **Internal carotid stenosis** occasionally leads to episodic insufficiency of the circulation to one half of the brain with transient hemiplegia, and sometimes transient loss of vision in the eye on the side of the stenosis. Such attacks may be indistinguishable from epilepsy except by the involvement of vision or their precipitation by the sudden assumption of the upright position.

(viii) **Ménière's disease** causes episodic vertigo, almost always with vomiting, and normally lasting several hours. In severe attacks there may be some clouding of consciousness, but the vertiginous sensation is usually vividly remembered. During an attack the patient resists any attempt to move the head because this aggravates his sickening giddiness. Increasing deafness and persistent tinnitus complete the syndrome.

IS THE EPILEPSY SYMPTOMATIC?

Epilepsy is a non-specific response of the brain to an injurious agent, be it mechanical, chemical, bacterial or metabolic. A large number of conditions can thus give rise to fits and space-occupying lesion is only one. Most often no overt cause is found and the diagnosis remains "idiopathic" epilepsy, although there is probably an underlying structural abnormality in most cases, perhaps resulting from minor birth trauma.

Idiopathic epilepsy usually begins in childhood and it is when a patient suffers his first fit in adult life that suspicions are aroused regarding underlying organic disease. When fits are focal there is even greater likelihood of a local lesion. However, brain tumours more often cause non-focal attacks than focal, whilst focal attacks, especially of temporal lobe origin, are frequently found in idiopathic epilepsy.

There is nothing characteristic therefore about the epilepsy due to tumour to distinguish it from either idiopathic or other symptomatic epilepsy. In all forms the frequency of attacks varies widely, with long remissions, sometimes of years, occurring unaccountably or as a response to anticonvulsant drugs. Attacks may be frequent for a few months and then disappear although the tumour continues to grow. Sometimes epilepsy persists but the pattern changes as the tumour grows into fresh areas of the brain.

Epilepsy first appearing in adult life is always suspicious of a brain tumour or some other acquired organic lesion, and preliminary tests (Chapter 5) should always be carried out. If all of these are negative, and there are no physical signs pointing either to a focal lesion or to raised pressure, it is probably not worthwhile proceeding to contrast radiological investigations, provided the patient can be kept under outpatient observation. No cause is found in the majority of cases of epilepsy of late onset but this should not deter the clinician from investigating every case as far as it seems to deserve.

Other causes of symptomatic epilepsy are legion and would take too much space to list here. Perhaps the condition most often confused with tumour is cerebral arteriosclerosis, especially as dementia and hemiplegia may also occur.

A NOTE ON NOMENCLATURE

Epilepsy carries a stigma second only to that of mental illness, and especially feared because it precludes so many types of employment. Euphemisms are therefore often used by patients and tend to be employed loosely even by doctors, to their own confusion.

Convulsions, fits, attacks, blackouts, dysrhythmic episodes and seizures can all mean the same. The terms grand mal, generalised epilepsy and major fits are all used to describe what have been described here under non-focal attacks. But the terms are imprecise; some contend that "major" means only that consciousness is lost, some that "grand mal" should be restricted to classical generalised convulsions with tongue biting and incontinence, whilst "generalised" does not specify whether the fit began in one area or was general from the start. "Minor" epilepsy is an even more vague term, whilst "petit mal" has a strictly limited application. Partial epilepsy is used by some to describe any attack which does not become generalised.

Status epilepticus refers to a succession of attacks of a generalised nature (though the onset may be focal) in which one attack follows another without return of consciousness between them. A dangerous state of affairs with an appreciable mortality, it may develop out of the very first fit a patient suffers, especially if the lesion is frontal; once it has happened it is liable to be repeated if that individual suffers further fits in the future and may be precipitated by sudden withdrawal of anticonvulsants (for treatment see p. 268).

Epilepsia partialis continuans is status epilepticus confined locally, to the face or fingers or foot usually, and may continue for hours or days without impairment of consciousness or any serious threat to life.

To summarise, epilepsy is a very common manifestation of disease in the nervous system; it is often the first evidence of a brain tumour, though very few people with epilepsy have a tumour; it more commonly heralds an abscess than a hæmatoma. The two important questions to answer are: has the patient had an epileptic fit?, and is there any indication of which part of the brain was primarily affected?

Dysphasia (Language disorders)

Language is largely dependent on the left temporal lobe in right-handed persons, and also in most who are left-handed. Dominance of either hemisphere appears to be less marked in true left-handers who may suffer dysphasia from lesions on either side, but they tend to recover more rapidly as the other side asserts itself. The right hemisphere is seldom dominant, but if the left brain is severely damaged in early childhood the right side of the brain seems able to assume responsibility for language function.

The various aspects of language function, speaking, reading, writing and listening are special cases of sensorimotor activity, with motor function represented anterior to sensory. Although mixed types of disorder are most common, predominantly motor or sensory defects can be recognised in many instances and are sometimes regarded as special varieties of apraxia or agnosia.

Motor dysphasia is both the most frequent and the most obvious type, the patient being unable either to utter words which he has in his mind, or to think of the correct words to express himself. Commonly only the names of certain objects or people are inaccessible whilst the patient is able to explain what an object is used for, indicating both that he has recognised it and has no difficulty in making sentence constructions using other words (nominal dysphasia). Indeed purely nominal dysphasia may not be immediately obvious, particularly if the patient is not allowed to get beyond the exchange of clichés which is often the limit of daily contact with the doctor in hospital. These he may manage perfectly, but when asked to name a series of objects the defect is soon obvious, although he may name the first two or three correctly, mispronounce the next two names (paraphasia) and then be unable to name any more.

Perseveration is exhibited by many dysphasic patients, the name of one object correctly given being reproduced as the name for succeeding objects. It may be indicative of general mental clouding rather than of specific language disorder.

Dysgraphia is also a motor defect in language function, but is seldom the only one; more often the ability to write survives the loss of the spoken word. Wrong words, misspellings and perseveration all appear before the writing is reduced to a meaningless scribble.

Sensory dysphasia comprises the inability to understand spoken or written words and commands. Reading aloud may still be possible but without comprehension. As with motor defects this may be obvious only on direct testing, in the early stages, by giving a number of commands in rapid succession; perseveration of response may then be observed. If sensory dysphasia is present in addition to motor the patient is unaware of his mistakes when he speaks; this aggravates the motor disability and the almost speechless and largely inaccessible state which results is termed *global aphasia*. The words aphasia and dysphasia are loosely used in practice, without implying that aphasia means total inability to speak; likewise agraphia, dysgraphia; alexia, dyslexia.

The great value of dysphasia as a localising sign makes its recognition important. Two conditions may simulate it.

(i) **Mental confusion** leads to inappropriate responses to questions and commands, and it may be impossible for even a skilled observer to decide whether language function is disturbed. The dysphasic patient will usually make a guess which is near the mark, or in some other way indicate that he has recognised but cannot name an object, thus giving the impression that he is trying to co-operate. It is curious that dysphasia seldom makes a man taciturn, and the prolix splutterings of the dysphasic patient making unnecessary conversations are characteristic.

(ii) **Dysarthria** due to bulbar palsy or cerebellar lesions causes slurred speech which may be difficult to understand, but a moment's thought will prevent this being mistaken for dysphasia. Confusion is less likely to arise if reference is made to disorders of *language* rather than of speech.

Parietal spatial disorders

The non-dominant, right parietal lobe is necessary for the correct appreciation of the image of a man's own body, and his orientation in extra-personal space. With this lobe damaged a patient may neglect his limbs, in particular the left ones; he forgets where they are and allows them to lie in bizarre positions; even if the arms are not weak he fails to bring both into use for bimanual skills. If extrapersonal space is incorrectly perceived there will be difficulty in getting around even in familiar surroundings, wrong turnings taken in moving from room to room in a man's own house, an inability to recognise common landmarks or follow simple routes in the street. Asked to draw a map of the ward, or a clock, or to copy diagrams, he may be quite unable to do so, or else execute only a wobbly outline more fitting for a four-year-old child.

The patient with a lesion in the left (dominant) parieto-temporal lobe may be unable to recognise parts of his own body, to distinguish between his different fingers, between left and right limbs or even between his own limbs and those of the examiner. Inability to calculate, which involves the correct arrangement of serial symbols in space, is another sequel (dyscalculia) with left-sided lesions.

The implications of these disorders of the mind and the insight they give into the way in which we relate to our surroundings are fascinating. But as a localising sign they indicate no more than a lesion in the right parietal region, which will often be suspected already from the homonymous hemianopia usually accompanying these curious distortions of perception.

Anosmia

Anterior fossa masses may damage the olfactory bulbs and tracts giving anosmia on one or both sides. Unilateral loss is much more significant, but even this can be due to abnormalities in the nose which must be excluded. Bilateral anosmia is a common and often permanent sequel of head injury which should be excluded before attributing anosmia to a local expanding lesion. Raised intracranial pressure over a long period may also impair olfactory function bilaterally.

Homonymous hemianopia

Interruption of the visual pathway anywhere from the optic tracts to the calcarine cortex will lead to complete or partial loss of the opposite visual field, homonymous hemianopia (fig. 6). The temporal half of vision is lost in one eye and the nasal half in the other; whichever eye is used the same half (either left or right) of the field will be lost. The projection is reversed, horizontally and vertically, right-sided lesions causing left hemianopia and a high lesion (parietal) giving loss of the lower quadrant, a low lesion (temporal) an upper quadrantic hemianopia. Most lesions involve the optic radiations, which being spread out over a wide area are susceptible to damage from a wide range of lesions. A lesion in the calcarine cortex itself, which is rare, spares the macula; this is only likely to be appreciated if the fields are plotted on a perimeter or screen.

Confrontation can be used to test fields roughly, the patient fixing his eyes on those of the examiner who brings in his fingers from the periphery of the fields. He compares the patient's field with his own, whilst watching the patient's eyes for any failure to fix which will falsify the result. If visual acuity is impaired a torch or waving white card or handkerchief may be used to plot a crude field which may nonetheless be invaluable; the inexperienced too readily accept the excuse that vision is too poor for field testing, or that the patient is too drowsy or uncooperative. In the latter event the reaction to menace from the two sides may be compared. Parietal lesions may give only an *attention* hemianopia; when objects are simultaneously presented in both right and left visual fields only one is attended to; if the same stimulus is then applied again, in the defective field alone, it is immediately seen.

More accurate records of the visual fields in co-operative patients with adequate vision are obtained with the *perimeter* or tangent *screen* (of Bjerrum). Small white objects, 1–5 mm. in diameter, are moved into the field against a black background marked in degrees, and the field mapped on a chart. Different isopters are drawn, expressed as object size over distance from the screen, and a defect which is not apparent with a large object may be obvious when a small one is used. The size of the blind spot and of any scotomata (islands of visual loss) can be charted in addition to the peripheral field; and because the conditions are reproducible, serial examinations made over weeks or years can be accurately compared (fig. 7).

Like dysphasia this is so important a localising sign that no effort should be spared in the attempt to elicit it. Homonymous hemianopia is occasionally produced by parasellar lesions involving the optic tract,

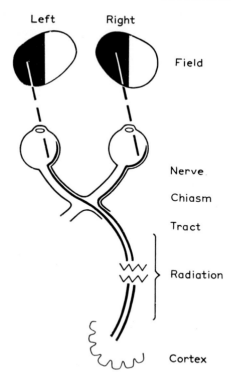

(Right sided lesion)

(*a*) Lesions of the optic tract, radiation or cortex cause hemianopia on the opposite side.

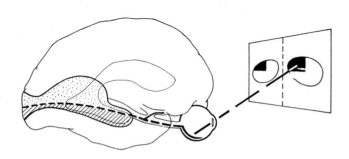

(Right temporal lobe lesion)

(*b*) Lesions affecting only the lower part of these pathways cause hemianopia in only the upper part of the affected field.

FIG. 6 Homonymous hemianopia

but there will usually be other signs of a lesion in this region. It may also be misleading when due to posterior cerebral artery occlusion due to a

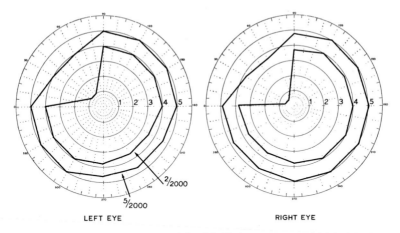

LEFT EYE   RIGHT EYE

FIG. 7 Visual field chart

From Bjerrum screen: patient–screen distance = 2 metres. The quadrant defect barely shown on the 5/2000 isopter is obvious when a smaller object (2 mm.) is used.

tentorial cone or basilar artery thrombosis—again conditions which normally declare themselves by obvious local signs.

Hemiplegia

This sensorimotor disturbance is less valuable as a localising feature because it may be produced by a lesion anywhere on the pyramidal pathway from the cortex, through the internal capsule, cerebral peduncles and pons, to the medullary pyramids (fig. 8). When due to a lesion of the cortex or the subcortical pathways the paralysis seldom affects the whole of one side equally; only the face may be involved but more often both face and arm are weak, or the leg alone. Lower down in the pathway the fibres for face, arm and leg are so closely packed together that a lesion tends to produce a relatively total hemiplegia. Concomitant dysphasia, hemianopia or focal epilepsy indicate that the lesion is above the tentorium.

The severity of hemiplegia ranges from complete paralysis to mild increase in tone, first noticed in the forearm pronators and reflected in tendon hyperreflexia; there is an extensor plantar reflex (Babinski response), and absence or easy tiring of the abdominal reflexes on that side. Weakness due to a hemisphere lesion usually affects fine peripheral movements initially, whilst gross proximal movements of the shoulder and hip remain unaffected. This too is the pattern of recovery, proximal before distal, gross before fine movements.

When cortical sensation is deranged there is loss of *two-point discrimination*, the ability to discern that a double touch or pain stimulus is in fact made up of two discrete points. The distance between them which can be detected varies widely on different parts of the body, being most fine on the finger tips, most crude on the back of the trunk; the normal side is the standard for comparison. *Astereognosis* is the inability to

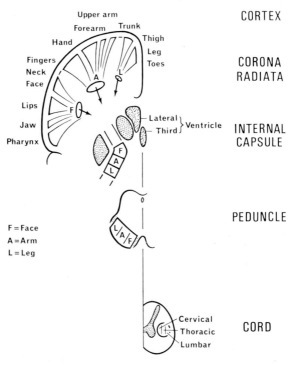

FIG. 8 Cortico-spinal tract

appreciate differences in texture of materials and weight, and to recognise an object from feeling its shape or character. Even when astereognosis occurs without any weakness it may seriously limit the use of fingers and hand which will be capable of fine movements only when under direct vision. When *joint position sense* is lost the patient is unaware of the state of his joints or even the location of his limb, and this renders a limb almost useless although muscle strength remains unimpaired. Complex movements depend as much on sensory guidance as on motor control, and sensory hemiplegia is a crippling condition. When a limb is found to be obviously powerful on simple testing, yet the patient protests that it is useless, he may be wrongly suspected of exaggerating the disability.

Centrally Placed Supratentorial Tumours
Anterior part of third ventricle

In the cavity of the ventricle tumours usually produce only increased pressure, by occluding the foramen of Monro (fig. 3). Because the commonest lesion, a colloid cyst, is sometimes mobile in the ventricle the obstruction may be intermittent with sudden **episodes of headache** of the utmost severity, hydrocephalic attacks; **drop attacks** also occur (p. 28).

Above the ventricle, in the corpus callosum or septum pellucidum, tumours cause the most profound **dementia,** much more severe than is common either from increased pressure or from unilateral frontal tumours. Drowsiness and repeated yawning are frequent and the patient may become mentally inaccessible even though there is no increase in intracranial pressure. Hemiplegia is sometimes bilateral, but occasionally affects the two sides alternately, probably due to pressure on the anterior cerebral arteries. **Alternating hemiplegia,** which is sometimes mistakenly suspected of being hysterical, may also be produced by parasagittal lesions involving the medial surfaces of both hemispheres and by lesions in the brain stem or at the foramen magnum where the pyramidal fibres for the two sides are contiguous.

Lateral to the third ventricle lie the basal ganglia, involvement of which may give symptomatic **Parkinsonism** characterised by extrapyramidal rigidity of a cog-wheel (as distinct from clasp-knife pyramidal type), paucity of movement, occasionally involuntary movements. The internal capsule is very close and there may be **hemiplegia** which involves all parts of the one side, for the fibres are closely crowded together here; there may be a capsular **hemianopia** in addition. **Hydrocephalus** results from block of the foramen of Monro.

Below the ventricle lies the tuber cinereum, disorders of which cause **endocrine imbalance** with obesity or wasting and occasionally precocious puberty; the wasting state may be mistaken for anorexia nervosa.

Sellar and parasellar tumours

Chiasmal compression is a most important condition to recognise because it is frequently possible to save sight by surgical intervention if this is done in time. Careful plotting of the visual fields is essential (p. 35) because certain patterns of field defect are associated with pressure from different directions although these patterns are seldom pure for long. They take time to develop, and are frequently incomplete at the stage when it is most important to detect a tumour, whilst later the involvement of other parts of the tracts may lead to a mixture of more than one type of field defect. What matters is to realise that the location of the lesion is chiasmal.

Central pressure from below, as from tumour growing out of the sella, causes bitemporal hemianopia which appears first in the upper quadrant (fig. 9). If pressure begins further forwards, one eye alone may

BITEMPORAL HEMIANOPIA

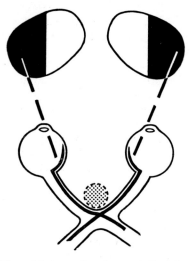

(*a*) Anterior chiasmal lesions affect the nasal fibres from each retina.

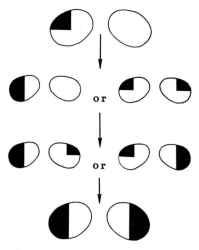

(*b*) Pressure from below the chiasm (e.g. pituitary tumour) affects first the upper field; according to the direction of tumour growth, bitemporal hemianopia may be evolved in different ways.

FIG. 9 Bitemporal hemianopia

become blind from optic nerve pressure, if further back the optic tract may be affected initially resulting in a homonymous defect. The length of the nerve and tract vary a great deal, pre-fixed (short nerve) and post-fixed chiasms being recognised as anatomical variations, so that conclusions about whether a compressing mass is anterior or posterior cannot be too confident.

Visual acuity is not always tested as part of the examination of the cranial nerves; patients can go blind unnoticed if their remarks about not seeing the print too well go unverified. Standard test types should be used; they allow repeated observations to be made over a period of time, provided that the same glasses are worn (if any are) on each occasion. If distant and near vision are both tested errors of refraction will be detected. Papillœdema and retinal lesions, as well as opacities in the media, must be excluded before ascribing failing vision to a lesion of the visual pathways.

Endocrine abnormalities can result from interference with the anterior or posterior pituitary itself, or from involvement of the hypothalamic nuclei, or the portal vessels and nerve fibres in the pituitary stalk. Hypogonadism, hypothyroidism and adrenocortical deficiency result in varying degrees, diabetes insipidus, obesity and dwarfism (p. 144).

Cavernous sinus syndromes develop from lateral spread involving the third to sixth cranial nerves, which are in the lateral wall of the sinus. Clinically recognisable thrombosis of the sinus with congestion of the conjunctiva seldom occurs though some degree of *proptosis* may appear. *Fifth* nerve dysfunction shows itself as facial pain, usually of the first division (forehead), a local sensation quite clearly distinguishable from headache. Loss of sensation over the trigeminal distribution is less common, but corneal anæsthesia, often the first sign, will go undetected unless specifically tested for. *Oculomotor* palsy is commoner than fourth or sixth nerve weakness, and may begin with squint, a dilated unreactive pupil or ptosis; eventually all three features develop. *Diplopia* is the earliest sign of imbalance of the external ocular muscles, and before it is sufficiently marked for two images to be appreciated the complaint is of *blurring* of vision, which is corrected by closing one eye; this *latent* diplopia can be mistaken for visual failure. Diplopia will not develop if visual acuity is severely depressed in one eye, as it often is by lesions in this situation; complete ptosis likewise masks it.

Infratentorial tumours

It is less easy to be sure that a tumour lies in the posterior fossa than to know that is must be above the tentorium. Manifestations of radies pressure usually dominate the clinical picture from an early stage, and need relief before the appearance of any localising signs. This is partly due to the smaller size of this compartment of the skull but also to the readiness with which the CSF pathways become blocked by masses in this situation.

Many of these patients are children; two-thirds of intracranial tumours occurring under the age of fifteen are in the posterior fossa. In infancy papilloedema may not develop because the skull bones give way, resulting in prominent sutures and a wide **tight fontanelle;** an unusually **large head** is always suspicious (fig. 71). **Vomiting** is a very frequent symptom, and children can become cachexic and acidotic from daily vomiting over a period of time. The prominence of this complaint may be due to the frequency with which these lesions cause raised pressure or sometimes to involvement of the floor of the fourth ventricle. **Headache** from tumours in the posterior fossa is often confined to the occipital region and radiates down the neck; it may even favour the side of the tumour if this is in the cerebello-pontine angle. **Dementia** in adults with slowly growing tumours is quite common, and is probably secondary to internal hydrocephalus, though many patients with very high pressure and huge ventricles remain alert. Squint due to non-localising sixth nerve palsy is very common.

Signs of **foraminal coning** are important in pointing to a posterior fossa tumour (p. 56).

Central

Tumours of the vermis and fourth ventricle are apt to be silent in respect of local signs but are very liable to produce severe internal hydrocephalus and raised pressure. Nystagmus and limb ataxia are seldom seen, but **trunkal ataxia** may be disabling, the patient unable to stand or even to sit up in bed although the limbs can be moved gracefully. **Vomiting** as a sole sign, before there are signs of pressure, bespeaks involvement of the floor of the fourth ventricle which may also give nuclear facial palsy and respiratory irregularities.

Lateral

Ataxia of the limbs on one side, usually first noticed in walking, is often the presenting symptom. Even if the classical staggering wide-based gait is not obvious, unsteadiness may be detected by having the patient walk across the room and turn quickly; he will usually sway for a moment and need to steady up before he begins to walk again. Hopping on one foot may be more difficult on one side, and intention tremor may be detected when a finger or the big toe is aimed at a small target.

Nystagmus of cerebellar origin is slower and coarser when the eyes are deviated to the side of the lesion, indeed may only occur in this position. Rotatory or vertical nystagmus usually indicates invasion of the central pathways in the brain stem. Unsustained nystagmus at the extremes of deviation may be found in normal individuals, whilst patients taking high doses of epanutin for epilepsy may have both nystagmus and ataxia. *Middle ear disease* is probably the commonest cause of nystagmus, but this vestibular type is finer and less obviously lateralised than the cerebellar type and persists when gaze is not fixed; *recent head injury* is another frequent cause of vestibular nystagmus.

Dysarthria can result from a cerebellar defect, a special form of ataxia, or it may be due to bulbar palsy from a tumour spreading to the medulla or the issuing nerves. In either event this defect of phonation must be distinguished from disorders of language function, and from the slurred and indistinct speech of confused and drowsy patients, and that due to facial paralysis.

Cranial nerve palsies, other than the sixth palsy from pressure, may develop with any lateral cerebellar lesion but are most constant when the tumour is in the cerebello-pontine angle. *Deafness* is often the first sign; tuning fork tests will help to distinguish nerve and conduction types, but audiometry may be needed to assess mixed types of deafness (p. 155). *Vertigo* is a frequent complaint, and the function of the vestibular nerve may be tested objectively by the caloric reaction; absence of this reaction indicates that the nerve is dead, provided disease of the inner ear has been excluded (p. 155). *Facial palsy* may be hard to detect when slight, but diminished blink on one side is an early sign. The *bulbar nerves* (ix, x, xi, xii) are usually affected as a group as they lie close together on the jugular bulb; dysphagia and dysarthria result. *Fifth nerve irritation* occasionally gives rise to symptomatic trigeminal neuralgia, but this is much less common than facial anæsthesia which may at first be very limited, often to loss of corneal reflex only.

Transtentorial tumours

Lateral tumours either grow through the tentorial hiatus and lie alongside the brain stem both above and below the tent, or arise from the dura of the tent and expand in both directions, indenting the under surface of the occipital lobe and the upper surface of the cerebellar hemisphere. Palsies of the seventh and eighth **cranial nerves,** combined with lesions of the second and third; **hemianopia** or **dysphasia** associated with **cerebellar ataxia;** these are the kind of surprising combinations to which these tumours may give rise. Intracranial pressure may be very high, either from a block to upward flow through the cisterna ambiens or due to obstruction of the lateral venous sinus retarding venous drainage from the brain and perhaps impeding CSF absorption.

Central tumours exert their effects without encroaching functionally on either of the main compartments of the skull until late in their course. These arise in the region of the pineal gland or the tectal plate but eventually spread more widely, usually above the tent (to cause hemianopia or hemiplegia). Internal hydrocephalus from aqueduct obstruction develops early; and there are signs of **dysfunction of the third nerve nucleus**—the dilated, sluggishly reacting pupils, with impaired upward movement of the eyes and mild ptosis. This syndrome was for long believed to be pathognomonic of pineal tumours but it may also result from transtentorial herniation of the temporal lobe (p. 50).

FURTHER READING

Brain, W. R. (1961). *Brain*, **84,** 145–166. The neurology of language.
Hughes, B. (1954). *The Visual Fields*, Oxford Univ. Press.
Matthews, W. B. (1963). *Practical Neurology*. Blackwell, Oxford.
Penfield, W. and Jasper, H. (1954). *Epilepsy and the Functional Anatomy of the Human Brain*. Churchill, London.

CHAPTER 4

Clinical Diagnosis

Presenting syndromes
   Increased intracranial pressure with focal symptoms and signs
   Focal features alone
   Increased intracranial pressure alone

Evidence of brain shift
   Transtentorial herniation
   Foraminal Impaction

Intracranial space-occupying lesions may present with clinical evidence of increased pressure or with focal neurological disorders, or both, and the differential diagnosis varies with the type of presentation. Sometimes false localising signs complicate the problem of diagnosis, although properly evaluated these can be helpful by indicating the type of brain shift which has developed.

Presenting syndromes

When a patient has a combination of **raised pressure and focal CNS signs** there will be little doubt that he is suffering from an intracranial mass. Tumour may be distinguished in most instances from abscess or hæmatoma by the typical preceding history in the latter conditions, but the exclusion of hypertensive cerebrovascular disease with papillœdema is not easy. Neither a sudden onset nor spontaneous remission excludes tumour, and patients with tumour may have raised blood pressure either from pre-existing hypertension or as a reaction to raised intracranial pressure. There is no certain way to tell on clinical grounds alone, and inevitably a number of hypertensive patients must be investigated to exclude tumour.

   Focal signs without raised pressure opens a wider field of differential diagnosis. Confusion most often arises with cerebrovascular disease, cerebral atrophy and demyelinating disorders. In making the distinction from brain tumour a careful history is invaluable; the steadily progressive development of dysfunction which is confined to a single, even if extensive, area of the brain is suggestive of tumour. Probably all patients developing focal neurological signs which persist or progress should be investigated as brain tumour suspects, unless there are definite indications of vascular disease or demyelination in the form of previous episodes of transient disturbance of function in parts of the brain remote from that presently affected.

Raised pressure without focal signs is a more frequent and a more pressing situation. Likely causes are midline masses blocking CSF flow and causing internal hydrocephalus, silent slowly-growing lateral supratentorial masses (usually right frontal or temporal) and chronic bilateral subdural hæmatoma. Progressive *loss of vision* from papillœdema can occur with relatively little headache; no one is more tragic than the patient with a benign meningioma totally blind, carrying a bundle of spectacles successively prescribed. *Mental disorder* can so dominate the scene in these patients with pressure and no signs that they may be admitted to mental hospital without any suspicion of the underlying organic disease until the fundi are examined.

A number of patients with raised pressure alone appear to have no local lesion, and are diagnosed as suffering from the unexplained but not uncommon condition known as **pseudotumour cerebri** (syn. otitic hydrocephalus, serous meningitis, benign intracranial hypertension). It is commonest in young adults, women more than men; it may be associated with pregnancy or childbirth, sometimes with infections, especially of the ear. Headaches, seldom of great severity, are followed by diplopia due to sixth nerve weakness from raised intracranial pressure. There is severe papillœdema; in some cases obscurations of vision give way to blindness from consecutive atrophy. With all this evidence of severely raised intracranial pressure the general well-being of the patient is as surprising as it is characteristic.

The natural history is towards resolution but it may be many months before the papillœdema subsides completely. Lumbar puncture, sometimes done repeatedly as an aid to recovery, shows that the pressure fluctuates widely from day to day; a further curious feature is an abnormally low CSF protein (10–20 mg./100 ml.). Subtemporal decompression is sometimes needed to save sight; the defect in the bone may bulge intermittently for many months, further evidence of the prolonged course of this condition.

The association with otitis media led to the term otitic hydrocephalus and to the theory that it was due to thrombosis spreading from the lateral to the sagittal sinus with impaired absorption of CSF. But ventriculography never shows a dilated system, indeed the ventricles are small and give the impression of being squeezed tight by a swollen brain. The pathogenesis of this condition remains unexplained.

There are *other causes of raised pressure* than brain tumour; arterial hypertension, polycythæmia and chronic emphysema are among the more common. Each must be severe before it affects intracranial pressure, and is therefore obvious if a general clinical examination is conducted, as it should be in every case of suspected brain tumour.

Evidence of brain shift

In addition to primary localising signs there may be focal signs originating in structures remote from the site of the primary expanding lesion, the result of brain shifts and herniations. Such signs prove false or misleading only if it is assumed that they result from compression in the immediate neighbourhood of the tumour. Properly evaluated they can be of help in indicating, from the nature of the brain shift, whether a tumour is more likely to be above or below the tent. They are also a warning that the brain is dangerously compressed.

Sooner or later as pressure rises, the brain itself must move. The direction in which it does so depends on the site of the expanding lesion relative to the contours of the skull and the dural partitions which subdivide the cranial cavity. Part of the brain shifts from a compartment where pressure is rising to one where it is lower, and also into the larger subarachnoid spaces, cisterna ambiens and cisterna magna, from which the CSF can be displaced.

The tentorium is the most complete of the dural barriers and divides the posterior fossa from the supratentorial compartment (made up of the middle and anterior cranial fossæ). This division is complete but for the hiatus, which is filled by the brain stem and the narrow cisterna ambiens beside it (fig. 10). Masses above the tentorium push the brain stem and part of the cerebral hemisphere down through the tentorial hiatus, the only exit from this compartment; posterior fossa tumours drive the cerebellar tonsils and medulla through the foramen magnum. These comprise the two most important brain shifts; each puts a vital part of the brain in jeopardy.

Transtentorial herniation (syn. tentorial or temporal cone*)

PATHOLOGY

The medial part of the temporal lobe (the uncus and hippocampus) is packed down into the cisterna ambiens forming a hernia (fig. 11). The consequences of this herniation are several; the mid-brain is compressed from side to side.

The brain stem is also thrust downwards through the hiatus, suffering strains in its long axis, either longitudinal stretching or buckling. Brain stem dysfunction declares itself in decerebrate rigidity and in impaired alertness due to reticular formation involvement. The third nerves and posterior cerebral arteries, being fixed above, are stretched; the nerve may also be compressed against the unyielding petroclinoid ligament as well as being pushed down by the temporal herniation. Posterior

* The word "cone" was first applied to herniation of the cerebellum through the foramen magnum to form a cone-shaped plug of tissue. The verb "to cone" is common usage among neurosurgeons and neurologists to describe the development of clinical syndromes associated with transtentorial herniation or foraminal impaction.

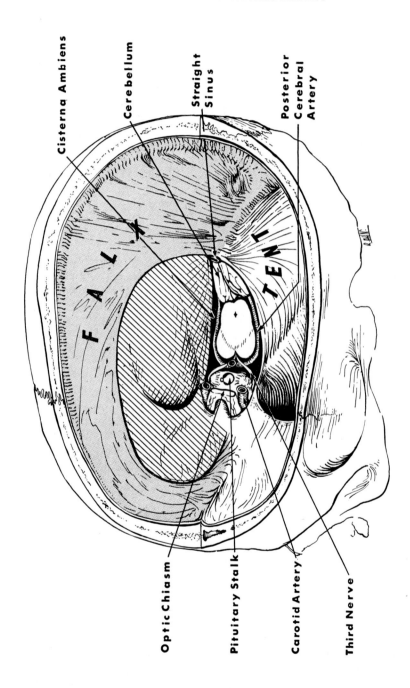

Cisterna Ambiens

Cerebellum

Straight Sinus

Posterior Cerebral Artery

FALX

TENT

Optic Chiasm

Pituitary Stalk

Carotid Artery

Third Nerve

cerebral artery occlusion results in hæmorrhagic infarction of the occipital lobe. The pituitary stalk may be angled across the dorsum sellæ, resulting in diabetes insipidus.

Not only are the nuclear masses and tracts of the brain stem distorted but so are their intrinsic vessels. This frequently results in local hæmorrhages which add to the disruption of function. These were previously

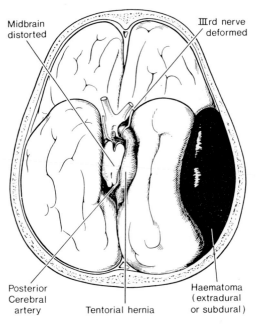

Fig. 11 Tentorial herniation of the medial part of the temporal lobe, causing dysfunction in the midbrain, the third nerve and the territory of the posterior cerebral artery. A temporal hæmatoma is shown for clarity but a mass in any situation above the tent can produce a hernia.

believed to result from venous congestion but are more likely due to tearing of the stretched arterioles and capillaries. Hæmorrhages are most striking after an acute compression which may not have had time to produce much tentorial herniation, whilst gross herniation and midbrain distortion without any hæmorrhage can occur in slowly developing compressions.

Fig. 10 (*facing*) Tentorial hiatus
The midbrain largely fills the hiatus but the cerebellum is visible behind, the third nerves and posterior cerebral arteries in front. The subarachnoid cisterna ambiens (in black) lies at the side of the midbrain, communicating with the cisterna interpeduncularis in front.
(*After Johnson.*)

CLINICAL

Acute tentorial cone

This critical condition is most often encountered by *physicians* in patients who have suffered cerebral hæmorrhage; a massive infarct followed by œdema, or necrotising encephalitis (p. 190); and by *surgeons* in association with rapidly accumulating extradural hæmatoma due to middle meningeal hæmorrhage. It can also develop as an acute-on-chronic episode in temporal lobe abscess and rapidly advancing malignant tumours above the tentorium.

Third nerve palsy on the side of the compression is most readily detected by dilatation of the pupil with loss of both the direct and consensual light reflexes (fig. 12). Other third nerve functions are difficult to test in these patients who are in coma or losing consciousness, but in the few who will co-operate some ptosis and loss of eye movement (especially upward) may be discovered. Relief of the compression frequently reverses the oculomotor palsy immediately, but it may recover only gradually over days or weeks. If the condition is not relieved the opposite pupil follows the course of the first one; recovery is rare once the condition has advanced to the stage of bilaterally fixed and dilated pupils.

Before ascribing a unilateral dilated pupil to tentorial herniation it is important to exclude other causes such as atropine drops, posterior communicating artery aneurysm and, after recent head injury, damage to the optic nerve which is the afferent path for the light reflex (fig. 11). In the last case the pupil will constrict normally when light is shone in the opposite eye (consensual reaction). Bilaterally fixed dilated pupils occur during epilepsy and this possibility must be considered when pupillary change and coma develop very suddenly: if due to epilepsy the pupils will usually recover quickly.

Decerebrate rigidity is a release phenomenon consisting of increased extensor tone in the limbs, often associated with neck retraction. The legs are straight at the knees with strong plantar flexion, the arms hyperpronated with the fists clenched and the elbows extended. Variations in tone are frequent, the posture often aggravated during the hyperpnœic phase of periodic respiration or by any sensory stimulus; this has given rise to the terms "decerebrate attacks" and "tonic mesencephalic fits". In mild instances this abnormal tonus may be assumed only when painful stimuli are applied to a limb; that limb alone may become decerebrate or the response may be generalised. This is evidence of a midbrain lesion and after a head injury may be due either to primary damage in this region or to secondary compression; the sequence of events and accompanying features will usually indicate which.

Slowing of the pulse to 50 per minute can occur in patients with compression who are quite alert. Such a rate may be normal in athletic subjects, and heart block can give even lower counts. Only in the context of supporting signs should bradycardia be ascribed to raised intracranial pressure.

The **blood pressure** may rise in response to increasing intracranial pressure, possibly as a result of reflexes which safeguard the supply of blood to the vital centres in the medulla. If the blood pressure is elevated

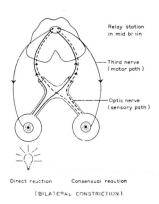

NORMAL LIGHT REFLEX

Relay station in mid brain

Third nerve (motor path)

Optic nerve (sensory path)

Direct reaction   Consensual reaction

(BILATERAL CONSTRICTION)

(a) Whichever eye is illuminated both pupils react by constriction.

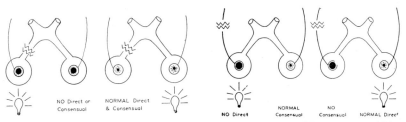

OPTIC NERVE LESION

NO Direct or Consensual   NORMAL Direct & Consensual

THIRD NERVE LESION

NO Direct   NORMAL Consensual   NO Consensual   NORMAL Direct

(b) Illumination of affected eye produces no reaction.

(c) Affected pupil fails to react whichever eye is illuminated.

(After Potter.)

Fig. 12 Pupillary light reflex (position of third nerve is diagrammatic). Both direct and consensual reactions must be tested to localise the lesion.

when a patient first presents, the diagnosis of hypertension with a vascular accident must also be considered.

Chronic tentorial cone

Any slowly growing supratentorial mass can give rise to this but the most striking examples have been due to chronic bilateral subdural hæmatoma.

Loss of conjugate upward gaze with bilateral ptosis is probably the result of compression of the dorsal midbrain. Ptosis is easily overlooked when the patient is in bed, but the wrinkled forehead and look of surprise (due to overaction of frontalis), with the eyes only partly open, is characteristic. If co-operation is poor, the eyes may be induced to turn up reflexly by touching the cornea, and a diminution in upward movement detected. Both ptosis and loss of upward movement are sometimes more marked on one side than the other. A tumour in the pineal region may be suspected, but dilated pupils reacting only sluggishly to light, common with a pineal tumour, are rarely a feature of a chronic cone.

A fluctuating conscious level, probably due to impairment of function in the midbrain reticular formation, is a striking feature. A patient who is drowsy and almost inaccessible may appear normally alert only a few hours later, and this cycle may be repeated many times without any obvious precipitating factors.

Ipsilateral hemiplegia, on the same side as a supratentorial mass, is due to pressure of the free edge of the tentorium against the opposite cerebral peduncle, producing the Kernohan–Woltman notch.

Homonymous hemianopia, from posterior cerebral artery compression, is not often detected clinically.

Occasionally a mass in the posterior fossa causes the upward displacement of the upper part of the vermis through the tentorial hiatus. This *upward transtentorial herniation* may compress the dorsal midbrain, and is encouraged by lowering the supratentorial pressure, by draining the lateral ventricles, without also lowering the infratentorial pressure by providing a bony decompression of the posterior fossa.

Foraminal Impaction
(syn. cerebellar or tonsillar cone)

PATHOLOGY

When pressure in the posterior fossa reaches critical levels the cerebellar tonsils crowd into the foramen magnum, and the medulla is compressed between them and the anterior bony margin (fig. 13). Normally the tonsils just reach the level of the foramen but with posterior fossa compression they are often found as low as the spine of the axis (second cervical vertebra).

CLINICAL

A foraminal cone may lead to apnœa with little or no warning with an acute compression, or it may develop as a late stage of a neglected tentorial cone.

Abnormal neck posture takes several forms. Probably due to vestibular imbalance a child may have a *head tilt* when he walks; this may

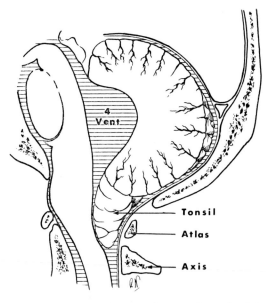

(a) Cerebellar tonsils driven between the posterior arch of the atlas and the medulla, which is compressed.

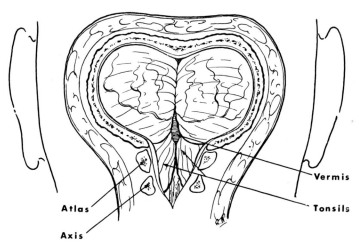

(b) Tip of tonsil is normally above the arch of the atlas; here it is at the level of the axis.

FIG. 13 Foraminal impaction

also occur with loss of vision in one eye, the head position being adjusted to bring the remaining eye into a central position. This head tilt is seldom noticed by the patient or his relatives.

Stiff neck, due to irritation of the dura around the foramen magnum by the structures stuffed tightly into it, may raise the question of meningitis. *Tingling in the arms* on extension of the neck is due to pressure on the cervical cord by the prolapsed plug in the foramen magnum, and some patients "black out" if they extend the neck too far; this movement probably raises pressure by completing the block to CSF circulation in addition to causing pressure directly on the medulla.

Abnormalities of respiratory rate and rhythm are danger signs in posterior fossa compression. A slow rate, say 9 breaths a minute, may be continued with complete regularity for days but this is uncommon. Periodic breathing is common. In its classical form (Cheyne–Stokes breathing) it consists of a crescendo of breaths of increasing depth and frequency followed by a period of total apnœa of up to a minute or so, probably until the accumulating carbon dioxide reaches a high enough level to stimulate the failing respiratory centre. Any irregularity of respiration should raise suspicion of a foraminal cone, which is probably the final stage of cerebral compression of whatever origin. When the mass is in the posterior fossa, however, apnœa is frequently quite sudden, without impaired consciousness or any other warning signs.

FURTHER READING

Adams, J. H. and Graham, D. I. (1976). The relationship between ventricular fluid pressure and the neuropathology of raised intracranial pressure. *Neuropathology and Applied Neurobiology,* **2,** 323–332.

Berg, L., Rosomoff, H. L., Aronson, N., Silbermann, M. and Pool, J. L. (1955). The significance of increased intracranial pressure without localising signs. *Archives of Neurology and Phychiatry (Chicago),* **74,** 498–506.

Greer, M. (1968). Management of benign intracranial hypertension (pseudo-tumour cerebri). *Clinical Neurosurgery,* **15,** 161–174. Williams and Wilkins, Baltimore.

Jennett, W. B. and Stern, W. E. (1960). Tentorial herniation, the midbrain and the pupil. *Journal of Neurosurgery,* **17,** 598–609.

Lysak, R. and Svien, H. J. (1966). Long-term follow-up on patients with diagnosis of pseudotumour cerebri. *Journal of Neurosurgery,* **25,** 288–297.

Plum, F. and Posner, J. B. (1972). *Diagnosis of Stupor and Coma.* 2nd edition. Davis, Philadelphia.

Thompson, R. K. and Malina, S. (1959). Dynamic axial brain stem distortion as a mechanism explaining the cardiorespiratory changes in increased intra-cranial pressure. *Journal of Neurosurgery,* **16,** 664–675.

CHAPTER 5

Preliminary Investigation

Search for primary disease

Plain X-rays of skull

Lumbar puncture

Electroencephalography (EEG)

Echo-encephalography

Radio-isotope tests

EMI (CAT) scanning

Several procedures can be employed to supplement the clinical assessment of patients suspected of harbouring an intracranial mass, some of them available in general hospitals or on an out-patient basis. These may dispense with the need to investigate the patient more elaborately if, for example, underlying disease is revealed which will account for the disorder in the nervous system. On the other hand the initial suspicion of a tumour may be strengthened, and there may be clear indications as to how best to plan neuroradiological investigation.

Search for primary disease

The range of conditions which may develop CNS complications is enormous. The commoner ones should be considered in many cases of suspected brain tumour, especially if the problem is one of focal signs without pressure. Evidence of cerebral *arterial disease* and hypertension is important, and a *source of cerebral emboli* such as auricular fibrillation or subacute bacterial endocarditis will suggest an alternative explanation for symptoms. Neurosyphilis still occurs and testing for the *Wasserman reaction* should be routine. *Infective foci* in the ears, sinuses or lungs, hydatid disease of the liver, cysticerci in the muscles—all will raise the possibility of CNS symptoms related to the spread of infected material or parasites to the brain.

Metastatic intracranial tumours are so common that a diligent search for a *primary extracranial tumour and other secondary tumours* is essential. Abdominal and pelvic examination, palpation of the breasts and of all gland fields, and a chest X-ray should be carried out in all patients suspected of having a brain tumour.

Plain (straight) skull X-rays

These are within the compass of any X-ray department and may yield invaluable information. The normal routine is to take three axial projections and one or both laterals. However, a recent survey suggests that in patients without physical signs (e.g. presenting with headache, dementia or epilepsy) a single lateral film is quite adequate for screening purposes; this will show the pituitary fossa, dorsum sellæ, state of the sutures, size of posterior fossa, angle of the clivus and the presence of calcification either above or below the tentorium. Other views, which may be indicated because of abnormalities seen in this lateral film, or because of certain physical signs are:

Postero-anterior (PA) to show the frontal region, sphenoidal wings and orbits.

Antero-posterior (AP) to show occipital region, foramen magnum, posterior clinoid processes and petrous bones.

Basal (occipito-mental) to show the petrous and sphenoid bones, foramen magnum, other basal foramina.

Special views are required for detailed examination of the internal auditory meati and the optic foramina.

INFORMATION FROM PLAIN FILMS

Evidence of raised intracranial pressure

The most common sign in adults is some **thinning of the dorsum sellæ** and **erosion of the posterior clinoids** (fig. 14); in the elderly some degree of decalcification of these structures is normal. Children develop **widening of the sutures,** which may occur up to the age of seven or eight (syn. diastosis, springing or starting of sutures) (fig. 15).

Digital markings (beaten silver appearance) of the vault, although often associated with long-standing pressure, are not uncommon in normal individuals under the age of 30 and should never be accepted alone as evidence of pressure. Dilatation of the third ventricle, due to internal hydrocephalus, may **enlarge the pituitary fossa** in addition to eroding the dorsum and the floor of the fossa is indistinct (fig. 14).

Intracranial calcification

Calcification in normal structures may enable their displacement by masses to be recognised. The *pineal* forms a stippled area like a flattened pea and immediately in front of it is a more densely calcified structure,

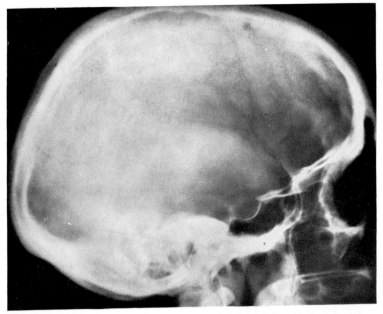

(*a*) Posterior clinoid processes (dorsum sellæ) eroded.

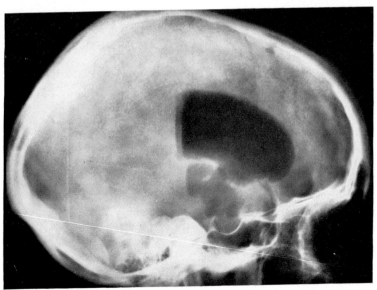

(*b*) Air ventriculogram shows dilated third ventricle in contact with sella.

FIG. 14 Raised intracranial pressure in an adult

the comma-shaped habenular commisure; both calcified structures displace together and are often loosely referred to as the calcified pineal. This calcification is seen increasingly frequently with age, up to 60% of patients over 20 years having a detectable shadow in the lateral view, but this is dense enough to be visible in the axial projections in only half as many. Calcification in a child under the age of 10 suggests a

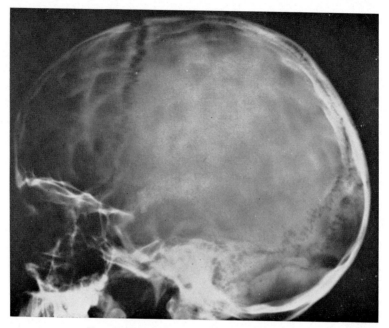

FIG. 15 Raised intracranial pressure in a child

Widened coronal suture, eroded dorsum sellæ digital impressions on the vault.
Note enlarged pituitary fossa and suprasellar calcification—craniopharyngioma.

pineal tumour. Lateral shift of the calcified pineal is significant provided the film is accurately centred; displacement in the lateral view is less easily interpreted although there are charts (Vastine and Kinney) which enable the normal range for any film to be calculated.

The **choroid plexus** of the lateral ventricle is less useful as a guide to brain shift because it is mobile in the ventricle and its position in relation to the skull varies with posture.

Calcification in the falx or tentorium adds to their rigidity and displacement is rarely seen. Other dural folds occasionally calcify, especially the petroclinoid ligament.

In the posterior fossa the **dentate nucleus** may occasionally calcify.

Non-tumorous pathological calcification includes cysticercosis, toxoplasmosis, tuberose sclerosis, hyperparathyroidism, congenital disorder of basal ganglia; atherosclerotic vessels, especially the carotid siphon, and aneurysms may develop small calcified arcs; the abnormal cerebral cortex in Sturges–Weber disease may calcify. It is important to be aware of the possibility of calcification in these various situations lest it be wrongly attributed to a tumour.

Calcification in a tumour is an unusual though valuable sign. Over half the cases of craniopharyngioma have fine flecking above the sella, best seen in the lateral (fig. 15) or Towne projection. About 40% of oligodendrogliomas calcify but this is a rare tumour (fig. 16a); the commoner ependymoma less often develops punctate shadows or streaks of calcium, but other gliomas rarely do. About a fifth of meningiomas throw a recognisable shadow which may be compact enough to outline the tumour (fig. 16b), apart from those with an exostosis which can be felt and seen (fig. 18a). Of the bone tumours which invade the skull the chordoma is the only one which is commonly calcified.

Altered bone density

Reduced density

Vault erosions are the most common and the most obvious. Areas where the bone is *normally* thin are sometimes mistakenly regarded as the seat of disease—the broad transverse grooves for the lateral sinuses, the parietal spider of diploic venous channels, thinning at the top of the coronal suture due to large arachnoid villi, and multiple pits with vascular grooves running to them.

Abnormal vault erosions fall into the following groups:

1. Single scalloped defects, often with a dense margin of condensed bone—dermoids or lipomas of the skull.

2. Multiple punched-out areas, usually less than 1 cm. diameter each —secondary carcinoma or multiple myeloma (fig. 17a).

3. Single irregular erosion without surrounding bone reaction— epithelioma of scalp, eosinophilic granuloma, secondary carcinoma.

4. Erosion with areas of hyperostosis or irregular sclerosis—meningioma or fibrous dysplasia (fig. 17b).

Basal erosions are less easy to detect, as the occipito-mental projection of the skull is technically difficult to take and the bony contour is normally very irregular with a wide variation in the disposition and size of the various foramina. Chordoma and nasopharyngeal carcinoma are the tumours which most often cause destructive lesions in this region; the petrous bone may be irregularly eroded by infective cholesteatoma or show a rounded translucency due to a primary pearly tumour. Thinning of the greater wing of the sphenoid by meningioma

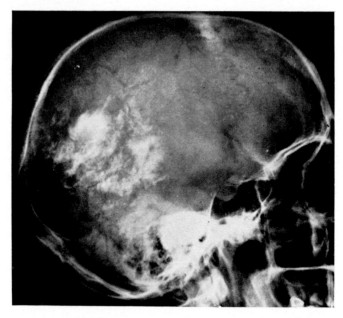

(*a*) Parietal oligodendroglioma.

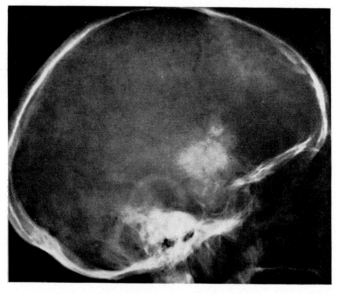

(*b*) Sphenoidal wing meningioma

Fig. 16 Calcification in tumour

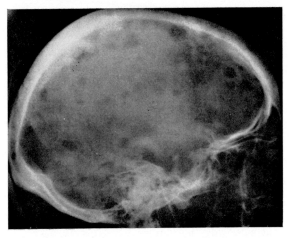

(*a*) Multiple punched out areas—secondary carcinoma.

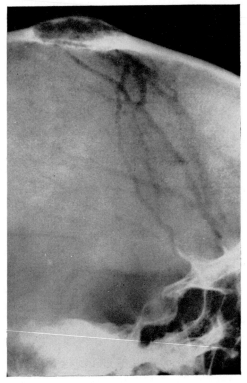

(*b*) Expansion of the vault with sclerosis, associated with dilated vascular channels—meningioma.

FIG. 17 Skull erosion

is best appreciated in the straight PA view which projects this area through the orbit.

Increased density

This is much less common and is usually due to meningioma which may produce hyperostosis; a local thickening projects from the outer table, an exostosis (fig. 18a), or from the inner table, an endostosis. In the sphenoid wing, however, meningioma usually provokes only dense sclerosis without expansion of bone or any externally visible swelling (fig. 18b). Fibrous dysplasia and Paget's disease, the only common imitators, both tend to be more widespread and deforming.

Enlargement of intracranial cavities, foramina, canals

In cases of chronic subdural hæmatoma in children the *whole vault* on one side, but especially the temporal fossa, may be bulged out and larger than the normal side. The opposite effect results from hemispheral atrophy, either congenital or as a consequence of infantile hemiplegia from vascular occlusion; the affected side of the skull is then smaller, the petrous bone high and horizontal (and an angiogram may show that the vessels are also smaller).

Enlargement of the *pituitary fossa* is an invaluable sign, readily recognised on lateral films. The upper limit of normal is about 10 mm. in the AP axis and the same in depth. *Optic canals* and *internal auditory meati* enlarge if harbouring tumours, but special views are needed to show them, and tomography may be helpful.

Lumbar puncture

This is apt to be carried out rather too readily, perhaps because it is the one laboratory method which requires neither special skill nor unusual equipment. Yet it is by no means always harmless and the information it yields is often meagre.

Raised pressure may be detected on lumbar puncture, but it should not be. If there is papillœdema a lumbar puncture should not be done. A high lumbar puncture pressure is, however, sometimes found in the absence of swelling of the discs; this alone should not be accepted as evidence of raised pressure unless the observation is very reliable— the pressure measured with the patient horizontal, fully relaxed and the legs extended so that the thighs are not pressing on the abdomen. Patients are sometimes referred for further investigation on account of raised lumbar puncture pressure which proves to have been measured in the sitting position, and was therefore misleadingly high.

Lumbar puncture is dangerous in patients with raised intracranial pressure in whom herniations and brain shifts are already established. The removal of CSF from below allows the brain stem to move caudally through the tentorial hiatus and the foramen magnum. The patient may die suddenly while the needle is still in place, but more often coning is delayed for several hours, even until the next day. Continual leakage

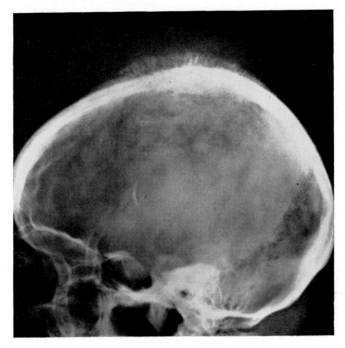

(*a*) Sun-ray appearance associated with a palpable lump—meningioma.

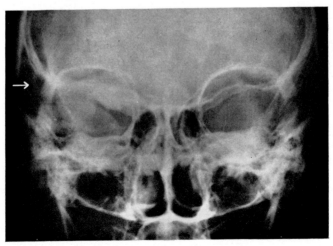

(*b*) Thickening and sclerosis of sphenoidal wing—meningioma.

FIG. 18 Skull hyperostosis

of CSF through the puncture hole in the lumbar dura decompresses the system long after the needle has been withdrawn. This leakage is believed to occur even in patients without raised pressure, and may explain the severe headache which sometimes follows lumbar puncture and which is associated with a low CSF pressure. The possibility of its occurrence means that even "careful" lumbar puncture, using a fine needle and letting off only a small amount of fluid, is not without risk; once the theca has been punctured the situation is out of control.

A **raised protein** level is the most frequent abnormality of the CSF in patients with tumours; about 70% have more than 45 mg. per 100 ml., but less than half of these have more than 100 mg. protein. Apart from neurinomas, which usually give very high levels (400 mg. or more) there is little difference between the tendency of various tumour types to increase the protein. Site may be more important—intraventricular and paraventricular tumours have high levels, and if a large area of tumour abuts on the subarachnoid space the protein is more likely to be raised. The finding of a high CSF protein in a patient suffering from a non-specific symptom, such as epilepsy or dementia, indicates the need to investigate the case exhaustively as there is likely to be an underlying organic lesion.

Xanthochromia of the CSF may be an unexpected finding and raise the possibility of a vascular lesion or of head injury; subdural or subcortical hæmatoma may first be suspected on this account.

Pleocytosis does not always mean an infective lesion, though it often does. Tuberculous meningitis, which can closely simulate a tumour clinically, gives up to 500 lymphocytes as a rule, although when the onset is very acute as many as 1,000 polymorphs may be found. Brain abscess causes only a mild reaction, 100 cells or so, unless complicated by frank meningitis. Encephalitis is suspected when a small number of cells are associated with high protein and low sugar.

Tumours give rise to cells in the CSF in about 10% of cases; about half of those that do are gliomas. Although less than 50 cells is the rule, up to 1,000 cells, either polymorphs or lymphocytes, can occur, probably due to necrosis in a malignant glioma close to the ventricles or subarachnoid pathways. Tumour cells can occasionally be recognised in the CSF when it is centrifuged and the deposit stained after fixation in formalin; in routine counts these are usually reported as large mononuclear or bizarre white cells. Medulloblastoma, malignant glioma or metastasis (especially meningitis carcinomatosa) are the most likely to shed cells into the CSF but it is unusual to be able to identify the cell type in the fluid.

Electroencephalogram (EEG)

As a preliminary screening test this has the virtues of being both painless and entirely free from risk; moreover it can be performed on outpatients. Electrodes can be applied to the scalp using a rubber harness, or they may be stuck on with collodion which is rapidly dried with an air gun. Good contact is essential because the low voltage of the electrical activity of the brain (less than a tenth of that of the ECG) calls for such a degree of amplification that artefacts are readily recorded. The array (or montage) of electrodes may vary but most centres now use the internationally agreed "10/20" system which is based

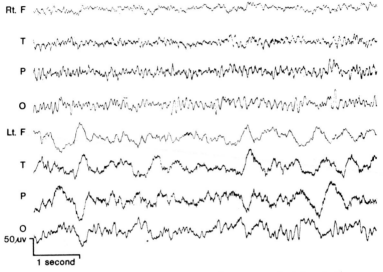

Rt. F

T

P

O

Lt. F

T

P

O

50 μV

1 second

(a) *Left hemisphere lesion:* right side shows normal alpha rhythm (8 Hz), most marked posteriorly; left side is slow with delta activity (< 4Hz) but some alpha remains in occipital lead.

FIG. 19 EEG recordings (only 8 channels displayed from 16 channel record)

on a percentage of the nasion-inion distance and the sagittal/skull base distance.

The normal frequency is 8–11 Hz* known as the alpha rhythm; this is most consistently found in the occipital region when the eyes are closed and the mind is relaxing; it is normally replaced by desynchronised or random activity when the eyes are open or the subject engages in active thinking, such as doing mental arithmetic (fig. 19a). The alpha rhythm would thus seem to be an idling rhythm and its failure to disappear (or block) on eye-opening suggests a lesion on that side of the brain.

The source of the normal waves is not understood, but focal abnormalities are usually regarded as having an origin in disturbed cerebral cortex close to the lesion. Tumours on or near the cortex may cause local slow waves, either theta (4–7 Hz) or delta (less than 4 Hz) (fig. 19b).

* Hz = Hertz = cycles per second.

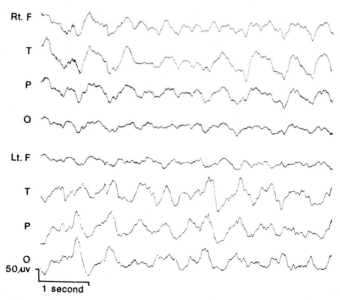

(*b*) *Coma record:* slow waves in all leads with no normal frequencies persisting.

FIG. 19 (*contd.*)

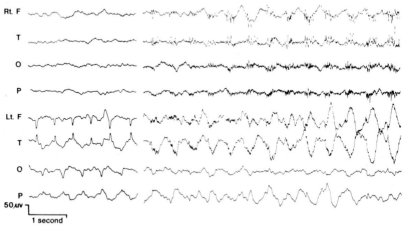

(*c*) *Focal spikes* most marked in left frontal and temporal leads in unconscious patient: a minute later right sided facial twitching produces bursts of muscle spikes in *right* fronto-temporal leads, associated with high voltage activity in *left* fronto-temporal leads. Note phase reversal between left frontal and temporal channels, denoting origin of abnormal activity near electrode common to these two leads.

FIG. 19 (*contd.*)

More accurate localisation is possible if phase reversals are seen, waves in opposite directions occurring simultaneously in two channels which share a common electrode, under which the maximum abnormality is assumed to be located. Supratentorial tumours may show such abnormalities and the EEG may provide the only localising evidence on which to base a decision about which side angiography should be carried out; a less localised but definite abnormality may provide the additional evidence required to justify further investigation in a patient presenting with no definite signs of an intracranial lesion but with suggestive symptoms. Intracranial infections often produce a very dramatic abnormality and emergency EEG can be of value in such instances. A supratentorial abscess, commonly produces local delta waves of unusual slowness (<0.5 Hz) and of high amplitude, an appearance rarely produced by any other lesion. Acute encephalitis produces widespread delta and theta activity, whilst subacute encephalitis has a characteristic record (p. 191).

The EEG will not diagnose epilepsy, apart from idiopathic petit mal in children. The decision that a given clinical episode was epileptic cannot be made from a subsequent record unless an attack happens to be repeated during the recording; even so there are occasional seizures which are electrically silent. However, there are features in some resting records which suggest an underlying epileptic disturbance; when these are diffusely distributed the presumption is that the condition is constitutional rather than due to a local acquired lesion, though the latter can give rise to bilateral secondary electrical disturbances. Moreover many normal subjects, who never had a fit in their lives, have resting records of "epileptic" type. When, however, surgical intervention for epilepsy is considered then the EEG assumes an important role in localising the electrical abnormality (p. 339).

The limitations of the EEG must be fully appreciated if it is not to be misleading; a high degree of skill both in recording and interpretation are essential and the investigation is better not done if these are not available. Even with the best technique no abnormality may be found in the presence of a large tumour. When the patient is very drowsy or in coma, from whatever cause, a non-specific slowing of the record in all channels is usual and may mask local abnormalities. Young children have an unstable record which may not become fully mature until the age of 10 or 12.

Echo-encephalography

Displacement of the midline structure above the tentorium can be detected by reflecting sound vibrations off them from each side of the skull in turn. This uses the principle of ASDIC employed for submarine detection and by bats and porpoises in direction finding. Short pulses of high frequency and low energy sound waves are generated using portable equipment and running off mains electricity supply. A small probe is held to the scalp, making good contact through a coupling fluid smeared on to the skin. The same probe detects its own echoes from the various tissue interfaces of the head. The time taken for the

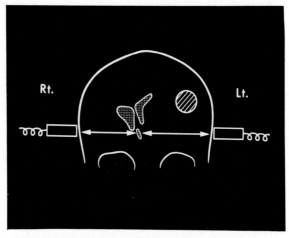

(*a*) Probe applied in turn to the temporal scalp on each side in a case of left-sided mass causing shift to the right.

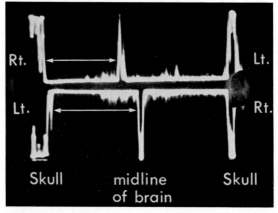

(*b*) Polaroid print of oscilloscope trace, indicating midline closer to right side of the skull.

FIG. 20 Echo-encephalography

echoes to return from various interfaces of the brain (the third ventricle, the septum pellucidum and the vessels, the membranes and the CSF of the longitudinal fissure) can be detected, and enable the distance of these structures from the probe to be compared from identical spots on each side of the head in turn (fig. 20). A shift of midline structures to one side of more than 0·5 to 1·0 cm. can be detected and the ventricular size and site may be distinguished.

Although only available for supratentorial lesions this method is of value chiefly because of its simplicity. No indication is given about the reason for the displacement, nor whether the lesion is anterior or posterior, high or low; its use is in demonstrating the need for further investigation. The risks are nil, for the kind of vibrations used are of such low energy that no damage occurs in the tissues through which they pass.

Use of radio-isotopes in diagnosis

The distribution of gamma emitting isotopes within the brain can be detected through the intact skull, using scintillation detectors; these are activated by the gamma emission and the pulses of electrical energy produced are amplified and counted, and the result displayed on a chart. Three quite distinct types of investigation are possible: *brain scanning* in which the static distribution of an intravenously injected isotope in the brain is mapped out in order to localise lesions such as tumours, abscesses and infarcts; measurements of *cerebral circulation* in which the behaviour of isotope in the blood supply to the brain is detected; and *isotope ventriculography* in which the distribution and flow of CSF is determined after injections into the ventricle or subarachnoid space. The term "isotope encephalography" is confusing because it has been used by different authors for brain scanning and for CSF studies.

Brain scanning

Various isotopes are available and new ones are being sought and tried, particularly those with a short half-life which enable the dose to be increased and statistics of counting improved without exceeding a safe radiation dosage to the body as a whole. The most commonly used is technetium (Tc^{99m}) which has a six hour half-life; with it a scan can be arranged and completed within a few hours. Scanning begins at an interval after injection which is appropriate to the isotope used, and at present most machines produce a lateral and an axial view of the intracranial activity; however, multiple detectors ranged in a halo round the head are being developed in an attempt to give a three dimensional localisation of areas of increased uptake. The gamma camera can give rapid serial views of the uptake and distribution of isotope, thus adding the fourth dimension—time.

The physico-chemical abnormalities which determine the accumulation or exclusion of isotope from pathological areas is not yet understood, but seem likely to be related to alterations in the blood-brain barrier. To a large extent therefore the method remains empirical, and its discriminative value has still to be assessed. It is of most use in detecting supratentorial lesions, but with optimal collimation lesions can be shown the posterior fossa. Meningiomas have the densest uptake, but this does not seem to relate to vascularity; metastases usually show clearly, and the demonstration of more than one area of increased uptake may be of considerable help in management; gliomas can usually be recognised although they do not as a rule show up as strikingly as meningiomas or metastases unless they are rapidly growing. Abscesses, infarcts and hæmatomas may show up satisfactorily. Brain scanning carries a negligible risk and can be done on out-patients; it is therefore of great value as a primary screening procedure, and it may save the patient the need for the more elaborate and unpleasant neuro-radiological investigations with their associated risks. More and more patients are being managed without any other neuroradiological investigations but it is important to recognise the limitations of isotope scanning. Only angiography will indicate the site and size of feeding vessels or circumferential arteries around a tumour; only ventriculo-graphy will show the anatomy of a blockage of the CSF pathways and the exact relationship of a tumour to intraventricular structures. Moreover, the reliability of a negative scan in excluding different types of lesion remains uncertain. Whilst it is considerably less informative than EMI scanning, it is much less expensive and is likely to remain more readily available.

Measurements of the cerebral circulation

The brain is more critically dependent on the integrity of the circula-tion than any other organ in the body. Neurones are uniquely vulner-able to ischæmia; cerebral ischæmia is the penultimate common path by which most types of brain damage are caused, whether due to head injury, space-occupying lesion, blockage of a main arterial trunk or sudden loss of perfusion pressure due to a fall in cardiac output. There is therefore concern about the cerebral circulation in many conditions other than those due to occlusive vascular lesions. But only recently, with the application of radioactive isotopes to this field, has it become a practical possibility to measure the cerebral blood flow in patients with brain disease.

The outstanding characteristic of the microcirculation in the brain is the efficiency of its autoregulation, which ensures a constancy of flow under widely varying conditions. Regulation depends chiefly on altera-tion of arteriolar diameter, and flow is critically dependent on the arterial tension of carbon dioxide and of oxygen (P_aCO_2 and P_aO_2), less so on arterial blood pressure. When cerebral blood flow is being measured these factors must be known and if comparisons are made between cerebral blood flow in one patient on two different occasions these other factors must be shown to have been the same on each occasion; this applies most particularly to the P_aCO_2. Accurate estimates of the regional cerebral blood flow (r CBF) can now be made using gamma emitting isotopes. With inert and freely diffusible isotopes the rate of disappearance of the radioactivity from the brain will depend only on the blood flow, and by using gases which are excreted into the air by the lungs during one circulation the re-introduction of radioactivity into the brain by re-circulation is avoided. The blood flow in ml./100 gm./min. can be calculated from the exponential curve of clearance from the brain, and different parts of the brain can be compared by using multiple dectors; but the geometry of collimators and the high energy of the isotope limits the degree of resolution because some overlap between adjacent detectors cannot be avoided.

This technique originally involved injection of isotope into the carotid artery in the course of angiography or of carotid surgery. In the latter context this remains a useful method (p. 205), but the inhalation technique is now used for the investigation of patients in wards and out-patients; it is atraumatic and can therefore be done repeatedly so that changes due to pathological progression or recovery, of the effects of drugs can be recorded.

Isotope ventriculography

The route and speed of circulation of the CSF may be investigated by injecting tracers into the lumbar theca or the ventricles, and scanning repeatedly over the succeeding hours or days. Normally after lumbar injection most of the radioactivity has reached the basal (intracranial) cisterns within an hour; by 12–24 hours most of the activity is around the superior longitudinal sinus, and no activity is recorded at any stage in the ventricles. Various types of hydrocephalus may be distinguished by the finding of abnormal distribution of isotope (pp. 320, 325).

EMI scan (computerised transaxial tomography)

This method of obtaining a density picture of a series of horizontal slices of the intracranial cavity has revolutionised the investigation of the brain. A narrow beam of X-rays is shot through the head from a succession of positions on an arc, the X-ray source being advanced 1° successively; a computer solves the equations necessary to calculate the density of over 2000 separate squares on the matrix of the cross-section of the brain being examined. The density is different for brain, CSF, haematoma, infarcted brain, œdema and tumour. This method therefore provides not only localisation but indication of the pathological process; in this regard it is superior to any previous method. It also shows the ventricular system and therefore allows brain shift and ventricular dilatation to be recognised. Its most useful characteristic is that it entails no risk whatever, which distinguishes it from all the techniques of contrast radiology, which carry some hazard. However, the patient must keep his head absolutely still for a period of 4 minutes, and this may require an anaesthetic in a child, or in a confused adult.

The only limitation on the use of the EMI scan is its limited availability; due to its capital cost it may be some time before every centre has a machine. But even when one is installed its very versatility can quickly lead to over-demand, because it is likely to be called on not only for the investigation of cases which hitherto have required contrast radiology, but also for the investigation of many patients who would previously not have been considered for serious investigation at all, because of the risk involved. It is not possible to indicate here what use may be appropriate in different places, nor would it be useful to have an atlas of appearances when the technique is advancing so rapidly.

FURTHER READING

Di Chiro, G., Ashburn, W. L. and Briner, W. H. (1968). Technetium (99m) serum albumin for cisternography. *Arch. Neurol.*, **19**, 218–227.

Di Chiro, G., Ashburn, W. L. and Grove, A. S. (1968). Which radioisotopes for brain scanning? *Neurology* (Minneap) **18**, 225–236.

Duffy, G. P. (1969). Lumbar puncture in the presence of raised intracranial pressure. *Brit. med. J.*, **1**, 407–409.

El Batata, M. (1968). Cytology of CSF in the diagnosis of malignancy. *J. Neurosurg.* **28**, 317–326.

Ford, R. and Ambrose, J. (1963). Echo-encephalography. *Brain*, **86**, 189–196.

Hill, D. and Driver, M. V. (1962). Chapter in *Recent Advances in Neurology and Neuropsychiatry*, ed. Brain, W. R. London: Churchill.

Joynt, R. J. Cape, C. A., Knott, J. R. (1965). Significance of focal delta activity in adult EEG. *Arch. Neurol.*, **12**, 631–638.

McMenemy, W. H. and Cumings, J. N. (1959). The value of the examination of the CSF in the diagnosis of intracranial tumour. *J. Clin. Path.*, **12**, 400–411.

Oldendorf, W. H. (1967). Detection of brain tumours using radioisotopes. *Bull. Los. Ang. Neurol Soc.*, **32**, 220–233.

CHAPTER 6

Contrast Radiology

Introduction

Carotid angiography

Vertebral angiography

Ventriculography

Air encephalography

Only the closest co-operation between surgeon and radiologist will lead to conspicuous success in this field. Without it inappropriate or unnecessary investigations may be carried out, adding only information which is unhelpful and at the price to the patient of added discomfort and possibly of increased risk. The problem of the particular patient should be kept in mind during the performance of each test because with critically ill patients a decision may have to be made whether to persist with or abandon an examination at a certain stage; the right course can be followed only if the radiologist has a clear idea of what information is required, and what can be dispensed with if circumstances are difficult.

The introduction of the EMI scan has greatly reduced the need for contrast radiology, except for vascular lesions such as aneurysms and malformations. However, there will be many centres without access to EMI scanning for some years to come; and there may be problems of access to the scanner, or in getting satisfactory prints. It is therefore important to retain the repertoire of traditional contrast investigations —and the indications given are those applying when EMI scanning is not available or unsuccessful.

Carotid Angiography

Angiography is now so ordinary a procedure that it is becoming available outside special centres. But the interpretation of the films is

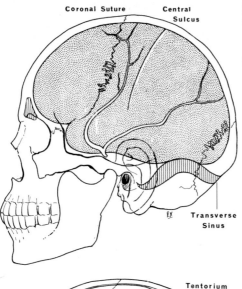

Coronal Suture   **Central Sulcus**

Transverse Sinus

Fɪɢ. 21 Relationship between skull anatomy and underlying structures.

(*a*) Upper part of central sulcus (Rolandic fissure) lies ½ in. posterior to the mid-point of the arc between nasion and inion. Floor of middle fossa is at the level of the zygoma.

Frontal *lobe* is anterior to central sulcus: frontal *bone* is anterior to coronal suture. Middle meningeal artery soon divides into anterior and posterior branches.

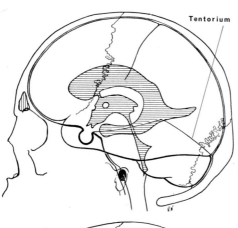

Tentorium

(*b*) Tentorium is not a straight line from torcula to posterior clinoid, but is in fact *a tent*, rising medially to a ridge; one result is that the occipital lobe overlies the cerebellum laterally.

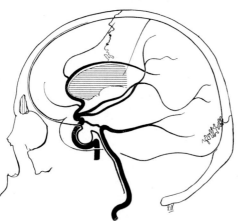

(*c*) Calloso-marginal artery is closely applied to the roof of the lateral ventricle.

Posterior communicating artery connects the carotid and basilar systems.

not always straightforward or easy and patients may not always benefit from the availability of angiography in isolation from the other techniques of neuroradiology, and without surgical facilities at hand.

Carotid injections display the vessels in the territories of the anterior and middle cerebral arteries, and sometimes of the posterior cerebral also. Supratentorial masses can be expected to produce abnormalities, particularly if situated in the anterior two-thirds of the hemisphere; posterior fossa and transtentorial lesions do not usually disclose their presence except indirectly, by producing hydrocephalic stretching of the pericallosal artery.

TECHNIQUE

This is frequently done under *local anæsthesia* with suitable premedication but it can be an unpleasant procedure which few patients submit to a second time without some protest. The needling can be painful and prolonged on occasions, whilst the inevitable sudden hot flush in the head and neck when the contrast is injected is vividly described and remembered by most patients. In addition, the elaborate apparatus, lead screens and masked figures, the click and thud of exposure and cassette changer, all make for a somewhat alarming experience. Some centres use general anæsthesia as a routine, others confine its use to children and difficult patients. With short-acting drugs and skilled anæsthetists there is probably little increased risk except in patients with rapidly advancing brain compression but the neuroleptanalgesic drugs (see p. 101) are making angiography under local anæsthesia more acceptable.

Once the needle is inserted into the common carotid artery separate injections of 8–12 ml. of 76% Urografin or 45% Hypaque are made for the lateral and axial projections. Films taken towards the end of injection and then at 2 second intervals show the arterial, capillary and venous phases of the circulation. The sequence of filling can be studied in greater detail with *rapid serial angiography* in which two or more films are taken every second for twelve seconds.

COMPLICATIONS

Hæmatoma in the neck is seldom alarming if a finger is kept firmly on the puncture point for five minutes after withdrawing the needle, but it is important to ascertain before the procedure that long-term anticoagulants are not being administered. Tracheal deviation and respiratory embarrassment occasionally develop, but the extravasation can usually be encouraged to disperse into the mediastinum by sitting the patient up. However, endotracheal tubes and a tracheostomy set should be available. Because of the possibility of this complication it is always

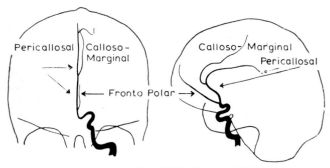

ANTERIOR CEREBRAL ARTERY

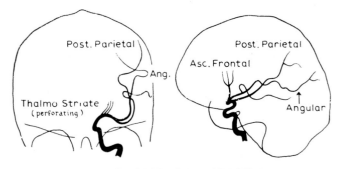

MIDDLE CEREBRAL ARTERY

(*a*) Anterior and middle cerebral arteries separately displayed, with
the internal carotid. The anterior cerebral becomes the pericallosal
artery after the anterior communicating branch.

FIG. 22 Anatomy of the carotid angiograms

advisable to admit out-patients to hospital for the night following
angiography, even when this has been done under local anæsthesia.

Sensitivity to iodine is rarely seen with Urografin or Hypaque, but
if there is an allergic or asthmatic history it is wise to do a preliminary
skin test. Reactions include allergic rash, bronchospasm and cardiorespiratory failure.

Renal damage may delay the excretion of the contrast medium which
can further add to the damage, and the method is contraindicated in
patients with advanced renal disease.

Development or aggravation of CNS signs is reported with widely
varying frequency, which probably reflects variations in the skill of the
operator, in the concentration and volume of contrast injected and in
the care with which signs are sought. Probably many patients with

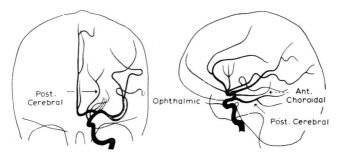

(b) Complete arterial tree—anterior and middle cerebral branches and also vessels arising directly from the carotid (ophthalmic, anterior choroidal and posterior cerebral).
Posterior cerebral fills in about one-third of carotid angiograms via posterior communicating artery.

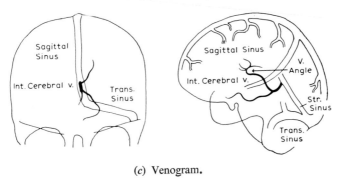

(c) Venogram.

FIG. 22 (contd.)

hemiplegia or dysphasia have a temporary increase in signs for a few hours after angiography, but it is seldom noticed; occasionally when hemiplegia is produced or seriously worsened it persists. Several factors may contribute to this: needling by chance through an atheromatous plaque may set free fragments as emboli into the cerebral circulation or inadvertent injection into the carotid sheath or subintimally can result in reflex spasm in cerebral vessels or in occlusion of the carotid itself. Systemic arterial hypotension, induced by anæsthesia or by the injection of contrast, may aggravate such a situation. If there is already occlusion of the opposite carotid artery, or of either of the vertebral arteries, any of these accidents may result in an inadequate cerebral blood supply, and most complications have arisen in patients with arterial degeneration. The irritant effect of the contrast medium itself on cerebral vessels and the brain is much less marked than with earlier preparations, and it is probably safe to inject up to 100 ml. during one session.

Increased intracranial pressure is sometimes suspected after angiography, usually in patients already critically compressed. Œdema may increase around a malignant tumour, perhaps due to excess contrast medium (or large quantities of saline injected between films) acting on abnormal vessels with an altered blood-brain barrier.

An *epileptic fit* occasionally occurs as soon as contrast is injected. *Nausea* is often complained of immediately after the first injection, rarely after subsequent ones. *Syncope* can occur from the needle being in the carotid sinus, and calls for replacement of the needle. *Carotid aneurysms* and *carotico-jugular* (*arteriovenous*) *fistulæ* are rare late developments.

Complications are uncommon in experienced hands, but may occur in up to 10% of cases. The risk of their developing, the quality of films produced, and the amount of discomfort suffered by the patient under local anæsthesia, depend very largely on the skill of the operator and his team, skill which takes time to acquire and continued practice to maintain. There is little place for the occasional operator.

INFORMATION

Lateralisation of a supratentorial tumour depends mainly on displacement of the pericallosal artery from its normal mid-line situation in the AP view. Rotation of the head on the film, indicated by asymmetry in the relationship between the orbits or mastoid tips and the lateral skull vault, will falsify the appearance of displacement.

The more posteriorly placed a mass the less arterial shift it produces, and posterior parietal and occipital lesions may give none at all. The falx becomes deeper behind, and is fixed by its attachment to the tentorium, splinting the brain, but posterior tumours if infiltrating deeply can displace the deep cerebral veins. Other tumours which fail to produce shift are those within the lateral ventricle which take up space in the cavity, and those which are bilateral and balanced.

Localisation of a mass to one part of one supratentorial compartment depends on the pattern of lateral displacement, on local stretching of vessels and on abnormal tumour vessels (when they fill) (fig. 23).

AP axial view. Displacement of the pericallosal is most marked with *frontal* masses which cause this vessel to be bowed; maximal shift may be high or low according to the site of the tumour. *Temporal or anterior parietal* masses cause a step-like, straight shift as the falx remains in the midline, together with the upper and more posterior part of the artery and its branches. Elevation of the anterior cerebral artery indicates a large *suprasellar* mass, whilst *anterior temporal or posterior subfrontal lesions* lift up the corresponding part of the middle cerebral artery. Medial displacement of the middle cerebral vessels suggest a *surface Sylvian tumour*.

Lateral view. Frontal masses frequently produce no displacement in spite of striking shift in the AP view. *Parietal* masses depress and *temporal* masses elevate the middle cerebral leash. *Subfrontal or anterior temporal* tumours uncurl the carotid siphon and displace the first part

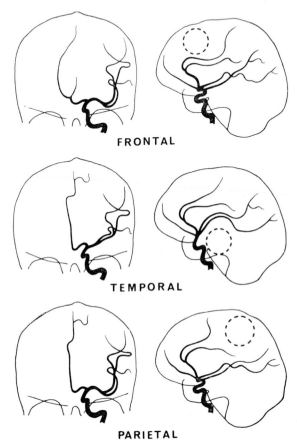

FRONTAL

TEMPORAL

PARIETAL

AP views are most informative—frontal and parietal tumours seldom cause striking displacements in the lateral projection. The more posteriorly placed a tumour the less the lateral displacement (AP view); occipital tumours may cause no abnormality in either view.

Fig. 23 Tumour localisation by vessel displacement

of the anterior cerebral backwards and upwards. Local stretching of vessels around a tumour is most often seen in the mid-parietal region, but the local variation in vessel pattern is such that this appearance needs to be striking before it is diagnostic.

When **tumour vessels** fill much more information is available; not only is the *site* much more accurately determined, but the *size* may be indicated (fig. 35). This is never safe to guess from the degree of lateral displacement because a small tumour or abscess may cause extensive cerebral swelling and brain shift. The *vascularity* and the *disposition of main feeding vessels* to the tumour may help in planning surgical approach.

In certain cases the *pathological nature* of the tumour may be suggested by the type of tumour vessels seen and the circulation time but a firm diagnosis must never be made on this basis (fig. 30). The suspicion of a certain type of tumour may be heightened by its situation, taking account of the predisposition for particular sites; for example olfactory groove or sphenoidal wing meningiomas give rise to typical displacement, but even so may be mimicked by other tumours chancing to occur in these situations. The only way to establish the pathological nature of a tumour in the brain, is by histological examination. It is seldom wise to assume that a patient has a maligannt tumour on the basis of angiographic appearances alone, without a biopsy.

INDICATIONS

For *clinically lateralised cerebral lesions* angiography is the investigation of choice and often the only one needed. Not only does it carry less risk in the presence of raised pressure than either air ventriculography or air encephalography, but it may also exclude obliterative arterial disease both in the extracranial and intracranial arteries, and subdural hæmatoma, which are perhaps the commonest differential diagnoses.

For *raised pressure without localising features* a right carotid angiogram is sometimes carried out as an initial screening test, because of its comparative safety, to exclude a silent hemisphere tumour. Not only can lateral displacement be excluded but hydrocephalic bowing of the pericallosal artery may be seen in the lateral view (fig. 32a).

LIMITATIONS

Angiography will not usually disclose *midline* lesions, and often fails to show *intraventricular* masses unless they are vascular, because neither usually causes lateral shift. A *small* tumour, unless giving rise to œdema and shift, may not cause any abnormality. Tumours in the *parieto-occipital region* seldom shift the pericallosal artery laterally, and may also fail to show any abnormality on the lateral view; they are supplied mainly by the posterior cerebral artery which fills (via the posterior communicating artery) in only about a third of carotid angiograms.

Vertebral angiography

This is much less widely employed in tumour diagnosis but has certain specific applications. It is more difficult to carry out, as witnessed by the number of techniques developed. An anterior approach, similar to that used for the carotid, entails puncturing the vessel *in its bony canal*; cervical nerve roots are liable to be hit by the needle, and for this reason a general anæsthetic is advisable. Needling the artery in its transverse course *on the atlas* is a technical feat mastered by a few radiologists, but it carries the risk of injecting dye into the subarachnoid space. *Retrograde catheterisation* via the brachial or femoral arteries is the most reliable and least traumatic method, but *retrograde injection* after percutaneous puncture of brachial or subclavian artery avoids even the small risk of a catheter dislodging part of an atheromatous plaque. Injections of 30 ml. of 50% hypaque are required for this technique, and better contrast results if intrathoracic pressure is temporarily raised during the injection to discourage reflux into the aorta.

When the posterior cerebral artery does not fill on carotid angiography a vertebral angiogram may show up a posteriorly placed tumour which has failed to displace the pericallosal laterally. Even when carotid angiography has demonstrated a tumour on the borderland of posterior cerebral territory, vertebral filling may show that the lesion is much bigger than was at first thought and give a fuller and more accurate idea of its size and vascularity.

For posterior fossa tumours angiography has not so far been fully explored in regard to vessel displacements but vascular tumours such as angiomas and hæmangioblastnmas show up well. Recurrences of these tumours are better shown than by ventriculography which can be difficult to interpret if the posterior fossa has been previously explored.

Ventriculography

The replacement of ventricular CSF by air through a burr hole was the first contrast method ever used. With the development of angiography, and more recently the EMI scan, ventriculography is now used only in limited circumstances—most often when a block in the ventricular system has to be localised. Positive contrast media, either oil or water soluble, are more commonly used than air because the technique is both safer and gives better visualisation of the ventricular system.

TECHNIQUE

A single burr hole is usually adequate, but if there is a block of both foramina of Monro then only the side injected may fill. A frontal burr hole, on the coronal sture 3 cm. from the midline, is most useful; this is usually placed on the non-dominant side unless there are reasons to put it on the other side. (the ventricle is frequently obliterated on the side of a large supratentorial tumour). It is most convenient to place a catheter in the ventricle so that the injection of contrast (whether air or positive material) can be done in the X-ray room. When a burr hole made weeks or months previously is to be used, a track must be made through the sear with a pointed tenotome prior to introducing eithera blunt brain cannula or a catheter. In infants a sharp needle passed through the fontanelle dispenses with the need for a burr hole. Once the contrast is injected the patient's head is put in a series of positions in order to visualise different parts of the system. It should be known from the provisional diagnosis just what is required of the investigation, and it is seldom that a complete visualisation of the system is required or indeed advisable.

COMPLICATIONS

The risk from the burr hole is small, but *infection* and *haemorrhage* can develop. The latter results either from cortical contusion or from collapse of a hydrocephalic brain, allowing subdural or extradural collection of blood. Occasionally a fit is precipitated. More important are the results of altering the balance of intracranial dynamics, when there is already raised intracranial pressure. These are much less common when fluid contrast rather than air is used. If air is employed then large volumes should never be injected, particularly in hydrocephalic infants. Small bubbles can be moved around the ventricular system by changing the head position. Headache and vomiting developing soon after ventriculography may indicate that tentorial or foraminal coning is occurring and if air has been the medium then the ventricles should be tapped to let air escape. If a definitive operation is required then it should be carried out on the same day after air ventriculography, because there is otherwise a real risk of irreversible compression despite the tapping of the ventricle. Even when immediate operation is performed the brain is often found to be tight and the patient is in less than the ideal condition as a result of an air ventriculogram.

The irritant effect of positive contrast media seems seldom to cause a problem. However, care must be taken to use appropriate concentrations of water soluble contrast or else there may be a sudden collapse, or fits may be precipitated. Oily contrast may give rise to arachnoiditis if it escapes into the subarachnoid space or the spinal theca but this has seldom been reported. The possibility of oily media completing a CSF block, for example in the aqueduct, should be considered. In the event that a complete aqueduct stenosis is demonstrated by oil then it is advisable to proceed with a short-circuiting operation on the same day, or alternatively to set up external ventricular drainage until definitive surgery can be arranged.

INFORMATION

The **burr hole** itself can yield important information, such as the thickness of the skull, whether the brain tension is high or not, and the size and position of the ventricles can be roughly guessed from the depth at which the cannula reaches fluid. The CSF pressure can be measured before air is injected. Occasionally the diagnosis is made directly by the discovery of a subdural hæmorrhage or by the needle encountering tumour before entering the ventricle.

Lateralisation of supratentorial masses depends on observing shift to right or left of the lateral or third ventricles. Diffuse infiltrating tumours may give no shift, nor may bilateral masses but the latter usually do give marked deformities of the ventricle. Posterior fossa lesions may shift the aqueduct or fourth ventricle to one side but these structures are not always clearly visualised.

Localisation of supratentorial masses rests largely on the nature of the ventricular shift; from this it is usually possible to say whether a tumour is frontal, temporal, parietal or occipital, perhaps also whether it is likely to be high or low. Seldom is there any clue about size because the most gross shifts can occur from small tumours which cause extensive œdema. However, when a tumour is near to or in the cavity of a ventricle and is producing a filling defect, more accurate localisation is possible and the size may be estimated (fig. 24). Apart from these paraventricular tumours, ventriculography does not usually give as much information as a carotid angiogram when this demonstrates tumour vessels. Nor does it provide information about the pathological nature of the tumour. One exception is the infrequent paraventricular cholesteatoma (epidermoid) which takes up air into its interstices giving a highly characteristic appearance (fig. 41).

Displacement of the fourth ventricle and aqueduct enable the approximate position of posterior fossa tumours to be deduced; these structures are pushed back and up by brain stem tumours, forwards by a vermis mass and to the side by a lateral cerebellar or angle tumour (fig. 25).

Blocks to CSF flow within the ventricular system are detected by failure of contrast to pass from one part to the next, together with dilatation of the system above the obstruction.

Ventricular dilatation can result from non-obstructive lesions, notably cerebral atrophy. When generalised symmetrical dilatation is due to atrophy excessive amounts of air may be seen in the cortical sulci and the pressure is not raised. Unilateral dilatation subsequent to infarction is less easy to differentiate from tumour because the septum may be displaced to either the dilated side or the other. The ventricle on the side of a hemisphere tumour is usually the smaller of the two and the septum is never deflected towards a tumour.

INDICATIONS

Lateralised supratentorial lesions may require ventriculography when other investigations are inconclusive; this is most likely to occur with bilateral frontal lesions or with intraventricular tumours. Basal ganglia tumours may also be difficult to delineate in relation to the ventricle without actually visualising the ventricular cavity. In infants (unless an EMI scan is available) suspected masses and hydrocephalus are best

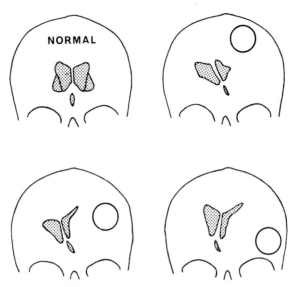

(a) AP views—high and low tumours cause different angulation of displaced ventricles.

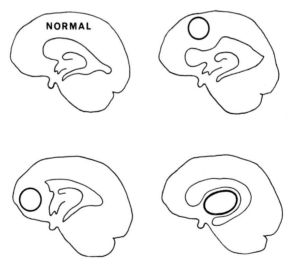

(b) Lateral views—tumours close to the ventricle may produce a filling defect; bottom right is a thalamic tumour causing hydrocephalus by obstructing the foramen of Monro, and encroaching on the *floor* of the body of the ventricle and the *roof* of the temporal horn.

FIG. 24 Abnormalities of the lateral ventricles shown by air studies

(*After Sutton.*)

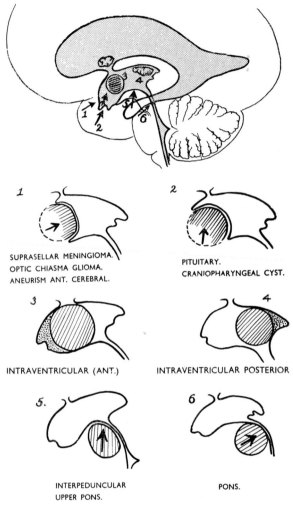

(*a*) By antero-inferior lesions.

FIG. 25 Deformities of midline ventricular pathways

investigated by a bubble ventriculogram for which neither burr holes or an anaesthetic are needed. Angiograms are difficult both to perform and to interpret in the first year of life. Suspected lesions in the 3rd ventricle, brain stem or posterior fossa, are well shown by this method, unless there is a complete block to the flow of CSF. Hydrocephalus, from whatever cause at whatever age will likely require ventriculography to establish the site of the block.

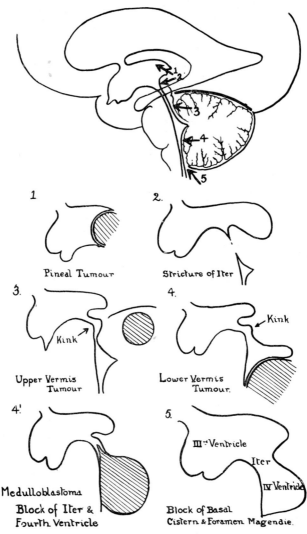

1 Pineal Tumour

2. Stricture of Iter

3. Upper Vermis Tumour Kink

4. Lower Vermis Tumour. Kink

4'. Medulloblastoma Block of Iter & Fourth Ventricle

5. III™ Ventricle Iter IV Ventricle Block of Basal Cistern & Foramen Magendie.

(*b*) By posterio-superior lesions.

Fig. 25 (*contd.*) Deformities of midline ventricular pathways

(*From Twining.*)

Air encephalography

The attraction of this method is that no special equipment is needed and a burr hole is avoided. Until recently its use was confined to the investigation of patients with unlocalised symptoms such as epilepsy or dementia, without signs of pressure. Because of the danger of precipitating coning air encephalography has until recently been regarded as contraindicated whenever pressure was raised or a brain tumour seriously suspected. But air encephalography using the fractional technique is now used with increasing frequency in some centres for localising certain tumours, provided certain safeguards are strictly observed; the most important is a surgeon prepared to proceed with operation immediately if necessary.

TECHNIQUE

The patient is seated for the first part of this procedure and, except in children, local anæsthesia suffices. General anæsthesia calls for a special chair and harness to support the limp patient in the upright position. When done under local anæsthetic it is important not to give as pre-medication drugs which can cause postural hypotension because the patient may faint when he is sat up.

Lumbar puncture is performed with the patient seated, his head resting against the film holder and the neck flexed at the correct angle to encourage the air to enter the ventricular system. Without allowing any CSF to escape 7 to 10 ml. of air are injected; lateral films taken after this injection should show air in the fourth ventricle and aqueduct. More air is then injected, up to 25–30 ml. in all, and about 15–20 ml. of CSF withdrawn. Further small amounts of air are injected until various structures are adequately outlined, and the air is moved around the head by positioning until the examination is complete. The final injections of air are usually made with the head more extended to encourage filling of the subarachnoid cisterns, and the subarachnoid space over the cortex.

Sometimes no air can be induced to enter the ventricles. This is commoner in unskilled hands and also when the examination is attempted within a few days of lumbar puncture after which the cisterns collapse, preventing air from readily entering the fourth ventricle. Even the most experienced fail to fill the ventricles in about 5% of cases; half of these subsequently prove to have some abnormality, a third having a brain tumour. It is important therefore to repeat the investigation, but not for about a week; the chances of filling the ventricles may be increased by giving 30 gm. of urea by mouth an hour or so before the examination—this shrinks the brain whilst leaving the cisterns distended.

COMPLICATIONS

Some **headache,** which may be severe, is usually complained of when air enters the cisterns and vomiting may also occur. The patient may faint either when the needle is put in or when air is injected; although this sometimes necessitates abandoning the procedure, such a decision should not be made too precipitately as often it is easy to resuscitate the patient and continue. It is important not to confuse a simple faint with an episode of coning, which of course has quite a different significance.

The risk of **coning** associated with lumbar puncture in the presence of raised intracranial pressure applies equally to puncture for encephalography. Nonetheless since the introduction of the fractional method, using small amounts of air, there have been strong claims that this investigation is safe even when there is high pressure. Those who recommend it stress the need for a meticulous technique, injecting some air before letting off any CSF so that the brain stem will not move caudally and cone, and many insist on a preliminary burr hole in case there is need for urgent ventricular tapping. All agree that if a mass is demonstrated it must be operated on without delay, immediately the investigation is complete.

Headache with pyrexia and some degree of meningism occurs after some encephalograms, and the CSF may have an increase in the number of cells; this reaction to the air is harmless, and should not be mistaken for infective meningitis which is exceptionally rare.

INFORMATION

Lateralisation and localisation of masses from **ventricular displacement** depends on the same principles as in ventriculography, but additional information is gained from abnormalities of the **subarachnoid cisterns** (fig 25). The cisterna magna and ambiens and the lateral recesses of the pontine cistern may be distorted by posterior fossa lesions; a pituitary tumour may be partly outlined by air in the chiasmatic cistern and the degree of suprasellar extension judged (fig. 36). **Blocks to CSF flow** are not as satisfactorily demonstrated by this technique as by others. Failure of air to flow upwards into the ventricles may be due to functional obstruction, and confirmation cannot be sought from dilatation of the segment above the block, as it can during ventriculography.

A **"failed"** encephalogram (no ventricular filling) may nonetheless give valuable information. The cisterns may be adequately seen and their normality may exclude the condition under suspicion. If the callosal cistern is well visualised and is not stretched the absence of marked hydrocephalus is established. The tonsils of the cerebellum are sometimes seen in a normal situation and posterior fossa compression largely ruled out. Although every attempt should be made to fill the ventricles, the information which is available from an "unsuccessful" examination should not be ignored.

Dilated ventricles and large amounts of air over the surface of the cortex, may raise suspicion of cerebral **atrophy**; but the amount of surface air is normally so variable that this alone should never be the basis of a diagnosis of atrophy.

INDICATIONS

Epilepsy and suspected *cerebral atrophy*, without localising signs or evidence of raised pressure, make up the majority of cases investigated

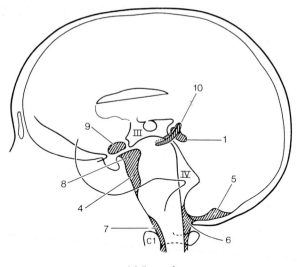

(*a*) Lateral

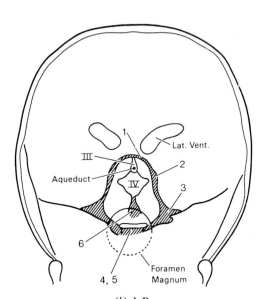

(*b*) A.P.

1. C. venal magnæ cerebri (Galeni).
2. C. ambiens.
3. C. ponto-cerebellaris.
4. C. pontis ⎱ (super-imposed in A.P. view.)
5. C. magna ⎰
6. Vallecula.
7. C. medullaris.
8. C. interpeduncularis.
9. C. chiasmatis.
10. C. ambiens (wings).

FIG. 26 Normal subarachnoid cisterns

by encephalography where EMI scanning is not available. *Parasellar tumours*, especially pituitary neoplasms, are well demarcated by this method; they seldom give rise to raised pressure, whilst cisternal filling gives more information than either ventriculography or angiography. Lesions of the *hemisphere without signs of pressure*, perhaps with inconclusive angiograms, may be demonstrated; and similarly *posterior fossa lesions* without pressure, such as atypical trigeminal neuralgia or Ménierè's disease. The limitations of its use for suspected posterior fossa tumours with signs of pressure have already been discussed.

Summary of Strategy of Investigation
Suspected Space-Occupying Lesion

All cases—plain skull X-ray/EMI scan
No cases—lumbar puncture

Suspected hemisphere lesion

Isotope scan ⎫
EEG   ⎬ aniography
If raised ICP—ventriculography
If normal ICP—air encephalography

Suspected posterior fossa lesion

Carotid angio (if no EMI) to exclude frontal lesion, to confirm hydrocephalus.
If raised ICP—ventriculography
If normal ICP—air encephalography

Suspected sellar or parasellar lesion

Bilateral carotid angio. to exclude aneurysm
Lumbar air encephalogram

Suspected lesion in third ventricle or aqueduct

If raised ICP—ventriculogram
If normal ICP—air encephalogram

FURTHER READING

El Batata, M. (1968). Cytology of CSF in the diagnosis of malignancy. *Journal of Neurosurgery*, **28**, 317–326.
Ford, R. and Ambrose, J. (1963). Echo-encephalography. *Brain*, **86**, 189–196.
Gowler, J., Bull, J. W. D., du Boulay, G. and Marhsall, J. (1975). Computerised anxial tomography with the EMI scanner *In: Advances in Technical Standards in Neurosurgery*. Ed. Krayenbuhl et al. (Vol. 2) Spring-Wien, New York.
Hellerstein, D. and Bickford, R. G. (1972). Electrical activity of the brain. In: *Scientific Foundations of Neurology*. pp. 327–341. Eds. Critchley, O'Leary and Jennett. Heinemann, London.

Klinger, M., Kazner, E., Grume, T. H., Amtenbrink, V., Graef, G., Hartmann, K. H., Hopman, H., Meese, W. and Vogel, B. (1975). Clinical experience with automatic midline echoencephalography: co-operative study of three neurosurgical clinics. *Journal of Neurology, Neurosurgery and Psychiatry*, **38**, 272–278.

McMenemy, W. H. and Cumings, J. N. (1959). The value of the examination of the CSF in the diagnosis of intracranial tumour. *Journal of Clinical Pathology*, **1**, 400–411.

Murphy, J. T., Gloor, P., Yamamoto, Y. L. and Feindel, W. (1967). A comparison of EEG and brain scan in supratentorial tumours. *New England Journal of Medicine*, **276**, 309–313.

Natelson, S. E., Sayers, M. P. and Hunt, W. E. (1972). Experiences with the technique and complication of Conray ventriculography. *Journal of Neurology, Neurosurgery and Psychiatry*, **35**, 264–269.

Newton, T. H. and Potts, D. G. (eds.) (1972). *Radiology of the Skull and Brain*. Vol. 1 The skull. Mosby, St. Louis.

Newton, T. H. and Potts, D. G. (1974). *Radiology of the Skull and Brain*, Vol. 2 Angiography. Mosby, St. Louis.

Rowan, J. O. (1972). Radioisotopes in diagnosis. *In: Scientific Foundations of Neurology*, p. 382–397. Eds. Critchley, O'Leary and Jennett. Heinemann, London.

Suberviola, P. D. and Greyson, N. D. (1975). Non-invasive screening for surgical intracranial lesions. *Journal of Neurology, Neurosurgery and Psychiatry*, **38**, 52–56.

CHAPTER 7

Treatment of Space-occupying Lesions

Operative approaches

Anæsthesia for intracranial operations

Non-operative reduction of intracranial pressure

Operative relief of intracranial pressure

Once a space-occupying lesion has been localised it remains to determine its pathological identity, and to manage the particular lesion appropriately. In some instances the history and investigation may leave little doubt as to the nature of the lesion, say temporal lobe abscess in a patient with chronic otitis, or meningioma when there are classical bone changes and angiographic appearances. Very often, however, the matter is nothing like so obvious and the final steps towards diagnosis are taken in the operating theatre, and the further management depends on the findings. Later chapters will deal in detail with the management of intracranial tumours, infections, and hæmorrhage, but here certain principles are outlined and certain measures described which may apply to any space-occupying lesion. They are concerned with the relief of intra-cranial pressure and the problems of access to the lesion such that at least a diagnosis is established; in favourable circumstances this will lead to effective treatment.

Operative Approaches

Exploratory burr holes

These are commonly made as an initial operative procedure to permit biopsy in order to determine the nature of an already accurately located mass. If the lesion is not well localised by neuroradiology then an exploratory burr hole is probably not wise and an exploratory open operation may be indicated. This initial burr hole must be so placed that a needle can be passed to the lesion without traversing vital areas of brain; and it must take account of what kind of skin flap and bone removal might be required if an open exploration should subsequently be required. The initial burr hole may form part of the flap and the direction of the skin incision is then vital (fig. 52, p. 251); or the burr hole may be placed so that it will lie in the middle of a flap and the skin incision should then lie approximately at right angles to the base of the flap.

Supratentorial exploration (fig. 27)

Before the surgeon can plan his approach to a lesion in this compartment of the skull he must have fairly precise information about its situation. The shape of the skin incision is also dictated by the need to preserve an adequate blood supply to the scalp flap, and by cosmetic considerations. When possible the incision is kept within the hair-line but if it must come down on the forehead it is usually least conspicuous if it remains strictly in the midline. For these reasons the scalp flap may be made larger than the bone flap, the size of which depends only on the region to be explored; the bone is cut between burr holes and turned down on a pedicle of periosteum (and of muscle in the temporal region).

The most commonly used flap is the frontal, which allows access to all of the brain in front of the central sulcus, enables a frontal lobectomy to be done as an internal decompression and is also used for approaching the optic chiasm and pituitary and suprasellar tumours. A satisfactory exposure of these basal structures is possible only by taking the lower limb of the flap well down across the supraorbital margin where medially it may open into the frontal sinus. Unless the sinus is infected no special precautions need be taken if it is opened, but some surgeons attempt to seal off the lower opening with a graft of temporal fascia. A coronal (bifrontal) bone flap is occasionally required for tumour surgery.

Posterior fossa exploration (fig. 28)

The whole of this compartment can be explored through a midline incision, so that pre-operative localisation is less vital. However, if a tumour is known to be situated far laterally, for example in the cerebellopontine angle, a lateral vertical incision allows a more direct approach. No skin or bone flap is used; instead sufficient of the occipital squama is nibbled away to form a craniectomy. Occasionally a large tumour in the posterior fossa can best be removed by a combined approach from above and below the tentorium; a small occipital bone flap is turned laterally and the tentorium divided (fig. 28b).

Anæsthesia

The neurosurgeon demands three conditions from an anæsthetic technique: that it should not increase intracranial pressure, that it should

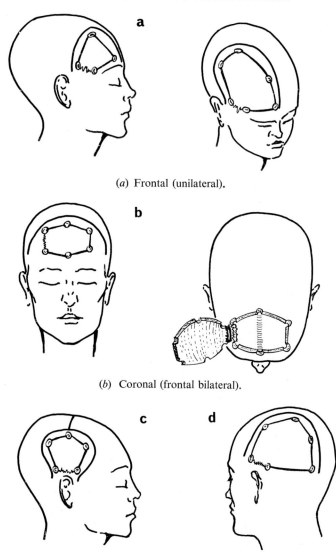

(*a*) Frontal (unilateral).

(*b*) Coronal (frontal bilateral).

(*c*) Lateral—split-ring incision allows access beyond the limits of the flap if necessary.

(*d*) Occipital.

Many variations are possible, limited only by cosmetic considerations and the need for a sufficiently wide base to assure viability. Flaps may be rectangular rather than rounded, and extra exposure can then be gained by extending one limb rather than a split-ring incision.

FIG. 27 Some commonly used supratentorial approaches

(*After Jefferson.*)

not impair cerebral oxygenation and that the patient should become responsive before leaving the operating theatre. These conditions are reliably met only by local anæsthesia, and this was indeed the method of choice until the introduction of the various new techniques in the 50's made general anæsthesia acceptable in most circumstances.

Intracranial pressure

Any degree of ventilatory insufficiency or obstruction will result in raised intracranial pressure, due to the vasodilatory effect of hypercapnia and hypoxia and due also to the transmission of raised central venous pressure to the intracranial venous sinuses. These factors are

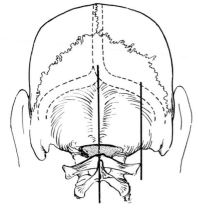

(a) Midline or paramedian incision allows sufficient access for most procedures; the incision may curve laterally at its upper end for further exposure (hockey stick incision).

(b) An additional occipital bone flap allows division of the lateral sinus and tentorium to improve access to difficult transtentorial tumours.

FIG. 28 Posterior fossa approaches

most reliably avoided if controlled respiration is employed so that the patient never strains; supplements of relaxant drugs must be given regularly because as soon as the patient does begin to "fight the pump" the brain will become tense, and will bulge if the skull is open. The only possible disadvantage of controlled respiration is the lack of natural respiration as a guide to the patient's condition when the surgeon is operating in the posterior fossa.

Even if ventilation is adequate and unimpeded the intracranial pressure may rise due to the direct effect of volatile anæsthetic agents on cerebral blood flow. This effect occurs with halothane, trichlorethylene and methoxyflurane, and is much more marked if there is an intracranial space-occupying lesion. Although this pressure rise may be temporary, damage can be done in certain critical situations; hyperventilation will mitigate this effect but it can be prevented only by avoiding these volatile agents, and supplementing nitrous oxide with a neuroleptanalgesic combination of drugs (p. 101).

Cerebral oxygenation

This depends on cerebral blood flow, oxygen saturation and the hæmoglobin level; all three factors may be impaired during operation under anæsthesia. Normally cerebral blood flow remains constant over a wide range of systemic blood pressure, but under anæsthesia autoregulation may be imperfect; moreover if intracranial pressure is raised the effect of a fall in blood pressure on perfusion pressure can be very significant (see p. 9). Factors which may lower the blood pressure are the induction dose of thiopentone and the initial or supplementary doses of d-tubocurarine; both halothane and methoxyflurane induce hypotension (and, as they also raise intracranial pressure, perfusion pressure may be markedly affected); when the patient is placed in the sitting position the blood pressure often falls abruptly and sometimes fails to return to normal levels; blood loss may contribute to hypotension at a later stage in any procedure. Patients already on treatment with hypotensive drugs have a labile blood pressure and are much more liable to develop falls in pressure in these various circumstances.

Induced hypotension is sometimes employed in an attempt to control blood loss or to reduce brain tension. Ganglion blocking agents are given intravenously and the tilt of the table used to achieve the right level of pressure. Conditions must be carefully controlled, and this should include continuous intra-arterial blood pressure monitoring; the degree and duration of hypotension must be carefully controlled.

Hypothermia has been employed to protect the brain from hypoxia associated with induced or accidental hypotension, or with temporary occlusion of intracranial or neck vessels. All these circumstances are most often encountered during surgery for ruptured aneurysms. The limit of conventional hypothermia is 28–29°C, because below this cardiac arrythmia or arrest may occur. At this temperature cerebral metabolism is reduced by 30–40%. Surface cooling either by the use of turbulent cold water in a bath or cold air in a cabinet may be used and is accelerated by drugs which prevent shivering (e.g. curare or chlorpromazine) and those which induce vasodilation in the skin (e.g. halothane).

Barbiturate protection shows promise, and depends likewise on reducing the demand for oxygen by depressing metabolism.

Recovery phase

Intracranial operations may be followed by intracamal hæmatomas, similar to those which develop after accidental trauma to the head.

The same rules apply in each situation, in that a deteriorating conscious level or developing signs signal cerebral compression and the need to open the skull urgently. But after an operation such signs may be the result of the intracranial surgery just completed, and unless the patient has been observed on leaving the theatre to be speaking, to have equal reactive pupils and to move all four limbs it may be impossible to judge whether signs, if first observed a few hours later, represent a newly developing complication. For this reason the anæsthetic technique should allow rapid recovery of consciousness.

Neuroleptanalgesia

This term is applied to combinations of a neuropletanalgesic drug (droperidol) with a narcotic analgesic (fentanyl or phenoperidine). These produce a quiet, inactive patient who will, however, respond rationally when spoken to; the respiratory depressant effect of these drugs is definite but with appropriate dosage is not serious. They are of great value for procedures such as angiography, stereotaxic surgery and burr holes in patients unlikely to tolerate only local anæsthesia. Because these drugs do not increase intracranial pressure, even in patients with space-occupying lesions, they may be more appropriate as supplements to nitrous-oxide oxygen anæsthesia than the volatile agents in patients with high pressure.

Position on the table

This can be crucial in achieving good operating conditions by ensuring there is no venous congestion. Care must be taken to ensure that venous return from the head is not obstructed by the neck being twisted; a lateral approach demands the full lateral position with kidney and chest rests to stabilise the patient. Occipital approaches require either the lateral, ¾-prone or fully prone position, and the hips and shoulders must then be built up with bridges or sandbags to keep the chest and abdomen free from pressure. Intracranial pressure can be further lowered by raising the head end of the table and dropping the feet, making sure that the patient is secured so that the head does not slip out of the head-rest.

The logical extension of this principle is to have the patient sitting up and this is commonly done for posterior fossa explorations (as well as for cervical laminectomies and operations on the trigeminal root via the middle fossa). *Air embolism* is a danger, however, due to air sucking into large muscle, diploic or emissary veins, or into an inadvertently opened dural venous sinus. Because the venous pressure is so low that no blood escapes, the surgeon may be unaware that he has opened venous channels. To minimise the risk of embolus the anæsthetist compresses the jugular veins intermittently during the opening of the wound and the surgeon promptly coagulates all vessels which bleed during compression. More continuous compression can be obtained by having the patient in a pressurised space suit. Once the wound opening is completed the danger period is past, provided all the veins have been closed off. It is unwise to use controlled respiration with a negative phase in the sitting position because air may be sucked in.

Air embolism is suspected if, during the opening of a wound in the sitting position, there is an unexplained alteration in respiratory rhythm, fall in the blood pressure or rise in the pulse rate. In this event the neck should immediately be squeezed in order to identify and coagulate any open veins; air bubbles may be seen coming out of open veins when the jugulars are compressed. Sometimes the first sign of this complication is a catastrophic fall in blood pressure or cardiac arrest. The patient must then be laid down on his left side, to keep air away from the opening of the pulmonary artery in the right ventricle. Air turbulence may be heard on auscultation and it may be possible to aspirate air from the heart; apart from this the management is that of cardiac arrest. Probably most cases which develop cardiac arrest could have been suspected (by a vigilant anæsthetist) of having an embolus at an earlier and more readily reversible stage.

Non-operative Relief of Raised Intracranial Pressure

Apart from avoiding conditions which may raise intracranial pressure there are a number of manœuvres which will reduce pressure and which may be employed not only by the anæsthetist in the operating theatre but also in the ward before or after operation. They are sometimes referred to as chemical methods of decompression.

Hypertonic solutions, given intravenously, depend for their effect on osmotic dehydration of the brain; as a result blood volume is increased and a diuresis induced. Reduction of intracranial pressure is evident within about 15 minutes of a rapid infusion and lasts for about 4–6 hours. A saturated solution of mannitol (20%) is most commonly used, but this must be kept in a warm cupboard to prevent crystallisation. The full dose is 500 ml. given over 20 minutes, but smaller amounts may be effective; it is preferable to urea (1·5 gms. per kg. body weight) which is locally irritant and which also requires some preparation immediately before injection. Frusemide may itself be effective, and if given 30 minutes before mannitol it will largely prevent the rise in blood pressure which is normally observed as the result of increase in blood volume. In the theatre mannitol may be given as a routine after induction of anæsthesia, so that its maximal effects are established by the time the bone flap is turned. However, in most situations a properly conducted anæsthetic with good positioning on the table and controlled respiration will give a sufficiently slack brain; there are even disadvantages in having the brain shrunk still further in that bridging veins may be torn and the olfactory nerves may be avulsed with resulting permanent anosmia.

Cortico-steroids are less rapid in action but their effects can be none-theless dramatic; moreover they can be maintained over weeks or months, and patients with inoperable tumours have remained improved over many months on a dosage of 2 mg. daily of betamethazone, only to develop symptoms again as soon as this drug is withdrawn. In acute situations a dose of 4 mg. 4 times a day is reduced to 2 mg. 3 times a day after 3 days and eventually to 2 mg. a day although sometimes employed as a routine post-operative measure to prevent œdema and brain swelling steroids are probably not useful in the treatment of head injuries.

Hyperventilation, by inducing cerebral vasoconstriction secondary to hypocapnia, reduces intracranial pressure within minutes. Anæsthetists frequently employ this as a routine measure but if unusually high levels of ventilation are maintained a degree of cerebral hypoxia can result.

Brain/Lung Interactions

Since Cheyne described periodic respiration it has been increasingly recognised that brain damage may affect not only the rate and rhythm of breathing but also the efficiency of pulmonary gas exchange. This latter may be affected by central respiratory depression, by respiratory com-plications of the unconscious state, and also, according to some reports, by ventilation, perfusion abnormalities in the lungs produced by neural influences acting either directly or through the cardiovascular system. Whatever the reasons for inadequate respiration the effects are similar for the brain, and they are particularly adverse if the brain is already damaged, or if there is already reduced intracranial elastance (page 6). Both hypercapnia and hypoxia cause cerebral vascular dilatation, which will raise intracranial pressure. But when there is significant hypoxia this will usually produce a degree of hyperventila-tion; the resulting hypocapnia causes cerebral vasoconstriction and this may additionally threaten cerebral oxygenation, even though the ICP may have been reduced by the hyperventilation. This will likewise be the case when a brain stem lesion causes central neurogenic hyper-ventilation; this is now believed to be a rare condition, and most hyperventilating patients are found to be primarily hypoxic.

Awareness of the deleterious effect of respiratory insufficiency on the brain has led to great care being taken in the course of neurosurgical operations to avoid conditions which are not only bad for the brain but which also, by producing 'a tight brain', make the surgeon's task more difficult. It has also led to increased attention to the respiratory care not only of post-operative patients but of all unconscious patients. Enthusiasm has sometimes overtaken understanding in this complex field and there are still divided opinions about the place and value of controlled ventilation for unconscious brain damaged patients, par-ticularly those who have recently sustained a head injury. No-one disputes the importance of maintaining a clear airway at all times (page 234). If, once this is established, the PaO_2 is less than 70 mmHg. despite efficient delivery of oxygen there is needed to consider control (assisted) ventilation *to correct hypoxia*. Another reason advanced for controlled ventilation is in order *to eliminate the work of breathing* in the patient who is maintaining an adequate PaO_2 only by hyperventilation, or who has neurogenic hyperventilation. In these instances controlled ventilation may be recommended in order to *reduce* rather than to increase ventilation, in order to benefit the brain by reducing the vasoconstriction of hypocapnia. But the reason most often advanced in support of controlled ventilation is that hyperventilation can be used to *reduce intracranial pressure*. The question is whether the patient has significantly raised pressure; and if he has whether there may not be a possible threat to cerebral oxygenation in seeking to reduce ICP by producing a reduced cerebral blood flow. There are other possible disadvantages to controlled ventilation, carried out over a period of several days; one is the effects on the lungs, including the possibility of infection, particularly if tracheostomy becomes necessary. Another is that the clinician is deprived of most clinical indications of the state of brain function, and so cannot judge whether the patient is improving or, more significantly, is showing evidence of developing intracranial complications. Whatever the theoretical case for its value it must be appreciated that in large series of similarly severely brain damaged patients there is no good evidence that outcome is better when controlled ventilation is used routinely than when it is reserved only for those circumstances which clearly require it. That will usually be in patients with associated chest injuries or specific pulmonary complications. If controlled ventilation is used for these purposes then the $PaCO_2$ should not mormally be lower than 30 mmHg., in order to avoid undue cerebral vasoconstriction.

Surgical Means of Reducing Intracranial Pressure

Internal decompression can be produced by removing part of the tumour, or by sacrificing healthy but relatively dispensable brain tissue by performing frontal, occipital or temporal lobectomy; ("frontal" lobectomy entails removing only the anterior half of the frontal lobe, in front of the Sylvian fissure). These two methods may be combined, when a lobectomy is carried out across tumour, part of which is taken with the lobe, but leaving as much of it as invades areas of the brain which could not be removed without causing serious disability. If the tumour is slowly-growing an internal decompression can give a patient several years of useful life before symptoms recur.

For posterior fossa pressure a *suboccipital* decomposition is done, removing the occipital squama, the posterior rim of foramen magnum and usually the arch of the atlas; this ensures relief of pressure on the medulla by prolapsing cerebellar tonsils. So thick is the muscle and scalp in this region that it may be almost impossible after some years to feel the bone defect at all.

Posterior fossa tumours often present with severely raised pressure, If there is acute headache, or slowing and periodicity of respiration, no time should be lost in providing a decompression, even if radiological investigations are incomplete and the exact location of the tumour is unknown. An apnœic patient may begin to breathe again as soon as the posterior rim of the foramen magnum and the arch of the atlas are removed. If the tumour is not immediately obvious, or conditions are not favourable for its removal, the wound can be closed leaving the dura open. Investigations can then be completed in safety and the tumour removed at a properly planned second operation. Such "blind" decompression is less often required now that myodil ventriculography is available for investigating these severely compressed patients.

Short-circuiting procedures relieve obstructive hydrocephalus resulting from tumours in the posterior fossa, in the pineal region and around the foramen of Monro. Many of these tumours are inaccessible, others can be removed only partially, and a tube may effectively bypass the block. If the tumour happens to be radiosensitive, and symptoms are mostly due to the hydrocephalus, very successful results can follow the combination of radiation therapy with short-circuiting or diversion of CSF; the various procedures are described in Chapter 17 (p. 321).

When operation cannot be performed immediately; pressure is relieved temporarily by tapping the ventricle through a burr hole. If repeated ventricular tapping becomes necessary it is preferable to employ continuous *ventricular drainage*, using a rubber or polythene catheter. This runs from the lateral ventricle through the burr hole to a sterile transfusion bottle attached to the bed head, the height of the loop of tubing being fixed at 150 mm. above the head; CSF will siphon over whenever the pressure exceeds this. A patient who is very ill with high pressure may be in a better condition for operation after 24 hours continuous drainage, but there is a small risk of infection if it is continued for long; another danger is upward herniation of the cerebellum through the tentorial hiatus (p. 52). Normal pressure is sometimes reduced by lumbar puncture drainage often during operations involving access to deeply placed structures.

FURTHER READING

Fitch, W. and MacDowall, D. G. (1970). Hazards of anæsthesia in patients with space-occupying lesions. In: *International Anaesthesiology Clinics*, 7, Ed. McDowall. Little, Brown, Boston.
Gillen, H. W. (1968). Symptomatology of cerebral gas embolism. *Neurology* (Minneapolis) **18,** 507–512.
Hancock, D. O. (1963). The fate of replaced bone flaps. *Journal of Neurosurgery,* **20,** 983–984.

Hunter, A. R. (1970). Scientific contributions to neurosurgical anæsthesia. In: *International Anaesthesiology Clinics*, **7**, Ed McDowall, Little, Brown, Boston.

Jennett, W. B., Barker, J., Fitch, W. and McDowall, D. G. (1969) Effect of anæsthesia on intracranial pressure in patients with space-occupying lesions. *Lancet*, **i**, 61–64.

Lundberg, N., Kjallquist, A., Kullberg, G., Poulen, G. and Sundborg, G. (1974). Non-operative management of intracranial hypertension. In: *Advances in Technical Standards in Neurosurgery*, Eds. Krayenbuhl et al. (Vol. 1) Springer-Wien, New York.

Lundberg, N., Ponten, U. and Brock, M. (eds.) (1975). Discussion on Longterm Controlled Ventilation in Intracranial Hypertension. In: *Intracranial Pressure*, **II**, Springer-Verlag, Berlin.

McDowall, D. G. and Norman, J. B. (eds.) (1976). Symposium on neurosurgical anæsthesia, In: *British Journal of Anaesthesia*, **48**, 717–804.

Schurmann, K., Brock, M., Reulen, H.-J., and Voth, D. (eds.) (1973). Advances in Neurosurgery 1. *Brain Edema: pathophysiology and therapy*. Springer-Verlag, Berlin.

CHAPTER 8

Post-operative Care and Complications

Intracranial clot

Pyrexia and infection

Epilepsy

Care of the eyes

An intracranial operation is a planned head injury, and the complications are similar. Comments here will be limited to those aspects of these complications that apply to the postoperative period, but the reader should refer to Chapters 13, 14 for details of monitoring, of the diagnosis and treatment of intracranial hæmatoma, and for a discussion of epilepsy after trauma or intracranial surgery.

Intracranial clot

Every neurosurgeon fears this complication, which may spoil the best operation; it may deprive the patient of some function which was carefully preserved at operation a few hours before or it may prove fatal. Unfortunately it is the best operations which are most liable to be followed by this complication; the cavity left by the partial resection of an infiltrating tumour is soon obliterated by swollen brain around it but the walls of the empty space left when a benign tumour (e.g. meningioma) has been removed can readily bleed, as may the overlying dura which strips away from the bone to sag into the cavity. Before closing the skull the surgeon must meticulously stop all bleeding, having ensured that the blood pressure has regained its normal level if it has been low. Observation of the patient over the next two days is directed primarily at detecting clot formation; to establish a base-line as soon as possible the anæsthetist is encouraged to have the patient answering simple questions and moving limbs to command before he leaves the operating theatre. Any subsequent change in conscious level, power of the limbs or size of the pupils must then be explained in terms of secondary changes—hæmorrhage, infarction or œdema, and not put down to some vague effect of the operation. A clot may form within hours of leaving the theatre, and the patient who is allowed to "sleep off" his operation, with either long-acting anæesthetic agents or post-operative sedation, may never wake up. Discomfort after craniotomy is seldom great and can be alleviated without masking changes in the conscious level by codeine, aspirin or other simple analgesics.

The signs looked for after a **supratentorial** operation are those sought after head injury (p. 232)—deteriorating conscious level, larger ipsilateral pupil, hemiplegia, decerebrate rigidity, rising blood pressure and falling pulse rate with stertorous periodic respiration. Observations of pulse, blood pressure, pupil reaction and conscious level must be made at least hourly for 24 hours, and longer if there is any doubt about progress, however unkind it may appear to the patient or his relatives. Sometimes a relapse is gradual and delayed till the second or third day; œdema rather than clot may be suspected. Post-operative monitoring of ICP may help to distinguish between deterioration from a hæmatoma or that due to infarction; pressure does not rise for 24 hours or so after infarction, if it does at all. EMI scanning or angiography may be useful, but can be difficult to interpret in the early post-operative period—and if any doubt remains the flap must be re-opened.

Clot may be extradural or intradural, or both, and a single sizeable bleeding point is less often found than a general ooze. The brain is frequently œdematous after this second handling within a few days; if the bone flap is at all difficult to replace comfortably it is best left out and stored in deep freeze; it can be replaced, after a few weeks or months. Suturing galea a second time at this early stage is difficult; it is best to insert only a few stitches and rely on more deeply placed skin sutures than usual, and these should lie between the original skin suture marks. Infection is a risk after re-opening; local antibiotics during closure and a systemic course for five days are probably wise precautions.

Posterior fossa hæmatomas are more treacherous because there may be little warning before terminal apnœa. Continual complaint of headache, especially if accompanied by vomiting, should raise suspicion, but the respiratory rate is the most critical index; a persisting fall below 16 per minute calls for a most careful review of all aspects of the case and inspection of the wound to see if it is tight and bulging. Even more than with supratentorial hæmatomas the slightest suspicion of a clot calls for investigation, and for operation if doubt remains.

Pyrexia and infection

Early pyrexia is unlikely to be due to infection. Moderate levels (up to 38°C) in the first 48 hours may reasonably be ascribed to *reaction to blood* at the operation site or in the subarachnoid space. Hyperpyrexia may occur following operations in the region of the upper brain stem and hypothalamus; this calls for vigorous treatment (p. 242).

Delayed pyrexia, after the third day, must be presumed to indicate infection and the most likely sites must be systematically searched.

THE WOUND

Some surgeons inspect operation wounds routinely on the first or second day; blood-soaked dressings, which are an excellent culture medium for bacteria, are removed. A wound which is distended by blood or CSF overlying a bone flap may be aspirated using either a sharp needle put in through the centre of the flap or a blunt cannula through the suture line; often the distension proves to be mostly air.

The occurrence of pyrexia calls for inspection of the wound whether this is routine or not. **Stitch abscesses** rarely form with flaps because the sutures are removed on the third day, the deep galeal layer taking all the tension off the skin; posterior fossa stitches are left 10 days and do have time to become infected. The affected stitch should be removed to allow the pus to come out and a culture taken to identify the organisms and test their sensitivity to antibiotics. Occasionally a **cellulitis** of the wound develops, calling for systemic antibiotics. The dura is an excellent barrier to infection and provided it is intact meningitis and brain abscess very rarely develop from superficial infections.

Prophylactic antibiotics are sometimes recommended but there is little evidence of their efficacy. However, in circumstances known to carry a risk of infection a topical spray and a five-day course of claxacillin and ampicillin is probably wise. These include all operations in which the frontal sinuses have been opened, those which were prolonged (contamination rises abruptly after about four hours), and wounds which were re-opened for any reason.

CSF leak carries the threat of meningitis; rhinorrhœa may follow the removal of a basal anterior fossa tumour, whilst CSF may leak directly from a posterior fossa wound when the dura has been left open. Every effort must be made to stop the leak by keeping the pressure low with repeated lumbar punctures and elevation of the head of the bed; an additional skin stitch may be needed where the leak is occurring, followed by a plastic sealing. Pressurised antibiotic sprays should not be used too close to a leaking wound; a jet may distend it and carry in contaminants.

MENINGITIS

Blood in the CSF may produce meningism and pyrexia at an early stage, but if these develop later meningitis must be suspected and a lumbar puncture promptly done. Even though the fluid is bloodstained the pathologist must be urged to count the cells because meningitis may be diagnosed if there is a marked excess of white cells compared with the normal number for the amount of blood contamination (one white cell per thousand red cells). Probably one to two hundred excess leucocytes can be accepted as a reaction to blood spilt at operation, but more than this are best regarded as evidence of infection. The fluid should be cultured, as should every aspirate in the early post-operative days even when no infection is suspected; treatment with intrathecal and systemic antibiotics should not await bacteriological confirmation (p. 187).

ABSCESS

The operative cavity is occasionally the site of a late intracranial abscess, weeks or months after recovery. Although this may be due to a foreign body, such as a stitch or fragment of cotton wool, it may develop with no such provocation. There may be repeated mild attacks of meningitis due to leakage of infected material, or the patient may present with raised pressure and signs of a local mass. This may suggest tumour recurrence but occurs too soon after operation for this possibility to be seriously considered. Treatment is by burr hole aspiration in the first instance as for brain abscess of other origin (p. 180).

OSTEOMYELITIS

Infection of the bone flap is suspected when a sinus forms with intermittent discharge of pus, often weeks or months after operation. The chronicity is typical whereas a brief episode of local infection, due to a loose deep suture, rapidly resolves once the offending stitch comes out.

Bone changes are difficult to detect radiologically but a frank sequestrum can be recognised as a relatively dense white shadow, and such a fragment must be removed before healing can be expected. If a sinus persists or recurs after local excision and removal of the granulation tissue, osteomyelitis must be presumed and the whole flap reopened. The inner surface of the bone is usually found to be "worm-eaten" for several centimetres from the region of the sinus, with granulation tissue filling the interstices of eroded bone and extending into the scalp (fig. 29). Nothing short of removal of the whole bone flap will ensure immediate and permanent wound healing unless the area of bone involvement is very local indeed and can be removed by nibbling. The diseased bone flap may be replaced several months later after boiling or sterilisation by gamma rays from a cobalt source, but if the bone is extensively destroyed some form of cranioplasty will be needed (p. 273).

Extracranial Infection

The chest and the bladder are frequent sites of infection in a patient who is unconscious for any period, and as specific complaints will not be made active efforts must be made to exclude these if pyrexia develops. The management of chest complications is dealt with in relation to head injury (p. 241).

mirror night and morning and to report immediately if there is any redness, regardless of the presence of pain or discomfort.

When *facial palsy* accompanies trigeminal anæsthesia the risks of keratitis are very high because the eye cannot be closed efficiently. In these circumstances a prophylactic tarsorraphy is required, stitching the lids together in the lateral third of the palpebral fissure being sufficient protection as a rule. No anæsthetic is needed for this simple operation as the area is already insensitive. The lid margin is made raw by slicing off a thin margin of the edge and a single mattress suture of nylon is tied over thin rubber tubing. This should be left in for 14–18 days, after which the closure is normally secure but if it comes apart the stitch is simply replaced after freshening the lid margin again.

Once keratitis develops treatment must be instituted without delay, and patients should be told where they can receive this in an emergency. When there is no ulceration the frequent instillation of drops of 10% albucid or of penicillin, and atropine if the patient is not elderly, with gentle closure of middle of the lids with strapping, should be tried for 24–48 hours. If there is not rapid improvement, or ulceration develops, tarsorraphy must be performed immediately, and usually a more extensive one than is done prophylactically. Once the acute inflammation settles it is easy to snip it partly open with sharp scissors (without an anæsthetic).

FURTHER READING

Balch, R. E. (1967). Wound infections complicating neurosurgical procedures. *Journal of Neurosurgery*, **26**, 41–45.

Bell, D. S. (1969). Danger of treatment of status epilepticus with Diazepam. *British Medical Journal*, **1**, 159–162.

Cabral, R., King, T. T., Scott, D. F. (1976). Incidence of post-operative epilepsy after a transtentorial approach to accoustic nerve tumours. *Journal of Neurology, Neurosurgery and Psychiatry*, **39**, 663–665.

Editorial (1967). Status epilepticus: a medical emergency. *British Medical Journal*, **3**, 63–64.

Logue, V. (1974). Surgery for supratentorial meningiomas. *Journal of Neurology, Neurosurgery and Psychiatry*, **37**, 1277.

Price, D. J. E. and Sleigh, J. D. (1970). Control of infection due to Elebsiella ærogenes in a neurosurgical unit by the withdrawal of all antibiotics. *Lancet*, **ii**, 1213–1215.

Purpura, D. P., Penry, J. K. and Walter, R. D. (eds.) (1975). Advances In Neurology. Volume 8: *Neurosurgical Management of the Epilepsies*. Raven Press, New York.

Wallis, W., Kutt, H. and MacDowell, F. (1968). Intravenous diphenylhydrantoin in the treatment of acute repetitive seizures. *Neurology* (Minneapolis), **18**, 513–525.

Wright, R. L. (1966). A survey of possible ætiological agents in post-operative craniotomy infections. *Journal of Neurosurgery*, **25**, 125–132.

II: Particular Intracranial Lesions

CHAPTER 9

Intracranial Tumours

Management
    Surgery
    Radiotherapy
    Chemotherapy

Classification

Glioma
    Astrocytoma
    Ependymoma
    Oligodendroglioma
    Management
        cerebral astrocytoma
        cerebellar gliomas
        other astrocytomas

Medulloblastoma

Meningioma

Pituitary tumours

Neuroma

Metastatic tumours

Vascular tumours

Congenital tumours
    Teratoma (pineal)
    Cholesteatoma (epidermoid)
    Dermoid
    Chordoma

Orbital tumours

Suspected tumour recurrence

Only when an anatomical diagnosis has been made, from clinical and radiological evidence, are the pathological possibilities considered and arranged in order of likelihood. This order will depend chiefly on a knowledge of the tendency of different tumours to favour certain sites, to occur at various ages and to evolve symptomatically according to characteristic patterns.

Benign and malignant primary tumours are less clearly contrasted in the cranium than elsewhere in the body because brain tumours rarely metastasise outside the nervous system. The **concept of malignancy** depends therefore on other aspects of tumour behaviour such as *rate of growth* and the tendency to *infiltrate diffusely*, as contrasted with a tendency to remain circumscribed.

Whatever its nature the *location* of an intracranial tumour is critical for many reasons: involvement of vital centres may threaten life directly or limit surgical accessibility: hydrocephalus may result from a small tumour blocking CSF flow: brain shifts and herniations, which vary with the site of the mass, may dominate the clinical picture and constitute the chief immediate danger to the patient. The paradox can arise of a small, discrete and slowly-growing mass having a relentless course because it lies in a vital site such as the hypothalamus or medulla, whilst a large and histologically malignant tumour (e.g. some pineal tumours) which is equally irremovable may be compatible with long survival, if producing only symptoms due to obstructive hydrocephalus, which can be relieved by short-circuiting procedures. It is impossible to separate the nature from the location of a tumour when discussing its clinical significance and prognosis.

A surgeon's natural reaction to a tumour is to remove the whole of it. Such a straightforward solution is not always possible in the brain, where loss of function may be too high a price to pay for radical surgery.

Judging the benefits of treatment for brain tumours is difficult because crude survival rates are unsatisfactory, and the quality as well as the length of survival needs to be examined critically. Most neurosurgeons have had the experience of a patient living for years, mentally or physically crippled, after surgical endeavours which in retrospect were over-ambitious. Yet if no risks are taken a patient may be denied his only chance of cure, and surgery that is too timorous can carry as high an ultimate mortality and morbidity as that which is too bold.

Radiation treatment, and more recently, chemotherapy are also available for dealing with intracranial tumours; however, the susceptibility of the still functioning brain, which surrounds and often traverses the tumour, places limitations on their use, as it does on the application of conventional surgical methods.

Improvements are slowly occurring with all three methods—surgery, radiation and chemotherapy; there are now clinical trials to find out what combinations of these are most effective. It is hoped that by using combined modality therapy it may be possible to achieve additive or synergistic effects without increasing the side effects. For example, even incomplete surgical removal almost always reduces tumour bulk by a greater proportion than either radiation or chemotherapy ever can; it is therefore logical to use these as means of dealing with residual tumour, in the hope of achieving long term survival. Their use for palliation of inoperable tumours aims at a different objective—and it is in this context that the quality of survival has to be balanced with the mere increase in surgical time.

Before dealing with the characteristics and management of specific tumours the general principles governing the use of these three methods, will be outlined.

SURGICAL PRINCIPLES

The technical feasibility of completely removing a tumour depends on many factors. The tumour may be inaccessible except by causing irreparable local damage; it may share a blood supply with more distant vital structures; regardless of situation, it may be prohibitively vascular as are large angiomatous malformations; it may be infiltrative, like gliomas where no clear plane of cleavage from surrounding brain can be found. It is often impossible to decide about these factors without surgical exploration, although contrast radiology may reveal the size, blood supply and relation to vital structures of certain tumours.

Investigations may strongly suggest, but can never diagnose definitely, the pathological nature of the tumour; histological confirmation must be obtained before declaring a tumour irremovable on pathological grounds. Even if a tumour is removable a particular patient's interest may not always be best served by total resection, having regard to its rate of growth and the patient's natural expectation of life. A satisfactory alleviation can often be gained by partial removal with much less risk than a radical operation, and some tumours show little tendency to recur. Patients with a brain tumour are *managed* rather than *cured*; the success of treatment depends on always balancing the probable neurological morbidity of the measures employed with that expected from the natural course of the disease.

Palliative procedures

The wide range of useful procedures available for certain tumours which are irremovable contrasts with the rather bleak outlook for such growths elsewhere in the body. Properly planned palliative surgery can give the patient with a brain tumour many years of useful life even though complete removal is never attempted. Two main groups of symptoms call for palliation.

1. **Symptoms of raised intracranial pressure** always demand treatment unless the tumour is so malignant histologically or is so advanced in

causing unrecoverable defects as to be quite hopeless. Raised pressure constitutes a threat to life, and often to vision (from consecutive optic atrophy). The methods available for relieving it are described in Chapter 7 (p. 96).

2. **Symptoms of local brain dysfunction** respond less reliably to incomplete surgical measures, even to complete tumour removal. Recovery depends on how long-standing the defect in function is, and how much extra damage either to brain itself or to its blood supply is inflicted during operation. *Vision* recovers well when chiasmal compression is relieved unless marked optic atrophy is already established. *Hemiplegia* due to hemisphere involvement is usually at least partially improved when a tumorous cyst is evacuated; but the manipulation of a vascular infiltrative tumour often aggravates the paralysis, although this effect may be only temporary. *Epilepsy* may undergo a temporary or permanent remission following surgery, or the pattern of the seizures may be altered; but it is unwise ever to promise that the attacks will cease. *Cerebellar symptoms*, ataxia and vertigo, are often satisfactorily relieved by subtotal removal of a laterally placed tumour, even when a considerable part of the cerebellar hemisphere is sacrificed, provided that the dentate nucleus and vermis are left intact.

RADIOTHERAPY

The susceptibility of the normal brain tissue to irradiation limits the value of this mode of treatment. Another limitation is that the commonest malignant brain tumour, glioma of the cerebral hemisphere, is usually so widespread through the brain that high doses cannot be be concentrated on a localised area of residual tumour. Even with medulloblastoma, the most sensitive and the most successfully treated tumour, radiation of the whole brain and also the spinal canal is necessary—in this case because of the frequency of tumour dissemination along CSF pathways. The most common regime is to give 5–6,000 rads, at a rate of 1,000 rads a week. Measures designed to radiosensitise the tumour have not yet improved results. Localised tumours have been treated by implantation of radioactive seeds under X-ray control, and cystic tumours by the injection of radioactive solutions.

Complications

Radiotherapy does not usually cause any immediate upset and constitutional disturbances such as normally accompany irradiation of the thorax or abdomen are unusual. Some temporary *epilation* may occur, depending on dose, and occasionally this is permanent. Sometimes a rapidly growing tumour appears to swell during the early stages of a course of radiation, and it is wise to provide a decompression of some kind for such tumours before radiation is begun; such protection may be conferred by a course of steroids (p. 103).

The susceptibility of normal brain tissue to radiation is the factor limiting dosage, even when treating a sensitive tumour in a circumscribed situation, e.g. a pituitary adenoma. Because the effects of excessive radiation to an area of brain (*radionecrosis*) are not evident for a long time after treatment (at least 9 months and usually about 5 years) the importance of this risk was only gradually appreciated. Many patients died of recurrent tumour without living long enough to develop radionecrosis, whilst those that did succumb to an overdose of X-rays were often assumed to have died of recurrence. The affected tissue becomes ischæmic due to a fibrinoid necrosis in small vessels; the mechanism of the necrosis and the reason for the long latent period are unexplained. The hypothalamus is particularly vulnerable to X-rays, and is liable to be in the target area when the pituitary is irradiated; delayed radiation effects here are usually fatal. Elsewhere, however, there may be no more than the rather sudden re-appearance of symptoms similar to those originally caused by the tumour; these may as rapidly subside without treatment.

Now that the dangers of radionecrosis are appreciated and more refined methods are available there should be little risk of producing any additional damage by the irradiation of brain tumours.

CHEMOTHERAPY

Most known *cytotoxic drugs* have been tried for glioma. Administration has been by oral or intravenous route as well as by local intralesional and intracarotid injection. The Nitrosourea group (BCNU, CCNU, Methyl CCNU) are cell-cycle non-specific agents which are fat soluble and enter the brain well. These agents have shown promise in prospective clinical trials, with significant responses in up to 40% of patients with malignant glioma of the brain. The most striking results have been obtained using adjunctive chemotherapy in combined modality treatment in an attempt to achieve additive or synergistic effects without increasing toxicity. Radical surgery with radiotherapy and BCNU resulted in median survival of 40 weeks in a group of patients with malignant glioma contrasted with 17 weeks for those treated by surgery alone. At 18 months, nearly all patients who received only one or two modalities of treatment were dead, whereas 25% of those receiving surgery supplemented by radiotherapy and chemotherapy were alive. Further improvement in results may come from use of combinations of drugs for chemotherapy. Encouraging results have been reported from the use of adjunctive combination chemotherapy for medulloblastoma in children following surgery and radiotherapy. There is some evidence that intraventricular cytotoxic agents may prolong survival in carcinomatous meningitis. Systemic toxic effects of cytotoxic agents in the doses required for brain tumours are seldom marked, but marrow depression can occur. Toxic peripheral neuro-pathy occurs with some drugs, and brain necrosis sometimes develops after combined chemotherapy and radiotherapy.

Corticosteroids are widely used, often with dramatic effect, to control symptoms associated with brain tumour (p. 103). Whether they have a significant oncolytic effect on tumour grow thrather than simply con-trolling cerebral oedema in surrounding normal brain is not yet known.

Immunotherapy is another possible method of treatment for malignant cerebral neoplasms. There is increasing evidence that brain tumours are associated with immunological responses similar to those found in other solid tumours, and that the immune responses of patients harbouring glioma are depressed. Immunotherapy for glioma in man has been attempted unsuccessfully in a smaller number of patients. However, the anticipated hazard, allergic encephalomyelitis has not been en-countered. Augmentation of the immune response in patients with glioma may eventually prove an important further adjunctive therapy when conventional methods become effective in reducing residual tumour to a very small mass.

FURTHER READING

Batley, F. (1973). Radiotherapy of brain tumours. *Chapter in Neurological Surgery* (Vol. 3). Ed. J. R. Youmans, Sanders, Philadelphia.

Bloom, H. J. G. (1975). Combined modality therapy for intracranial tumours. *Cancer*, **3.**, 111.

Kramer, S. (1968). Hazards of therapuetic irradiation of the central nervous system. *In: Clinical Neurosurgery.* pp. 301–318, Williams and Wilkins, Baltimore.

Posner, J. B. and Shapiro, W. B. (1975). Brain tumour—current status of treatment and its complications. *Archives of Neurology*, **32**, 781–784.

Walker, M. D. (1975). Malignant brain tumours—a synopsis. *Cancer Journal for Clinicians*, **25**, 114.

Wilson, C. B. and Norell, H. A. (1973). Chemotherapy of brain tumours. *Chapter in Neurological Surgery* (Vol. 3). Ed. J. R. Youmans. Sanders, Philadelphia.

Classification of tumours

The natural history and gross anatomy of tumours claim most attention in the account which follows, and microscopic characteristics are dealt with only briefly. The cellular origin of many brain tumours remains controversial and there is no close correlation between minor histological differences and the clinical behaviour of tumours.

Even when *histological criteria* are considered alone there are diffi-culties in attaching useful or practically significant labels to many tumours. Well-differentiated tumours may recur relentlessly because their diffuseness defies total surgical resection. Any one tumour may not be homogeneous, histological sections from one part appearing more benign than from another. Diagnosis based on a relatively small biopsy is therefore less reliable than an autopsy study of the whole tumour. Furthermore tumours may change their character over a period of time, with increasing anaplasia, and difficulties are then encountered when a single name is sought for a tumour which has been observed in a patient over many years.

The published accounts of the frequency of different tumour types depends on the source of the series which is analysed, surgical series commonly containing more benign, and necropsy figures more malignant, tumours.

The approximate distribution of 1300 intracranial tumours encountered over 6 years in the Institute of Neurological Sciences, Glasgow was:

Neuro-ectodermal		60%
astrocytoma		
(all grades including glioblastoma)	44%	
ependymoma	3%	
oligodendroglioma . . .	2·5%	
medulloblastoma . . .	3%	
Metastatic		18%
Meningioma		10%
Pituitary		7·5%
Acoustic neuroma		3·5%

Neuro-ectodermal tumours arise from cells derived from the primitive neuroectoderm which is represented in the mature nervous system by the neuroglia, viz. astrocytes, oligodendrocytes and ependymal cells, and by nerve cells. The great majority of cerebral tumours arise from the neuroglial cells and are known collectively as the gliomas.

Glioma

The neuroglia is structurally the connective tissue of the nervous system and is found throughout the brain and spinal cord; gliomas, likewise, may be widely distributed. These tumours are most difficult to put in clear-cut categories which reflect a consistent natural history and even their accurate pathological classification is difficult because of the great histological variations that may occur within an individual tumour.

PATHOLOGY

For long the authoritative scheme of Bailey and Cushing (1926) was accepted. They held that the tumours fell into 14 discrete groups each derived from a different embryonic cell type. Most subsequent classifications have been based on this scheme although many attempts have been made to simplify it. Kernohan and Adson (1949) thus reduced the field to five main groups in four of which they believed that they could recognise four grades of malignancy, viz. astrocytoma grades 1–4, ependymoma grades 1–4, oligodendroglioma grades 1–4, neuroastrocytoma grades 1–4 (rarely encountered) and medulloblastoma (homogeneous group). The propriety of classifying the last two groups as gliomas may, however, be questioned as the most prominent cell types belong to the neuronal series of cells and not to the glial series. Furthermore as certain rare but highly characteristic histological types of tumour are not included their classification may be said to be oversimplified. Another criticism of this system is that if the grading of the tumour is based on a biopsy taken through a burrhole, it implies a much greater degree of accuracy than can legitimately be claimed, particularly if any prognostic significance is placed on a biopsy showing the features of a well-differentiated (grade 1) tumour. The nomenclature and classification used here is based on that put forward by Russell and Rubinstein (1971).

Astrocytoma

This is by far the commonest of the gliomas and includes a wide range of tumours from those composed of well-differentiated cells where the predominant cell type is very similar to particular types of astrocyte, e.g. fibrillary, protoplasmic, gemistocytic, to highly anaplastic tumours. The mature well-differentiated astrocytoma is equivalent to Kernohan's grade 1 while the anaplastic astrocytomas are equivalent to grades 2–4. All grades of anaplasia may be encountered, however, in different parts of the same tumour, and initially mature astrocytomas above the tentorium display a strong tendency to become anaplastic with the passage of time.

Diffuseness is often the chief characteristic of a well-differentiated astrocytoma and it is often impossible to define any edge to the tumour, the affected area of the brain simply being expanded, firm and often rather pale. Even on microscopic examination there is a very gradual transition from obvious tumour to normal brain. In this transitional zone the appearances may be very difficult to distinguish from reactive gliosis. In extreme examples of diffuse astrocytoma there may be no real tumour mass. More often, however, there is a fleshy or friable tumour of low cellularity within which there may be small cysts. Large cysts filled with clear yellow fluid, which clots when exposed to air, are of frequent occurrence in well-differentiated astrocytomas of the cerebellum, where tumour cells may be confined to a circumscribed mural nodule. Similar cysts are less frequently encountered in astrocytomas in the cerebral hemispheres.

Anaplastic astrocytomas are characterised by hæmorrhage, necrosis, rapid growth and the presence of poorly differentiated anaplastic and pleomorphic cells of astrocytic type. These tumours often seem to have a more clearly defined edge than mature astrocytomas though this is not necessarily borne out by microscopic examination. Cysts, when present, usually contain fluid which is turbid or even creamy and pus-like, the result of necrosis. Massive hæmorrhage giving rise to sudden clinical deterioration is unusual.

Anaplasia is of very frequent occurrence in astrocytoma and may develop at any stage in its life history. The more carefully it is sought, the more likely it is to be found and this is the principal reason why some pathologists are reluctant to apply a particular grade to an astrocytoma on the basis of a small biopsy. In the most anaplastic astrocytomas (equivalent to Kernohan's grade 4 astrocytoma) there are sheets of closely packed tumour cells the majority of which are usually small although there may also be numerous multinucleate giant cells in some tumours; there are also numerous mitotic figures, irregular areas of necrosis and hæmorrhage, and intense capillary endothelial hyperplasia. This formation of many new vessels results in small arteriovenous shunts which may be detected on angiography, and which account for the red veins sometimes seen at operation around this tumour. All intermediate grades between the mature and highly anaplastic variants (equivalent to Kernohan grade 2 and 3) occur, depending on the maturity of the tumour cells, their density, the mitotic rate and the presence or absence of glial fibrils, necrosis, hæmorrhage and vascular endothelial hyperplasia. Because of the great variations that may be present in any one tumour, a biopsy from one area may have the typical appearance of a mature tumour (grade 1) while a biopsy taken from a different area may show a highly anaplastic (grade 4) tumour.

When a glial tumour is highly anaplastic throughout it has been argued that the most appropriate term is glioblastoma multiforme but such a diagnosis can be established only when the entire tumour is available for microscopical examination.

The growing edge of a tumour may appear to be confined within a gyrus but sometimes the pia-arachnoid is invaded and a carpet of tumour spreads over the surface of the brain. More rarely the dura is involved, but only by malignant tumours. The ependyma may also be breached so that tumour occupies the ventricular cavity; seeding can occur in the subarachnoid or ventricular spaces (but is much less common than from an ependymoma or medulloblastoma) and may give rise to tumour cells in CSF and secondary blocks to CSF flow. Subarachnoid hæmorrhage, rare with any tumour, is most frequently found to come from an astrocytoma which abuts on CSF pathways.

Astrocytomas may occur in any age group but some types of mature fibrillary astrocytoma are particularly common in childhood. In the cerebellum and optic nerve these tumours are more benign than any other type of glioma. Even after incomplete removal they may stop growing, or even regress, leading to the suggestion that growth is arrested when the child reaches maturity, as with hamartomas.

Anaplastic change in an astrocytoma may also occur at any age but is more common in adults. Primary glioblastoma multiforme is, however, distinctly rare under the age of 30. These rapidly growing tumours occur mainly in the cerebral hemispheres, particularly in the temporal lobe, and are distinctly rare in the cerebellum and brain stem. In the latter site, astrocytomas are usually of the diffuse infiltrating type and are usually well-differentiated and slow growing.

Ependymoma

Over 50% are in children, mostly aged 8–15 years. Some 60% occur below the tent although ependymomas make up only 10% of posterior fossa tumours under the age of 12. The tumour normally grows from the floor of the fourth ventricle making total removal impossible but occasionally the tumour arises in the cerebello-pontine angle and spares the fourth ventricle; only 10% are cystic.

Supratentorial ependymomas are usually related to some part of the lateral ventricle and the lobulated tumour may develop a large cyst anteriorly which can eventually block the foramen of Monro. These tumours more often have radiologically visible calcification than the cerebellar ones. Another site is the posterior end of the third ventricle.

This red nodular tumour, tufty like a cauliflower, and firm because of the dense network of branching vessels, tends to conform to the shape of its surrounding. Histologically there are rosettes and solid clusters of cells. Metastasis by CSF pathways occasionally occurs from paraventricular growths and sometimes it appears to have been precipitated by operation. As with astrocytomas, ependymomas may become anaplastic as shown by the increased cellularity, necrosis and hæmorrhage.

Oligodendroglioma

This occurs superficially in the cerebral hemisphere, and may mushroom through the surface and become adherent to the dura and be mistaken for a meningioma. Mucoid cysts and necrosis occur, and there is a special liability to spontaneous hæmorrhage which may lead to sudden clinical deterioration. Calcification, related to vessel walls, is visible on X-ray as irregular strands over a wide area (fig. 15); over half of these tumours calcify. Widespread meningeal and ventricular metastases may develop, possibly precipitated by surgery; this event bears no relation to histological malignancy but depends more on the proximity of the tumour to CSF pathways. Microscopically there are uniform sheets of small polyhedral spaces (clear cytoplasm) containing round nuclei. In keeping with other gliomas this tumour may become anaplastic. Most cases are in adults.

CLINICAL

Diffuse astrocytoma of cerebral hemisphere

The greater part of one hemisphere is swollen and firmer than normal. The white matter is expanded and rubbery in consistency, and the affected brain retains its shape when cut into, staying stiffly open instead of falling together as normal brain does. A cannula is passed through the affected area at operation it is "gripped" by the tumour tissue.

The clinical history is often already a long one by the time the patient comes for investigation, perhaps several years after the onset of epilepsy. Gradually slight weakness of a limb appears, and there may be mild mental changes; eventually more definite hemiplegia develops, perhaps with signs of raised pressure. Angiography may show no abnormality until a late stage because so diffuse a process may fail to produce distortion of vessels and there is no pathological tumour circulation visible; usually a slight lateral shift is discovered which can be confirmed by air studies.

Surgery cannot help the patient with this tumour, except for a decompression when there is raised pressure; it is doubtful if radiation influences its course. When, therefore, a patient presents with a history of epilepsy, has no physical disability, but a slight lateral shift is found on X-ray, the question of management is difficult. Untreated the tumour may grow only slowly and the patient continue to live usefully for years, whereas operation may add to his disability without improving his prospects. An exception may therefore be made to the rule of verifying histologically every suspected brain tumour, provided the clinical history and radiological investigation leave no serious doubt about the tumour being diffuse and consequently irremovable. Moreover the recognition of this tumour histologically is not always easy, especially when only a fragment of tissue is recovered from a burr hole biopsy. In reaching a decision the particular needs of individual patients have to be sympathetically appraised. A semi-literate artisan, a practising barrister, a harassed young mother and a lonely old widow: each has very different requirements—reasons perhaps for wanting to postpone for a year or so any measure which might result in additional disabilities, or reasons for wanting to have the diagnosis confirmed beyond doubt and without delay. Such matters must be given due weight in reaching a decision both in regard to how far to investigate, and how vigorously to treat, a patient suspected of having this type of tumour.

Localised astrocytoma of cerebral hemisphere

Any region can be involved but the occipital pole is rarely affected; frontal tumours tend to cross the midline in the region of the corpus callosum, forming a "butterfly" tumour constricted in the middle. Only part of the tumour is in fact circumscribed, and elsewhere it blends with tough, expanded white matter like a diffuse tumour; the circumscribed area may be cystic. Localised astrocytomas in the cerebral hemispheres show a marked tendency to anaplastic change (p. 123); one series of astrocytomas, reported on surgical biopsy as benign, showed anaplasia in over 90% at subsequent autopsy, mostly years later.

According to the rate of growth the history of epilepsy, hemiplegia and raised pressure may spread over many years or be telescoped into months or even weeks. Worsening is sometimes associated with a cyst, and simple aspiration may reverse the clinical course for a time. Terminal deterioration is more often due to brain shifts developing than to any new event in the tumour itself.

EMI scanning is the investigation of choice in most of these patients presenting with epilepsy and hemiplegia, because not only will the site of the tumour be disclosed but it may be possible to recognise oedema and ventricular enlargement and displacement; cysts inside larger tumours can also be identified. Angiography will show the vascularity of the tumour, and the nature of this may indicate the likely nature of the tumour. Astrocytomas of intermediate degrees of anaplasia (equivalent to grades 2 and 3) usually show only local displacements without tumour circulation (abnormal vessels), whilst highly anaplastic tumours, including glioblastoma (equivalent to grade 4) often have an obvious tumour circulation (fig. 30). Glioblastoma vessels fill early, with veins already beginning to show on the arterial (first) film together with the small arteriovenous fistulæ which account for this rapid circulation. Tumour vessels are of widely varying size, some of them beaded or tortuous; the remainder of the brain sometimes appears relatively starved of blood vessels. By the venous phase all contrast has left the tumour, as distinct from the delayed emptying typical of a meningioma. An angioma has many of these characteristics but the vessels are larger and more regular, the veins usually enormous. A metastasis closely resembles a glioblastoma on angiography. *Air studies* may be of value (fig. 31).

Ependymoma and oligodendroglioma behave in a similar fashion to localised astrocytoma, and indeed may sometimes be distinguished only histologically (pp. 123–4). What follows about treatment applies alike to all supratentorial gliomas.

TREATMENT OF CEREBRAL GLIOMAS

This, the commonest single type of brain tumour, is unfortunately the least satisfactory to treat. Even those gliomas which at first appear circumscribed are generally discovered to merge indistinguishably with the brain at some point; many spread across the midline as well as extensively in the hemisphere in which they arise. Radical surgery is therefore misdirected zeal, for even hemispherectomy may not ensure complete eradication. As many of these tumours are slowly growing, however, limited surgical removal offers a fair prospect of palliation.

For a relatively circumscribed glioma in the frontal or occipital pole, or the right temporal lobe, a **lobectomy** will provide an internal decompression, and most of the tumour may be removed. The hope that a really small tumour in this situation may be found and totally removed is seldom realised because diagnosis in these clinically silent sites is not

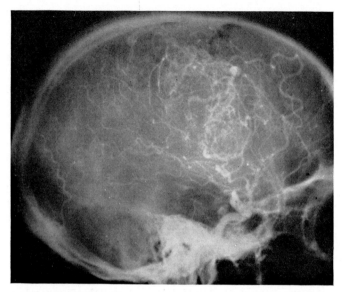

(*a*) Abnormal tumour vessels are filled early, when contrast is still in the carotid artery.

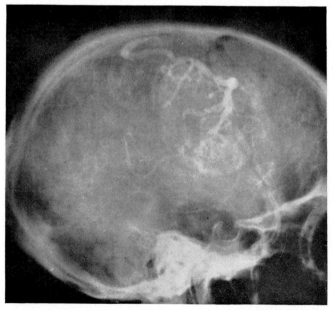

(*b*) Tumour veins are filling during the capillary phase.

FIG. 30 Glioblastoma, showing rapid circulation

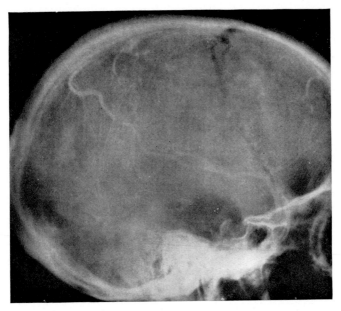

(*c*) By the venous phase the tumour is almost cleared of contrast.

Fig. 30 (*continued*)

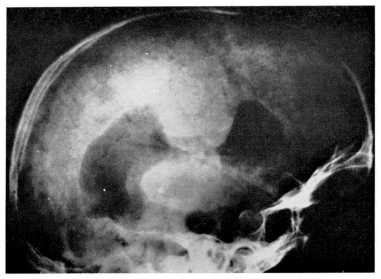

Fig. 31 Intraventricular glioma, causing a filling defect in the air
shadow of the lateral ventricle.

usually made until the tumour is large. If the tumour is near the central sulcus, in the posterior frontal or the parietal region, an extensive resection will likely cause hemiplegia if this has not already developed. When a tumour in this situation is causing raised pressure without severe hemiplegia a **limited "intracapsular" removal** is sometimes attempted. By keeping within the tumour substance the surgeon hopes to remove the centre of the tumour and reduce its bulk without endangering the surrounding and still functioning brain. But such a technique cannot be relied on to preserve function, because embarrassing bleeding may develop during the operation which can be controlled only by removing more tumour than was intended, and the operation then becomes a much more extensive one than was originally planned. The coagulation of a large vessel in the neighbourhood can be enough to precipitate hemiplegia or dysphasia.

When a glioma has already caused profound hemiplegia or dysphasia there is little hope of restoring function by operation unless there is a large cyst to be drained. Few people wish to see the lives of such seriously disabled patients prolonged by the simple relief of pressure; but before accepting such a case as hopeless it is essential to confirm the diagnosis, for should the tumour prove to be a meningioma the outlook is quite different.

A **burr hope biopsy** will usually provide enough tissue for a firm diagnosis, and also enables a cyst to be drained, whilst avoiding a major operation and external decompression. Clinical or radiological localisation must be reasonably precise if this method is to be successful. When the blunt brain cannula is advanced into a tumour a change of consistency can often be felt, and suction with a well-fitting 5 c.c. syringe will usually leave a small plug of tissue in the end of the needle. By smear or frozen section it should be possible to recognise a malignant tumour; the distinction between a metastasis and glioblastoma may not always be possible, nor is it very important at this stage. Very necrotic tissue, almost like pus, may be aspirated from a metastasis, less often from a glioblastoma; such material is often too degenerate for any cells to be recognised. Clear yellow fluid indicates a gliomatous cyst, even though no tissue can be aspirated from the wall. Sometimes biopsy is unsuccessful, either because the tumour is missed by the needle or because a firm tumour is encountered from which no material can be aspirated; this may be a meningioma and in these circumstances there is no option but to turn a bone flap and confirm the diagnosis directly. Biopsy through a burr hole may provoke bleeding in a vascular tumour and the patient's condition deteriorate rapidly afterwards. This danger is inherent in the method, which must therefore be employed only in circumstances that make it proper to accept such a risk. Because of this it is essential to have a pathologist available to give an immediate report, so that if the patient deteriorates a few hours later the surgeon is in a position to decide what action to take.

PROGNOSIS OF CEREBRAL GLIOMAS

In cerebral gliomas of the astrocytoma series the outlook depends on grade, site and age. In one series covering all sites in the brain 66% of grade I were alive at 3 years compared with less than 4% of grade IV (glioblastoma); there was little difference between grades II and III (15%). Most of the grade I tumours were the cystic cerebellar tumours of childhood; such benign tumours rarely occur in the cerebral hemispheres.

For gliomas of the cerebral hemisphere the median survival is 4–6 months; even with combined chemotherapy and radiotherapy this period averages 7 months, compared with 4 months for surgery alone.

However, every surgeon has a few patients who survive 5 years or more, and some with diffuse astrocytomas whose total history spans ten or twenty years before treatment. The duration of survival after operation may give a false notion of the natural history of a tumour, because surgery is somewhat arbitrarily timed in the course of the disease. Those tumours which will have a long survival cannot yet be recognised in advance, nor does their favourable course reflect particularly effective treatment—they are as likely to have had a burr hole biopsy and radiation as an extensive resection. Indeed of 13 patients in whom frontal lobectomies were believed to have totally extirpated a glioma, 11 were dead with recurrence within 3 years. Ependymomas behave like relatively favourable astrocytomas, oligodendrogliomas in much the same way.

Cerebellar astrocytoma and ependymoma

These are tumours of childhood. The astrocytoma is usually a well-differentiated fibrillary tumour, forming a cyst with a mural nodule; the rest of the cyst wall is made up of condensed non-tumorous tissue. Probably most originate near the midline, but spread into the hemisphere. A few astrocytomas and most ependymomas grow into the cavity of the fourth ventricle; they are mainly solid and may undergo anaplasia. Adults occasionally develop cerebellar astrocytomas, which then have the unfavourable characteristics of cerebral growths.

These children, commonly aged 6–12 years, present with signs of internal hydrocephalus—morning headache and vomiting. It is often possible to elicit an account of long-standing unsteadiness of gait, occasional vomiting without headache, and a head tilt. Chronic papilloedema, a biggish head, nystagmus and limb ataxia have usually developed by the time the surgeon sees the patient. Ventriculography confirms the diagnosis (fig. 32).

Cystic *astrocytoma* calls for removal of the mural nodule only, the rest of the wall of the cyst being non-tumorous. More solid tumours may have to be incompletely removed because of invasion of the floor of the fourth ventricle, although the outlook may still be good without radiation. However, recurrences after 30 years have been recorded,

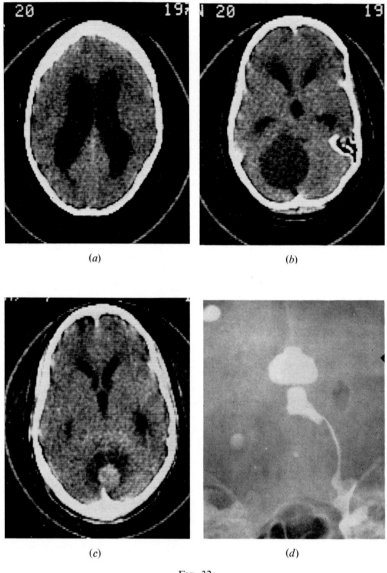

(a) (b)

(c) (d)

FIG. 32

(a) Hydrocephalus due to cystic cerebellar tumour which is seen in
(b) as low density mass.
(c) Cystic cerebellar tumour with solid mural nodule (showing as high
density zone).
(d) Myodil ventriculogram shows lateral displacement of the fourth
ventricle which is narrowed to a slit by tumour; dilated third
ventricle lies in the midline above the fourth (AP view).

sometimes with the histological appearance of the tumour indistinguishable from that removed years previously.

Ependymoma is rather less benign, because involvement of the floor of the fourth ventricle often limits tumour removal. It is relatively radiosensitive, however, and long survivals are possible if radiation is given to the site of any remnants of tumour; recurrences after many years can still occur, however.

Astrocytoma in other sites

In the *third ventricle* astrocytoma takes the form of a piloid growth in childhood. This dense white mass remains well-demarcated above, but below invades the hypothalamus producing endocrine disturbance—obesity, diabetes insipidus, and either infantilism or sexual precocity. The optic chiasma may be involved with subsequent visual failure, and eventually hydrocephalus supervenes from blockage of the foramen of Monro. Although this tumour remains histologically benign it is inaccessible because it involves vital structures; pressure may be temporarily relieved by ventriculocisternostomy but death usually follows within a year.

In the *basal ganglia* in adults local astrocytoma has the same tendency to anaplasia as in the hemisphere. Dense hemiplegia from involvement of the internal capsule may be associated with hydrocephalus from blockage of the foramen of Monro. Palliation may be achieved by X-ray treatment and short-circuit or shunt (p. 321).

In the *brain stem* an astrocytoma usually grows diffusely, expanding the pons, which retains its shape. This condition has been known in the past as "diffuse hypertrophy of the pons". Although most common in children aged 3–8 years, and fibrillary in type, it also occurs in adults and may undergo malignant change. Multiple cranial nerve palsies predominate over pyramidal signs, and evidence of raised pressure may never develop. In children personality and behavioural changes may be early signs. Biopsy is not feasible in this situation, and it is important to obtain diagnostic films of the aqueduct; myodil ventriculography or air encephalography are the most satisfactory methods, and as raised pressure is unusual the latter is quite safe. No treatment is possible and most patients die within a year.

In the *optic nerve* astrocytoma is also piloid and occurs in children, who often show stigmata of neurofibromatosis. It presents as an orbital tumour with proptosis and visual loss (p. 169).

FURTHER READING

Bucy, P. C. and Thieman, P. W. (1968). Astrocytoma of the cerebellum. *Archives of Neurology*, **19**, 14–19.
Elvidge, A. R. (1968). Survival in the astrocytoma series. *Journal of Neurosurgery*, **28**, 399–404

Fokes, E. C. and Earle, K. M. (1969). Ependymomas: clinical and pathological aspects. *Journal of Neurosurgery*, **30**, 585–594.

Gol, A. and McKissock, W. (1959). The cerebellar astrocytomas *Journal of Neurosurgery*, **16**, 287–295.

Jelsma, R. and Bucy, P. C. (1969). Glioblastoma multiforme: its treatment and some factors effecting survival. *Archives of Neurology*, **21**, 161–171.

Kricheef, I., Becker, M., Schneck, S. A. and Taveras, J. M. (1964). Intracranial ependymomas: factors influencing prognosis. *Journal of Neurosurgery*, **21**, 7–14.

Sarkari, N. B. S. and Bickerstaff, E. R. (1969). Relapsed and remissions in brain stem tumours. *British Medical Journal*, **2**, 21–23.

Weir, B. and Elvidge, A. R. (1968). Oligodendrogliomas. An analysis of 63 cases. *Journal of Neurosurgery*, **29**, 500–505.

Medulloblastoma

Tumours of the neurone series are much less common than gliomas. Tumours containing identifiable ganglion cells are extremely rare because medulloblastoma is the only frequently encountered tumour in this group.

PATHOLOGY

This highly malignant tumour forms a soft purplish mass which grows in the vermis of the cerebellum, invading the cavity of the fourth ventricle from the roof and obstructing the flow of CSF. It may spread up the cavity of the aqueduct to the third ventricle, and *seeding* may also occur in the subarachnoid space. This takes the form of grey sheets, tough with connective tissue, in the spinal arachnoid and over the convexity of the cerebral hemisphere. Distant *metastases* occasionally occur, when growth has breached the dura after operation; bones, lymph nodes and connective tissue of the trunk have been involved in reported cases. Microscopically the closely packed uniform round cells with frequent mitoses and occasional rosettes resemble no normal adult cells.

CLINICAL

This tumour of childhood is twice as frequent in boys as girls and is commonest between the ages of 6 and 10 years.

The clinical syndrome is remarkably similar from case to case. Morning vomiting, sometimes accompanied by headache, is followed after a few weeks by staggering gait. Lateralised cerebellar signs and nystagmus are unusual, but trunkal ataxia may be so severe that the child cannot sit up in bed and is quite unable to stand. Neck stiffness is common. Distant CNS signs suggest spread, directly or by seeding, to other parts of the nervous system.

This tumour does occasionally occur in young adults, affecting the cerebellar hemisphere. It behaves like a local cerebral astrocytoma without a tendency to seeding and with a better prognosis than the vermis tumour in children.

TREATMENT

Medulloblastoma is a consistently malignant tumour and 10–20% of children die within a month of operation; the average survival without radiation is about 6 months. As much tumour as possible is removed at operation as is compatible with avoiding serious post-operative deficit. Exploration is also essential to confirm the diagnosis because clinically and radiologically this tumour may be indistinguishable from astrocytomza and ependymoma. Radiation is the sheet anchor of treatment, and should be given as soon as the diagnosis is confirmed. Because of the tendency of this tumour to spread through the CSF pathways the whole neuraxis is treated, making a spade-like field of brain and spinal cord; for the same reason a CSF shunt should be avoided if possible. Of those who live long enough to have this radical radiation 25–40% are alive 5 years later. It is hoped that parallel and continuous chemotherapy for 2 years may improve this survival rate.

FURTHER READING

Smith, R. A., Lampe, I. and Kahn, E. (1961). The prognosis of medulloblastoma in children. *J. Neurosurg.*, **18**, 91–97.

Meningioma

The surgeon's interest in meningiomas springs from the prospect of total removal and cure in a number of cases. This accounts for a greater concern than may seem to be deserved by a tumour which makes up only a fifth of the intracranial growths seen.

PATHOLOGY

Causative factors

Preceding *trauma* is associated with several of these tumours, expecially those arising from the meninges of the vault. A relationship between trauma and neoplasia is always difficult to confirm, but cases are recorded of blows on the head followed years later by a meningioma the stalk of which lies exactly underneath the scalp scar. The association seems more frequent than chance would explain, and no such coincidence has been noticed with other and more common brain tumours.

An aggravating, rather than precipitating, factor is *pregnancy*. Patients with slowly growing and inaccessible tumours have suffered worsening of neurological signs in successive pregnancies, and sometimes also at the menses, with complete remission between these episodes.

Gross appearance

Regardless of histology meningiomas conform to two growth patterns. *Global* tumours are approximately spherical except where local rigid anatomy distorts this outline; they often arise from a small area of dura although more extensive secondary dural attachment may develop. *En plaque* growth implies a flat pancake of tumour, usually under an area of thickened and involved bone; this type is mainly confined to the pterion and bregma and tends to invade pia-arachnoid and blend intimately with the brain. Both types of tumour are firm, pink masses with a lobulated or finely nodular surface on which supplying vessels ramify. Most tumours are clearly demarcated from the brain, but limited invasion may occur without other evidence of malignancy or any great tendency to recur, provided a complete removal is affected. Some of the firmer tumours are gritty with flecks of calcification, a few are rock hard and may contain formed bone. Cysts are highly unusual, but when they occur are usually at one pole of the tumour between it and the brain. Multiple meningiomas, apparently unrelated, occur in 5–15% of patients with meningiomas examined at autopsy.

Bone changes

The great majority of meningiomas are related to the skull, of which the dura is the inner periosteum. Bone reacts to neighbouring tumour growth in different ways. Most often a conical overgrowth of bone butts into the base of the tumour; this *endostosis* is a non-specific reaction to periosteal stripping and increased vascularity and may contain no tumour. Bone reaction involving the outer table gives rise to a palpable lump on the skull—an *exostosis*. Even without obvious erosion tumour may invade the Haversian canals of the thickened, vascular bone and recurrence can stem from this source. Bone changes indicate both the site and the nature of the tumour in over a third of meningiomas, and it is of great importance to look specifically on plain films of the skull in the sites where meningiomas are known to occur; increased diploic venous channels and meningeal arterial grooves add supportive evidence; only a few meningiomas undergo sufficiently dense calcification to cast a shadow on X-ray (figs. 16b, 17b, 18).

Spread

Tumour may erode either hyperostotic or otherwise normal bone to form a mushroom of tumour under the scalp, but the galea prevents its further outward spread. Once bone is breached meningioma may spread to temporal muscle or invade the surrounding cavities of the orbit, air sinuses or the middle ear. Rarely an undifferentiated meningioma metastasises to viscera, but this is a pathological oddity not usually considered in managing patients with these essentially benign tumours.

Microscopic appearance

Arachnoid villi buried in dura give rise to these largely fibrous tumours, but whether they are essentially endothelial or mesothelial is an open question. Cushing's term "meningioma" was purposely chosen to avoid implicating any one theory of origin.

Many subgroups have been labelled by various authorities, but most show a preponderance either of whorls of spindle cells around central hyaline material which eventually calcifies, forming psammoma bodies; or of interlacing bundles of elongated fibroblasts with narrow nuclei. Some are angioblastic and may be indistinguishable histologically from a cerebellar hæmangioblastoma.

A sarcomatous variety occurs, particularly in children; it favours the posterior third of the parasagittal region in both children and adults.

Histological appearance has little to do with biological behaviour except for the sarcomatous type which is apt both to infiltrate and to recur. Tumours growing *en plaque* tend to invade pia-arachnoid, yet histologically they conform to no single pattern. The recurrence of a fifth of meningiomas, even after apparently adequate surgical removal, appears to result from a failure to perform a sufficiently radical operation rather than to a more malignant type of tumour.

CLINICAL

The site of the tumour determines not only the clinical features but also the surgical accessibility. Over 90% are supratentorial and over two-thirds of these are in the anterior half of the skull (fig. 32). Meningiomas are most common in adults, especially in middle-aged women, but occasionally occur in children. The frequency of tumours in the more commonly affected sites is approximately:

Parasagittal 25%

Convexity 20%

Anterior basal 40% — sphenoidal wing 20%, olfactory groove 10%, suprasellar 10%

Parasagittal

These arise in relation to the sagittal (superior longitudinal) sinus, most often in its *middle third* where they frequently cause focal epilepsy and later paralysis, both of which affect mainly the foot. This may lead to detection whilst the tumour is still quite small. *Anterior third* meningiomas tend to be bilateral and to cause only mental symptoms, so that the presence of a tumour is sometimes not suspected until it is so large that the patient is blind from papillœdema. Tumours arising primarily *from the falx* also favour the anterior third and tend to be bilateral, producing a similar syndrome. *At the bregma* a parasagittal meningioma often gives rise to marked exostosis, and a lump may have

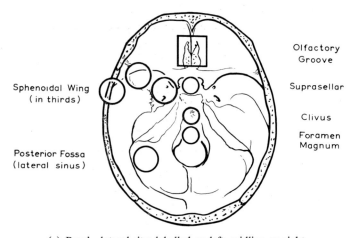

Olfactory Groove

Suprasellar

Clivus

Foramen Magnum

Sphenoidal Wing (in thirds)

Posterior Fossa (lateral sinus)

(*a*) Basal—lateral sites labelled on left, midline on right.

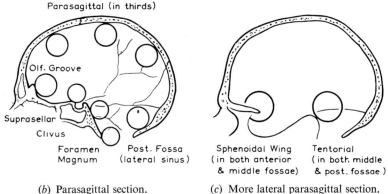

Parasagittal (in thirds)

Olf. Groove

Suprasellar

Clivus

Foramen Magnum

Post. Fossa (lateral sinus)

Sphenoidal Wing (in both anterior & middle fossae)

Tentorial (in both middle & post. fossae)

(*b*) Parasagittal section.   (*c*) More lateral parasagittal section.

FIG. 33 Meningioma—sites of predilection (excluding convexity tumours)

been noticed on the head since childhood. The intradural component of this hyperostotic tumour is usually *en plaque*, frequently bilateral and sometimes consists of only a carpet of tumour down both sides of the falx; no marked indentation of the brain occurs and there may be neither neurological disorder nor any evidence of raised ICP, unless this develops due to sinus obstruction by tumour. The few parasagittal meningiomas which develop in the *posterior third* of the sinus tend to grow large before papilloedema or hemianopia leads to their being detected; they tend to be sarcomatous.

Convexity

These are initially free of any sinus attachment, and more than 70% are frontal, anterior to the central sulcus; more than half arise from the region of the coronal suture. Like parasagittal tumours they may, if growing well in front of the central sulcus, remain silent until they become large. Further back they soon cause facio-brachial hemiplegia and focal epilepsy.

Anterior basal

Half of these arise from the **sphenoidal wing** and grow into both the anterior and middle fossæ of the skull (figs. 32, 33). At the *inner* end of the wing the cavernous sinus is involved with the nerves (3, 4, 5, 6) in its wall, as well as the optic nerve and carotid artery; proptosis often develops. At the *outer* end meningioma may take the form of a *global* tumour growing into the Sylvian fissure, causing temporal epilepsy, facial weakness and, on the left, dysphasia; or it may grow *en plaque* with little encroachment on the brain but forming a hyperostosis which causes proptosis and an obvious swelling in the temporal region.

Olfactory groove meningiomas usually grow bilaterally, the falx indenting the mass from above. With an anteriorly placed tumour there are usually no complaints until raised pressure asserts itself. Anosmia, the only localising sign, is rarely complained of, and will be detected only if the sense of smell is tested. More posteriorly placed tumours encroach on the optic nerve if unilateral, and this may result in a Foster Kennedy syndrome (atrophy in one fundus, papillœdema in the other). Mental symptoms are seldom striking until a late stage and epilepsy is not very common.

Suprasellar meningiomas arise from the tuberculum sellæ and compress the optic chiasm, leading to early diagnosis whilst the tumour is still quite small. Bitemporal hemianopia with optic atrophy may simulate a

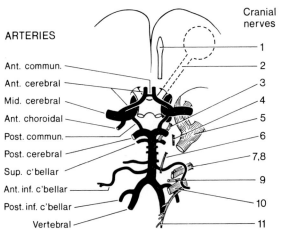

FIG. 34 Anatomy of base of skull, showing structures which may be involved by basal meningiomas

pituitary tumour, but endocrine symptoms are less constant and the sella is not ballooned, though minor bone changes can usually be detected.

Posterior fossa

Midline growths arise from the *basilar groove*, high ones on the clivus, low ones at the foramen magnum. Predictably these tend to give rise at an early stage to multiple cranial nerve palsies and long tract signs. Laterally, the commonest site is the *cerebello-pontine angle*, the tumour arising from the back of the petrous in relation to the sigmoid sinus. **Tentorial** meningiomas appear in most series as posterior fossa tumours, but at least half grow upwards as well as downwards. The confusing symptomatology of such a double tumour leads as a rule to late detection; raised pressure, cranial nerve palsies and ataxia suggest a posterior fossa tumour, but hemianopia and epilepsy may also develop.

Tumour remote from dura

Intraventricular meningiomas grow into the lateral ventricle, usually on the left side. Raised pressure may be accompanied by hemianopia and slight hemiplegia, but the angiogram usually shows no lateral shift; enlargement of the anterior choroidal artery which ends in tumour vessels may be seen.

Deep Sylvian tumours are presumed to arise from arachnoid condensations deep in the fissure, perhaps from the carotid sheath.

DIAGNOSIS

Plain X-rays are often of value in detecting meningiomas. Sphenoidal wing growths constantly produce changes, either erosion or dense hyperostosis, and a number of vault tumours do also. Large meningeal arteries running to a convexity tumour may make an obvious channel in the bone (figs. 16b, 17b, 18).

EMI scanning will show the tumour, encroachment into or displacement of the ventricles, and the degree of surrounding œdema.

Angiography can be most informative in supratentorial meningiomas, which show a tumour circulation more often than do glioblastomas; not only may the nature of the tumour be recognised but its vascularity can be assessed and the surgical approach planned. A ring of feeding vessels or of veins may outline the tumour; vessels entering the tumour are regular and often take on a sunray pattern. A blush in the capillary phase may give a striking picture of the entire tumour which persists after all the normal veins have emptied (fig. 35). Much of the blood supply of these tumours is derived from the external carotid circulation which is normally slower than the internal carotid circulation; the enlarged middle meningeal artery may be filled in the first film and be clearly seen to supply the tumour.

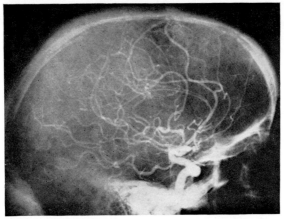

(a) Tumour vessels not yet filled but arteries surrounding the tumour suggest where it may lie.

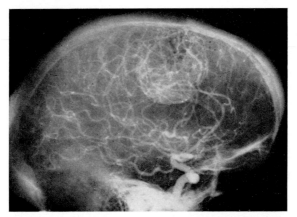

(b) Late arterial phase shows a dense network of tumour vessels.

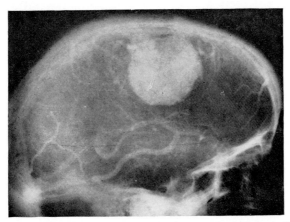

(c) Venous phase—contrast remains in the tumour which is outlined by a "blush."

Fig. 35 Meningioma, showing slow circulation

Meningiomas are generally thought of as benign because most are non-invasive and amitotic. Yet they may occur in situations, such as the cavernous sinus and the clivus, where total extirpation is impossible, and even accessible tumours sometimes present formidable technical problems by reason of their rich vascular attachments.

Convexity and parasagittal

The control of blood loss is the main pre-occupation during the removal of these tumours. Enlarged external carotid branches can give an unduly vascular scalp flap and hyperostotic bone bleeds freely when saw cuts are made. The dura over the tumour may pour blood when separated from bone, and there is still the inevitable bleeding from vessels in and around the tumour during removal. Because of this the removal may have to be done in two stages. The first procedure is limited to reflecting the bone flap and controlling hæmorrhage in the superficial layers. The second operation should ideally be performed within a week or so, before tissue planes have become firmly stuck. Hypothermia allows prolonged periods of controlled hypotension without risk to the brain, and this has made the surgery of these tumours less hazardous and staging is now seldom required.

Unless the growth has eroded completely through the skull the bone flap can be turned down off the underlying tumour; but if there is an endostosis or exostosis with obvious tumour invasion this part of the bone must be nibbled away before closure. When the area involved is large the whole bone flap may be removed and boiled before replacement, or the bone flap may be discarded and the defect made good by cranioplasty at a later date (p. 273).

There is no need to dissect dura off the base of the tumour, because this area of dura must be excised, and is best removed in one piece with the tumour. The dural incision encircles the base of the tumour which will then extrude whilst the remaining dura protects surrounding brain. If falx is involved a generous segment should be resected and the opposite side inspected.

There is no absolute need for the dural defect to be repaired, but a dural substitute is desirable to prevent the underlying brain becoming adherent to scalp or bone, which would make dissection tedious at any subsequent operation and may also predispose to epilepsy. Fascia lata from the thigh is the ideal material for permanent repair, and can be stitched in place. Temporary cover, until the second stage of tumour removal, or the replacement of a bone flap, is best given by a synthetic dural substitute; this produces no tissue reaction and is laid in place without suturing to the dural edge. There seems no advantage in using specially preserved dura removed from cadavers.

Involvement of the sagittal sinus presents a problem because division of the *patent* sinus in its posterior two-thirds is liable to be followed by congestion and hæmorrhagic infarction in part of the hemisphere. Care must be taken to shave tumour off the sinus as closely as possible if it is patent; but, if it is already blocked by tumour, it can safely be excised because collateral drainage channels will already have opened up. Sinus patency may be determined pre-operatively by sinograms (late phase of carotid arteriograms), or at operation by needling or catheterising the sinus; or radioactive material can be injected anteriorly and the emission counted further back. If a patent sinus is inadvertently opened it must be closed with stitches tied over a piece of muscle.

Anterior basal tumours

To prevent undue retraction in the confined spaces in which these tumours grow no attempt should be made to deliver them whole. The interior of the tumour is excavated, using suction if soft or the diathermy cutting loop if hard, and the remaining capsule then dissected free of surrounding structures. Radical excision of dura is not always feasible, but the area of tumour origin is burnt black in the hope of destroying all tumour remnants in it. If dura is sacrificed from the floor of the anterior fossa over the ethmoidal sinuses, a fascial patch from the thigh must be substituted to prevent CSF rhinorrhœa and the risk of meningitis.

Olfactory groove tumours should be totally removed although staging may be needed; the greatest hazard is damage to the anterior cerebral arteries which are closely applied to the posterior pole of the tumour and must be preserved at all costs.

Suprasellar tumours can be completely removed if small (<3 cm. diameter); larger tumours carry a risk of hypothalamic damage, and incomplete removal may be wise.

Inner sphenoidal wing tumours must often be incompletely removed because of their close relation to the carotid artery and cavernous sinus. *Global pterional* growths demand total removal, but the *en plaque* type are best left alone, once an angiogram has confirmed that there is no large intradural component. These are indolent tumours which may not shorten life, and bone involvement is so widespread and diffuse that complete extirpation is impossible, whilst partial removal seldom improves the proptosis or local swelling.

PROGNOSIS

This is good if the tumour is totally removed, though epilepsy often persists. However, a fifth of tumours regarded by surgeons as having been completely resected have been found to recur, usually within 5 years. Recurrence is probably more often due to inadequate removal rather than to a malignant tumour type, except for the small number of sarcomatous growths. The commonest sources of recurrence are an invaded venous sinus and transeptal spread (across tentorium or falx); parasagittal tumours are therefore the most likely to recur. Less often invaded bone is the site of recurrence, or dura in the region of the tumour base where a subdural carpet of tumour cells may spread beyond the naked eye limits of invasion. Occasionally a small nodule becomes detached and is overlooked, or there may be multiple tumours from the start.

Recurrence may re-enact the clinical evolution of the primary tumour but without any increase in intracranial pressure, the decompression from the previous operation remaining indrawn. Angiography is the most reliable way of demonstrating recurrence. "False recurrence" occurs from time to time, especially in ageing patients who have had convexity tumours removed years before; the re-appearance of hemiplegia is probably due to vascular insufficiency as arterial disease progresses and hits hardest an area already short of vessels.

The outlook for tumours not completely removed, because of their critical situation, may be quite good. Very long survivals are common, and little or no progress in the size of the tumour may be apparent over 10 years or more. Some meningiomas never declare themselves in life, and a third of one series of 300 intracranial tumours found incidently at post-mortem were meningiomas, mostly parasagittal. This must be remembered when assessing claims for radiotherapy restricting the growth of these tumours; an incompletely removed sarcomatous growth is certainly worth treating by radiation,

FURTHER READING

Crompton, R and Gautier-Smith, P. C. (1970). The prediction of recurrence in meningiomas. *Journal of Neurology, Neurosurgery and Psychiatry*, **33**, 80–87.

Gold, L. H. A., Kieffer, S. A. and Peterson, H. A. (1969). Intracranial meningiomas: a retrospective analysis of the diagnostic value of plain skull films. *Neurology* (Minneapolis), **19**, 873–878.

Logue, V (1975). Parasagittal meningiomas. In: *Advances in Technical Standards in Neurosurgery*. Eds Krayenbuhl et al. Springer Wien, New York.

Simpson, D (1957). The recurrence of intracranial meningiomas after surgical treatment. *Journal of Neurology Neurosurgery and Psychiatry*, **20**, 22–39.

Symposium (1975). Meningiomas—diagnostic and therapeutic problems. In: *Advances in Neurosurgery* (Vol. 2). Eds Keng et al. Springer, Berlin, New York.

Tytus, J. S., Laserjohn, J. T. and Reifel, E. (1967). Problem of malignancy in meningiomas. *Journal of Neurosurgery,* **27**, 551–557.

Pituitary region tumours

PATHOLOGY

Chromophobe adenoma

More than three-quarters of pituitary tumours are non-secreting adenomas of this type. Although histologically they conform to a pattern (polygonal cells arranged in alveoli or in rows in relation to intervascular connective tissue) their growth tendency varies widely. Most begin within the pituitary fossa and remain confined to it, ballooning up the diaphragma and enlarging the bony outlines of the sella. Others escape from the sella and some spread far, perhaps because the anatomy of the individual allows this, but more likely because some tumours have a disposition to spread. Extrasellar extension alters the symptomatology, poses problems in diagnosis and management and adds appreciably to the operative mortality. About 40% of chromophobe adenomas are cystic, usually containing <10 ml. of clear yellow fluid. Occasionally a tumour outstrips its blood supply and undergoes necrosis or hæmorrhagic infarction; this may be manifested clinically as pituitary apoplexy (p. 146).

Eosinophil adenoma

These tumours contain secreting cells, full of granules, and owe their clinical importance more to excessive growth hormone production than to bulk. Only occasionally do they grow large enough to compress the chiasm although the pituitary fossa is usually enlarged.

Craniopharyngioma (Rathké pouch tumour, suprasellar cyst)

These arise from a remnant of the buccal ectoderm of the pharyngeal pouch which forms the pars anterior of the pituitary. About 90% are cystic, at least in part, lined with squamous epithelium and containing dark brown fluid like engine oil, which is full of cholesterol crystals that shimmer in the light. Small intrasellar tumours do occur, but 50% are wholly suprasellar, causing no enlargement of the fossa, and growing mainly upwards towards the hypothalamus and third ventricle where they may cause hydrocephalus from obstruction of the foramen of Monro. Dumb-bell tumours, part in and part above the sella also occur. They are thin-walled and insinuate themselves into their surroundings, making total surgical removal difficult.

CLINICAL

Endocrine features

Some degree of pituitary insufficiency is common with all types of tumour of the pituitary gland itself. But it may be produced by other tumours adjacent to the sella which affect the pituitary stalk or the hypothalamus—through which the activities of the pituitary gland are controlled. It is an important feature to recognise because an endocrine crisis can readily be precipitated by various manœuvres in hospital if precautions are not taken. Endocrine excess is less common, and is less specific in relation to cell type than was previously thought; acromegaly or Cushing's syndrome may be produced by a tumour which to the pathologist is predominantly chromophobe.

The normal pituitary secretes trophic hormones and the clinical and biochemical aspects of pituitary deficiency mostly derive from the secondary deficiences in the target organs. The trophic hormones of most clinical significance are:

1. **Corticotrophin** (ACTH) stimulates the adrenal cortex to produce androgens, and glucocorticoids (cortisol); the latter acts as a feedback mechanism to reduce ACTH secretion by the pituitary. Aldosterone production is independent of pituitary control. Clinical features of Addison's disease do not occur with hypopituitarism, but stress (e.g. air encephalogram, operation or infection) may precipitate acute cortisol insufficiency—hypotension, hyponatræmia and coma; these can be prevented by prior injection of 100 mg. hydrocortisone.

Several tests are available for the integrity of the pituitary-adrenal axis:

1. *Urinary steroid excretion levels* (mg/24 hours)

	Male	Female
(a) Androgen products		
17-ketosteroids	10–20	5–15
(b) Glucocorticoid products		
17-ketogenic steroids	5–22	4–18
17-hydroxycorticosteroids . . .	3–12	1–9

2. *Plasma cortisol level*

Diurnal range = 7–25 μg/100 ml.: highest about 9 a.m., decreasing thereafter.

3. *Urinary cortisol (free)*

Normal level 100–150 μg/24 hrs.—raised in conditions of hyper-function.

4. *Corticotrophin stimulation* (tests adrenal reserve by response to ACTH)

Blood sample for cortisol; give 0·25 mg. Synacthen IM; cortisol level estimated at 30 minutes and should be both >7 μg greater than first sample, and >18 μg/100 ml.

5. *ACTH stimulation* (tests pituitary reserve by response to reduced plasma cortisol).

Insulin-induced hypoglycaemia (to < 40 mg./100 ml. blood sugar) is probably the simplest stimulus; this will usually require only 0·1 unit/Kg of insulin for patients who are hypopituitary, but up to 3 units/Kg body weight may be needed for acromegalics. Normally the cortisol should rise above 20 μg/100 ml., and the growth hormone above 20 μg/L.

2. **Gonadotrophins** (FSH and LH) are responsible for gonadal maturation at puberty and in the female for subsequent cyclical changes. Deficiency before puberty results in failure to develop secondary sex

characteristics: adult men have poor beard growth, women amenor-
rhoea, and both sexes loss of libido and deficient pubic and axillary
hair. Oestrogen and androgen production is low, with reduced urinary
17-keto-steroids. Plasma levels can be measured and the response to
gonadotrophin releasing hormone (Gn RH).

3. **Thyrotrophin** (TSH) maintains thyroxine production: secondary
myxoedema is often associated with normal blood cholesterol but
serum protein-bound iodine (PBI) is low ($<$4–8 μg/100 ml.) as is I^{131}
uptake ($<$20–55% in 24 hours). The latter is restored by 10 units TSH
for 3 days by IM injection, if low levels is due to hypopituitarism. Blood
levels of TSH are measurable and the response to TRH (200 μg)
(usually combined with Gn RH test); normal rise is to $>$2 μU/ml.
Plasma levels of thyroxine T_4, (5–12 μg/100 ml.) and Triodothyronine
T_3 (0·7–1·7 ng/ml.) are commonly measured now rather than PBI; also
the non-protein bound hormone (Free Thyroxine Index).

4. **Somatotrophin** (growth hormone) is produced by the eosinophil
cells. Deficiency before puberty combines with lack of gonadotrophin
to produce dwarfism and infantilism. Excess causes giantism before the
epiphyses are fused, and acromegaly after. Blood level is normally
$<$10 μg/L, but varies during the day and is put up by stress. Failure of
oral glucose to suppress level $<$5 μg/L is usual in acomegaly.

5. **Melanocyte Stimulating Hormone** (MSH)
Allied to ACTH, causes pigmentation in Addison's Disease and
Nelson's Syndrome.

6. **Prolactin**
Some tumours secrete this, but it is also released in hypothalamic
suppression.

Chromophobe adenoma

It is **chiasmal compression** which usually brings the patient to the
surgeon. Vision has commonly been failing for a year or more and a
characteristic bitemporal hemianopia may already have developed; it
is usually first evident in the upper quadrant of one side and progresses
variously (fig. 8): one eye may lose sight altogether before the other is
affected at all. In 5% the hemianopia is homonymous, implying compression of the optic tract rather than the chiasm; this tends to occur
when the chiasm is prefixed, i.e. the optic nerves are unusually short.
Early field defects are best detected by testing in detail on a screen
(fig. 6). Primary optic atrophy indicates long-standing compression
which may fail to recover after operative decompression of the
chiasm. Patients still present unduly late with pituitary tumours
because further investigations are not pursued for visual failure for
which no refractive error or ocular cause can be found. In most cases a
lateral skull X-ray would suggest the diagnosis.

"Hypopituitarism" is normally the first symptom, and may precede
visual symptoms by many years. Because its onset is so insidious, and

its separate components readily produced by many other conditions, a pituitary tumour is rarely suspected in the early stages before chiasmal compression develops. Gonadotrophins usually fail first in adults, and growth hormone in children; ACTH and TSH secretion are affected only later, and the deficiency is rarely as complete as in Simmond's syndrome.

It is important to recognise **extrasellar extension** because of its implications in management. Spread may be chiefly: *upward*, blocking the foramen of Monro and producing hydrocephalus and invading the hypothalamus; or *forwards* into the frontal lobes to give mental symptoms and anosmia; or *laterally* into the cavernous sinus causing palsies of 3, 4, 6, cranial nerves; or *subtemporally*, leading to epilepsy, hemiplegia and even dysphasia.

"Pituitary apoplexy", due to sudden necrosis or hæmorrhage, begins with abrupt headache, followed by rapid visual loss or diplopia due to ocular palsies. Confusion and even coma follow, and an endocrine crisis is precipitated. Lumbar puncture may show bloody or xanthochromic CSF and, with the story, suggest subarachnoid hæmorrhage from a rapidly enlarging internal carotid aneurysm. Angiography should always be done to exclude this possibility.

Enlargement of the pituitary fossa varies enormously according to the growth characters of the particular tumour. The earliest sign is usually a double contour to the floor in the lateral view. The normal depth of the sella is 8 mm. (max 12 mm.), and width 10·6 mm. (max. 16 mm.)—both measured in AP view. Some tumours arise in the stalk and have no effect on the sella, and one view is that these are ependymomas rather than adenomas. Usually there is equal increase in both the depth and antero-posterior diameter of the fossa with thinning of the floor; the dorsum may be levered back and the posterior clinoids isolated by erosion of the dorsum below them. These changes may be mimicked to some extent by most of the conditions which may be confused clinically with pituitary adenoma, and no single radiological sign is diagnostic.

Differential diagnosis, apart from other pituitary tumours, includes arachnoiditis and the empty sellar syndrome; of the many other conditions the most common can be grouped as follows:

1. *Suprasellar* meningioma and cholesteatoma, which less often produce endocrine features. When these do develop they are usually of recent onset in contrast to the many years history typical of adenoma.

2. *Infrasellar* masses, chordoma, mucocœle of the sphenoidal sinus, and optic were choma are distinguished by radiological appearances; widespread destruction with chordoma, bulging back of the anterior wall of the sella with mucocœle.

3. *Parasellar* masses, carotid aneurysm, inner third sphenoidal wing meningioma, are distinguished by angiography.

4. *Distant* tumours causing internal hydrocephalus, the dilated third ventricle invading the sella and eroding its bony margins.

Eosinophil adenoma

Excess of growth hormone produced by these tumours leads to gigantism before the epiphyses are fused and to acromegaly in adults. The sella may be greatly enlarged but this tumour less often extends beyond it to cause chiasmal compression than do chromophabe adenomas. Severe bitemporal headache is a common complaint and is believed to be due to stretching of the diaphragm sellæ; radiotherapy may dramatically relieve it, but it may also subside suddenly when field defects appear, suggesting that the tumour may have ruptured through the roof of the sella.

Acromegaly consists in a coarsening and enlargement of the facial features and the extremities and the typical appearance is immediately obvious. Soft tissue and bony components of this change can be recognised:

Soft tissue

1. Thick coarse skin and hair.
2. Deep voice with big tongue (causing slurred speech).
3. Huge hands and feet.
4. Carpal tunnel compression giving numbness and pain in fingers.

Objective assessment of these features can be made by measuring heel pad thickness on X-ray, skin fold thickness with calipeis and hand volume by displacement.

Bony

1. Huge frontal sinus.
2. Prognathic mandible with separation of teeth.
3. Broadening and flaring of terminal finger phalanges.
4. Thoracic kyphosis secondary to osteoporosis (causing backache).

Cushing's syndrome is due to excessive production of cortisol, either due to adrenal tumour or to adrenal hyperplasia secondary to excessive production of ACTH by the pituitary. Three quarters of cases are pituitary dependent and a third of these have a pituitary tumour; the rest are presumed to have basophil hyperplasia. Obesity, skin striae, hypertension and a variety of other features occur, and 50% untreated cases are fatal in five years. Following adrenalectomy for Cushing's syndrome some patients develop marked skin pigmentation with MSH overproduction associated with a pituitary adenoma (Nelson's syndrome). In both this condition and in pituitary-dependent Cushing's syndrome ACTH levels are abnormally high (normal 10–80 pg/ml. at 9 a.m., falling to 5–30 pg/ml. at midnight). These levels usually fall in response to dexamethasone when due to hyperplasia of the pituitary, but not when due to adenoma. When Cushing's is due to primary adrenal disorder ACTH levels are very low.

Craniopharyngioma (Rathké pouch cyst)

Although congenital in origin only half of these cysts present clinically under the age of 20; some declare themselves only in old age, when mental symptoms predominate due to arteriosclerotic changes superimposed on chronic hydrocephalus. In children, in whom this is the commonest non-gliomatous tumour, pressure symptoms tend to overshadow chiasmal compression; the combination of papilloedema and bitemporal hemianopia, when it occurs, is almost diagnostic. Failure to grow quickly enough, or delayed puberty, may be the only complaint or accompany other syndromes. Both thin (Lorraine pituitary dwarfs) and fat (Frohlich's adiposo-genital syndrome) clinical types occur and many teenage page boys with unbroken voices harbour one of these tumours. Diabetes insipidus is complained of by some. But serious visual loss can also occur, sometimes complete blindness, from a combination of primary and consecutive optic atrophy. The sella is normal radiologically in 50% of cases, but 75% have suprasellar calcification, more often finely speckled than dense (fig. 15).

TREATMENT

One or more of four different disorders produced by pituitary tumours may require treatment:

1. Chiasmal compression.
2. Hydrocephalus.
3. Endocrine excess.
4. Endocrine failure.

The methods available are surgery, radiation and hormone therapy.

Chiasmal compression (mostly chromophobe adenomas)

Surgery is favoured by most surgeons if vision is failing rapidly; there is no alternative in the presence of considerable extrasellar extension or raised intracranial pressure, or when there has been a recent episode of hæmorrhage or infarction. It is helpful to know the extent and direction of extrasellar spread of tumour before planning surgery; in most cases this information is best given by air encephalography with purposeful filling of the basal cisterns and third ventricle (fig. 35).

The **frontal approach** is still probably the most frequently used, and it involves turning a right-sided flap, opening the dura and retracting the frontal lobe; the olfactory tract is followed back to the optic nerve. The right side is traditionally recommended because the non-dominant

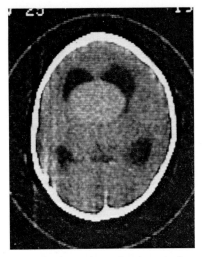

(*a*) Craniopharyngioma showing as a dense
    mass in the anterior horns of the lateral
    ventricles.

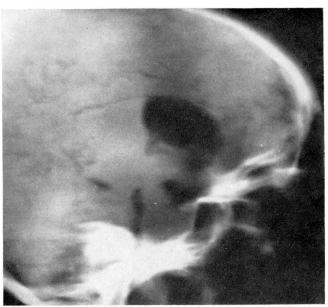

(*b*) Autotomography shows the suprasellar extension, outlined by the
interpeduncular cistern posteriorly and the chiasmatic cistern
anteriorly. Remnant of the third ventricle is seen immediately below the foramen of Monro, and is displaced upwards; tumour
has obliterated most of the ventricle (*see figs.* 25(*a*), 2, *p.* 89 *and
fig.* 26(*a*), *p.* 93).

FIG. 36 Pituitary adenoma, outlined by lumbar air encephalography

frontal lobe can be retracted without fear of producing dysphasia, and because it is somewhat easier for a right-handed surgeon to work from this side. Modern anæsthesia gives such good access with minimal retraction that these arguments are no longer compelling, and the side of the more severely affected eye, or on which there is more marked extrasellar extension, is preferred. Once the tumour is exposed, and before cutting into it, an aspirating needle is passed into it to confirm that the mass is not an aneurysm. Should the tumour prove cystic the aspiration of fluid may be enough to restore sight for a time, but it is advisable to dissect the capsule away from the optic nerves and remove such solid tumour as will come readily. Having cut a hole in the capsule a sucker is introduced into the tumour and a small spoon can be used to loosen tumour from capsule. The removal of capsule is necessarily incomplete in most instances, because the carotid arteries laterally, and the hypothalamus above and behind, must not be jeopardised by attempting to radical a resection. *Mortality* for this operation is less than 10% overall, being less for small intrasellar tumours but higher when there is marked extrasellar extension. Although replacement hormone therapy (*vide infra*) has reduced the risk of post-operative endocrine failure, fatal hypothalamic crisis from manipulations too near the third ventricle remains a hazard which only surgical skill and restraint can prevent. Hypothermia may reduce the risk of operating on these large and dangerous tumours, and can also prove useful post-operatively when hyperpyrexia is often a threat.

Improved vision results in about two-thirds of cases, a completely normal field being restored in half of these. For the rest the surgeon (and the patient) must be satisfied with preventing progressive blindness. The effect of operation on vision is often immediate, and seldom delayed more than a few weeks.

Recurrences occur in 10–20% of patients, usually within 5 years. Fortunately second and even third operations are frequently effective and carry no higher a mortality than the first. As the operation is acknowledged to be incomplete radiation is normally recommended after surgery unless the tumour is largely cystic or necrotic.

The **transphenoidal operation** was originally introduced by Cushing in order to avoid the hazards then associated with open craniotomy. With the development of the operating microscope it has now become the method of choice both for removal of the normal gland (hypophysectomy), and for intrasellar adenomas. With this method it is sometimes possible to achieve selective removal of the adenoma with preservation (or restoration) of normal pituitary function. Experienced surgeons are finding it possible to deal effectively with suprasellar extensions by the transphenoidal route, which has a lower mortality than trans-frontal surgery and a lower incidence of post-operative epilepsy. CSF rhinorrhoea rarely persists after skilful surgery, and infection is rare.

The route may be trans-ethmoidal, using a skin incision medial to the medial canthus. The ethmoid sinuses are first entered through the medial wall of the orbit—after the orbital periosteum and contents have been retracted laterally—and they lead on into the sphenoid sinus. The floor of the sella is then seen bulging into the roof of the sphenoid. The sella is opened and the pituitary removed, either *in toto* with its capsule or piecemeal. An alternative approach to the sphenoid is through the nostril by splitting the nasal septum and following the bony septum in the mid-line to the cavity of the sphenoid sinus.

Radiation, as primary treatment, naturally appeals to the patient because operation may be avoided. In special cases, when the threat

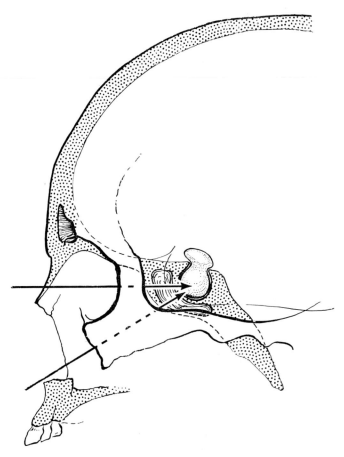

FIG. 37 Trans-sphenoidal approach to the pituitary

Either orbital (solid line) or nasal (dotted) routes to the sphenoidal sinus may be used.

to vision is slight or when the operative risks are high, the surgeon too may favour it. The question is whether it is sufficiently reliable, and safe for vision, to recommend in the first instance to most patients. Although improvement is usually obvious in three to four weeks, the beneficial effects of radiation may be delayed for months. Sight may even deteriorate temporarily, probably due to reactive swelling of the tumour. However, most tumours are radiosensitive as witnessed by improving visual fields, by reduced tumour size on repeated air encephalography and by the occasional post-radiation exploration which reveals no tumour at all. Operation is no more difficult after a course of radiation, and a trial of treatment is probably reasonable provided that the facilities allow weekly reviews of the visual fields and acuities, and there is agreement to accept surgery as soon as it is obvious that radiation is not proving effective. Some centres report almost 90% of chromophobe adenomas adequately treated by radiation without recourse to surgery. Large doses of radiation can be obtained locally with isotope implants

If vision is rapidly failing radiation is clearly unsuitable because it does not act quickly enough. Large extrasellar extensions pose problems for the therapist and force him to disperse his dose over a wider area with diminished effectiveness. Cystic and acutely necrotic tumours are probably resistant. The risk of late effects of radiation on the hypothalamus and optic chiasm cannot be ignored if radical dosage is employed, because these vulnerable areas are in the field of treatment when the target is the pituitary. The only solution is to reduce the dose to safer but less effective levels. But perhaps the strongest argument against using radiotherapy initially, without preliminary surgical exploration, is that the diagnosis is never confirmed. The differential diagnosis of chiasmal compression and of sellar enlargement is quite wide, and most of the alternatives are radioresistant, some of them very suitable for surgery (aneurysm, meningioma, mucocœle). Only exploration will confirm beyond doubt that the diagnosis is a pituitary adenoma.

Hydrocephalus (mostly craniopharyngiomas)

Surgery is essential if there is papillœdema. Whether a direct attack on the upward extension of the tumour is advisable depends on the nature of the tumour. Rathké cysts tend to be closely adherent to the anterior cerebral arteries and their vital branches to the hypothalamus; if the cyst wall is calcified and unyielding safe dissection may be impossible. In this event, even if a large cyst has been successfully aspirated, it is best to bypass the block by performing short-circuit or shunt (p. 321). As these tumours are often indolent for long periods a remission of years, even for life, may follow this comparatively simple manœuvre without any of the hazards of attempted removal. Radiation appears to restrain growth of the more active cysts.

Endocrine excess

Frequently eosinophil adenoma remains intrasellæ and transphenoidal removal is becoming the standard approach; removal of the adenoma with preservation of normal function is sometimes possible. For basophil hyperphasia hypophysectomy is required (p. 154).

Endocrine failure (all types of tumour)

Treatment may be required for acute or chronic deficiency and prophylactically to cover operation.

Acute deficiency results from sudden withdrawal of pituitary function due to *hæmorrhagic necrosis* in a pituitary tumour, to *hypophysectomy* or to *infarction* from obstetric hæmorrhage and subsequent prolonged hypotension. When there is already chronic deficiency an acute crisis may be precipitated in a number of ways, and these constitute the majority of cases of hypopituitary coma and collapse. Infection or subjection to surgical or radiological procedures cause stress to which the adrenal would normally react by producing cortisone in response to pituitary stimulus, and the failure to do so results in *hypotensive* collapse: vomiting or diarrhœa leads to salt depletion which the hypopituitary patient less readily restores and a sequence of *metabolic imbalance* follows: cold weather may precipitate *hypothermic* coma if secondary hypothyroidism is a prominent feature of the deficiency state, whilst starvation and vomiting can precipitate *hypoglycæmia*.

Prophylactic cortisone should always be given before a hypopituitary patient undergoes surgery or a major neuroradiological procedure. What factor constitutes the stress is unknown; general anæsthesia is one, aggravated by pre-operative starvation and by premedication with opiates or barbiturates, to which these patients are unduly sensitive; but collapse can also follow air encephalography or angiography under local anæsthesia. Nor is the severity of the pituitary deficiency, as indicated by laboratory tests, a reliable guide to the likelihood of a crisis; and it is wise to give 100 mg. hydrocortisone succinate intramuscularly an hour before any procedure to a patient who has clinical evidence of deficiency. Cortisone is rapidly metabolised; even if 50 mg. are given twice daily for a few days to cover stressful procedures there is no risk of permanent adrenal suppression, if these glands should still be active, nor any danger of delayed wound healing.

Once collapse or coma has occurred it is difficult to treat, and many patients with pituitary tumours probably die eventually from an endocrine crisis. Hydrocortisone succinate 100 mg. should be given intravenously without delay and 50 mg. intramuscularly six-hourly. If the blood pressure does not respond to cortisone in half an hour a noradrenaline infusion (4 ml. of 1 : 1000 to one litre of dextrose or dextrose saline) may be needed, the drip rate being adjusted to maintain a systolic pressure of 100 mm. Hg. or more. Blood electrolytes and glucose should be estimated, and the rectal temperature taken so that appropriate measures may be taken to correct whatever appears to be the main component of the collapse; the need for sugar and salt may be urgent, whilst recovery from hypothermic coma may follow warming slowly in a bath. A source of infection should always be sought and treated in crises otherwise unexplained.

Chronic deficiency, such as normally persists after operation in patients who had hypopituitrism before surgery, calls for replacement therapy. How much will be needed by any patient is not predictable—even after hypophysectomy some patients can be weaned from cortisone completely. More benefit from cortisone 25–50 mg. daily and thyroxine 0·05–0·3 mg. daily, whilst men usually experience increased appetite and energy with fluomesterone 5–10 mg. daily, and some report improvement in impotence and the return of beard growth. Women concerned about loss of libido and dyspareunia from genital atrophy may benefit from cyclical œstrogen therapy, e.g. ethinylœstradiol 0·02 mg. daily for 3 weeks in 4. Patients on replacement therapy should be warned of the risks of operations, infections and gastro-intestinal upsets; like diabetics they require increased replacement at such times when they are liable, possibly through ignorance or default, to have their vital drugs withdrawn.

Diabetes insipidus (DI) is more of a nuisance than a danger although if coma supervenes severe dehydration can result from the continued passage of large volumes of urine with inadequate intake. Polyuria may become evident only when cortisone replacement is begun; pre-operatively it can be distinguished from hysterical or compulsive water drinking by measuring the inability to produce concentrated urine, after 16–24 hours without fluid, which is rectified by a single dose of vasopressin. Specific gravity (SG) is an unreliable guide and the osmolality of the urine should be assessed; but in the first week or two post-operatively, when intake is controlled, a low SG ($<$1002) is diagnostic.

Diabetes insipidus may be treated by lypressin nasal spray, 3 to 8 applications daily. This can usually replace the inconvenient injections of vasopressin tannate. Some patients respond well to a thiazide diuretic, e.g. bendrofluazide 5 mg. daily, which may act by producing sodium depletion and stimulating formation of renin and angiotensin.

Hypophysectomy (removal or destruction of the normal pituitary gland) is now employed less often for hormone-dependent carcinomatosis (e.g. breast) than for diabetic retinopathy. Indications are florid retinopathy in diabetes of juvenile onset, associated with marked and rapid new vessel formation; and in more slowly progressive retinopathy in older patients if photocoagulation fails or if new vessels encroach on the optic disc.

The transsphenoidal approach using the microscope is now the usual method (p. 150). External radiation is a relatively ineffective alternative for producing total suppresion of the normal gland. Other means, such as implanted radioactive sources, the proton beam or large doses of œstrogens are now seldom used.

FURTHER READING

Elkington, S. G. and McKissock, W. (1967). Pitiutary adenoma: results of combined aurgial and radiotherapeutic treatment of 260 patients. *British Medical Journal*, **1**, 263–266.

Hardy, J (1971). Trans-sphenoidal hypophysectomy. *Journal of Neurosurgery*, **34**, 582–594.

Hoff, J. T and Patterson, R. H. (1972). Craniopharyngiomas in children and adults. *Journal of Neurosurgery*, **36**, 299–302.

Jenkins, J. S. and Else, W. (1968) Pituitary-adrenal function tests in untreated pitiutary tumours. *Lancet*, **2**, 940–943.

Kjellberg, R. N., Shintani, A., Frantz, A. G. and Kliman, B. (1968). Proton beam therapy in acromegaly. *New England Journal of Medicine*, **278**.

Ray, B. S. and Patterson, R. H. (1971). Surgical experience with chromophobe adenomas of the pituitary gland. *Journal of Neurosurgery*, **34**, 726–729.

Rovit, R. L. and Duane, T. D. (1969). Cushings syndrome and pituitary tumours. Pathophysiology and ocular manifestations of ACTH-secreting pituitary adenomas. *American Journal of Medicine*, **46**, 416–427.

Sachdev, Y., Gomez-Pan, A., Tunbridge, W. M G., Duns, A., Weightman, D. R. and Hall, R. (1975). Bromocryptine therapy in acromegaly. *Lancet*, **ii**, 1164–1168.

Williams, R. A., Jacobs, H. S., Kurtz, A. B., Millar, J. G. B , Oakley, N W., Spathis, G. S., Sulway, M. J. and Nabbarro, J. D. N. (1975). The treatment of acromegaly with special reference to transphenoidal hypophysectomy, *Journal of Medicine* **173**, 79–98.

Wright, A. D., Hill, D. M., Lowy, Clara and Fraser, R. T. (1970). Mortality in acromegaly *Journal of Medicine* **39**, 153.

Wise, B L. (1966). Management of post-operative diabetes insipidus. *Journal of Neurosurgery*, **25**, 416–420.

Neuroma (Schwannoma)

Any cranial or spinal nerve may give rise to one of these circumscribed tumours, but most intracranial neuromas are on the acoustic nerve, a few on the fifth at the Gasserian ganglion. Various synonyms exist (neurilemmoma, neurofibroma, neurinoma) but it is now becoming generally accepted that the proliferating elements in these tumours are derived from Schwann cells. There is no evidence that they originate in the nerve fibres themselves, although fibres may be found running through some tumours. The cells tend to form pallisades in a reticulin network with xanthomatous change and fat-filled foam cells giving the gross appearance of yellow buttery material in many tumours.

Families with generalised neurofibromatosis (von Recklinghausen's disease) tend to develop bilateral acoustic neuromas, often at a younger age than is common with the solitary tumours which occur in middle age. Tumours associated with von Recklinghausen's disease are often more fibroblastic in their stroma, more neurofibromatous, than solitary tumours.

Acoustic neuroma

The early diagnosis of acoustic neuroma is of concern to the neuro-surgeon because complete removal is usually possible if the tumour is detected before it is too large. Operative mortality and morbidity increase steadily as the tumour grows in size.

PATHOLOGY

The growth arises on the vestibular division of the eighth cranial nerve, where the neuroglial sheath gives way to a neurilemmal one. This is just inside the internal auditory meatus (porus acousticus) which thus becomes enlarged to a funnel shape. These tumours are extremely slowly growing and although pea-sized tumours have occasionally been diagnosed and removed this is unusual. More often by the time the surgeon sees the patient the tumour has filled the cerebello-pontine angle and burrowed ventral to the midbrain and pons which are in-dented and distorted. Tumour may also grow up through the tentorial hiatus into the middle cranial fossa to involve the third and fifth nerves, and down to the foramen magnum where it impinges on the lower cranial nerves passing to their exit foramina. The seventh nerve is almost always carried up on to the antero-superior surface of the tumour, intimately adherent to the capsule. Very often an arachnoid cyst develops on the surface of the tumour and adds to the amount of space taken up in the posterior fossa. Less often the tumour itself is mainly cystic; there is often a very long remission of symptoms after releasing such an intrinsic tumour cyst.

CLINICAL

The development of the classical signs and symptoms is such a slow business, spread over several years, sometimes as many as twenty, that each new feature tends to be treated as a new condition, and the relation-ship between the separate components of the cerebello-pontine syn-drome may escape notice. Deafness, tinnitus and vertigo commonly take the patient to the E.N.T. surgeon; vestibular symptoms may be only temporary whilst unilateral deafness may not impress itself on a patient until he chances to rely on one ear, perhaps on the telephone. The differential diagnosis at this stage is wide, if there are no other signs, but by a variety of neuro-otological investigations it can usually be established that there is an eighth nerve lesion rather than disease in peripheral structures. Auditory and vestibular function are separately tested, although both are often affected.

Loss of hearing is crudely tested by the ability to hear the whispered voice at a certain distance, with the other ear masked. Conductive deafness can be detected by finding air conduction less good than bone conduction on tuning fork tests (Rinne); pure tone audiometry enables the degree of hearing loss for different frequencies to be charted in quantitative terms (decibels loss), and again bone and air conduction can be compared; recruitment can also be detected. This term describes the apparent increase in acuity in a deaf ear as loudness of sound stimuli increases, and is found in certain instances of end-organ damage but not with nerve lesions. The Bekesy audiometer is a more elaborate means of detecting recruitment. Speech audiometry speaks for itself; nerve lesions commonly impair appreciation of speech more profoundly than of pure tones.

Vestibular function is tested by examining spontaneous and induced nystagmus. This may be directly observed, or recorded electrically; this (electronystagmography) is a much more sensitive detector of nystagmus but an even greater advantage is the possibility of recording nystagmus with the eyes closed or in a dark room—that is without fixation. This manoeuvre aggravates vestibular nystagmus but largely obliterates both central nystagmus (due to lesions of the nerve, brain stem or cerebellum) and congenital nystagmus. Nystagmus may be induced by rotation, by static position change or by caloric stimulation of the semi-circular canals. These caloric tests enable the vestibular function on the two sides to be distinguished. Both hot (44°C) and cold (30°C) water may be used, and either increments of 0·2 ml. are used or a continuing flow of water; in the latter case the time till onset of nystagmus is recorded. Acoustic neuroma is usually associated with a dead labyrinth (no reaction) from a fairly early stage.

Cerebellar ataxia and nystagmus, sometimes with early cranial nerve palsies (5, 7, 9, 10, 11), next appear. Diminished corneal sensation is the most constant sign. Facial weakness is rarely marked before operation, but slight weakness may be detected by delayed or absent blinking on the affected side. Facial pain, which may take the form of trigeminal neuralgia, sometimes occurs. A persistent suboccipital ache with a stiff neck is a frequent, if somewhat non-specific, complaint. Raised pressure may lead to neurosurgical investigations before the typical syndrome has evolved. Chronic hydrocephalus with marked mental changes and no clear history of eighth nerve or cerebellar disorder is a frequent presentation in the elderly.

Other less common tumours which grow in the cerebello-pontine angle may closely mimic an acoustic neuroma. Cholesteatoma, meningioma and laterally-placed intrinsic cerebellar tumours such as hæmangioblastoma or ependymoma, may all be equally indolent on occasion. Usually it can be discovered in patients with these other tumours that eighth nerve symptoms were not the initial ones, and the patient may not be very deaf even when presenting with involvement of other nerves, or with raised pressure.

Wherever neuromas occur in the nervous system they commonly cause a great increase in CSF protein (often over 400 mg. per 100 ml.), sometimes accompanied by xanthochromia. But a normal CSF protein level does not exclude the diagnosis especially in the early stages.

Radiological changes in the petrous bone can be detected with care in 90% of cases, much more often than with other angle tumours. Widening of the internal auditory meatus and canal is the commonest feature, but there may be more widespread erosion of the petrous pyramid. These are best seen on Towne's, Stenver's and basal views.

When obvious plain film changes accompany a typical clinical syndrome there may be no real doubt about the nature of the tumour. The additional information about the size of the tumour, the degree of ventricular displacement and the extent of the internal hydrocephalus is most readily provided by EMI scanning, with Conray enhancement; if this is not available then ventriculography (fig. 38), or air encephalography can be employed. Positive contrast encephalography, using oily media, may indicate that the internal auditory canal is normal.

TREATMENT

The **total removal** of this tumour when it is large is a difficult operation and carries an appreciable mortality and morbidity because of brain stem damage. Operative *deaths* are due either to spreading brain stem dysfunction, from retraction œdema or interruption of blood supply, or to accumulation of blood clot in tumour cavity. A total *facial palsy* is regarded as inevitable by most surgeons, but earlier diagnosis and microsurgical techniques have reduced the incidence of this complication. Facio-hypoglossal anostomosis, done within the first 6 months after operation, will improve tone in facial muscles at rest and patients may learn to initiate simple movements. *Neuroparalytic keratitis* is a risk, due to the combination of facial palsy and corneal anæsthesia and preventive measures are begun immediately after operation (p. 112). A temporary *bulbar palsy* may necessitate naso-œsophageal feeding for some weeks after operation, and during this time there is a risk of aspiration pneumonia. *Ataxia* is often aggravated by operation, though this too is usually only temporary. The ultimate results are good although facial palsy and some degree of ataxia are frequently permanent disabilities. Much depends on the reaction of the individual patient to these disabilities, but many do return to work.

The attraction of the **subtotal (intracapsular) operation** is that these complications can usually be avoided, and the immediate result can be very satisfactory, provided that sufficient tumour is removed from the tentorial hiatus to allow CSF to circulate freely and restore normal intracranial pressure. If the patient is elderly, or has some intercurrent disease with an expectation of less than 5 years, this operation may suffice. Also if the tumour is found to be almost completely cystic, an intracapsular removal may reasonably be accepted because recurrence of a cystic tumour is usually delayed for very many years.

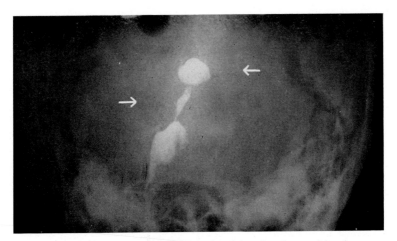

(a) Aqueduct (→) is displaced on the right; fourth ventricle also displaced and rotated (left side of floor pushed up); third ventricle (←) dilated but in normal midline position.

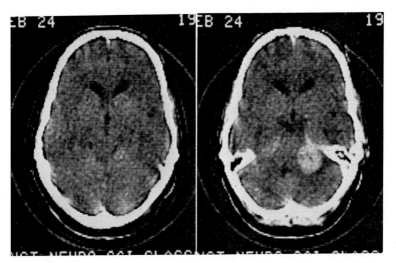

(b) EMI scan before enhancement.   (c) Same case after Conray injection.

FIG. 38 Acoustic neuroma

However, recurrence of local symptoms and of raised ICP is inevitable in most cases when only an intracapsular operation has been done. Having survived an initial intracapsular removal a patient requiring a second operation for recurrence faces a greater risk than that of initial total removal. Therefore if an acoustic neuroma is found in an otherwise healthy person, not of advanced years, total removal should be recommended; this applies even if the only complaint is of deafness, which surgery cannot improve.

Whichever operation is attempted the approach is the same, and the decision about the extent of the removal can be left until exploration has revealed the size and disposition of the tumour and the patient's reaction to operation. Staged procedures can be done, with an interval of a few weeks between the two operations. The second stage does not carry the high mortality rate associated with an operation repeated after several years; indeed by splitting this long and involved procedure into two shorter operations, and allowing raised intracranial pressure to resolve after the first stage, the hazards are appreciably reduced.

A paramedian incision half way between the midline and the mastoid brings the surgeon directly on to the tumour (fig. 28a). Access may be improved by the resection of the lateral third of the cerebellar hemisphere, and this does not appear to add to the post-operative disability. If the arachnoid of the cisterna magna is purposely opened CSF will escape during the operation from the fourth ventricle, and the pressure in the posterior fossa will remain low. The tumour is collapsed by spooning out its soft interior, and the slack capsule is then gently dissected free of its surroundings, taking care not to drag on the pons or on vessels entering it from the tumour. If during the dissection the respiration becomes irregular and the blood pressure fluctuates, it is wise not to persist in this direction but to turn to work on another part of the tumour. Later, when more of the bulk of the tumour has been removed, it may be safe to return to the previous danger zone. When tumour spreads far up through the tentorial hiatus, or anterior to the pons, the second stage may be facilitated by division of the tentorium (fig. 28).

The **dissecting microscope** is now routinely used when operating on this tumour, and this has reduced the frequency of damage to the brain stem and to the cranial nerves. The careful screening of patients with unilateral deafness using modern neuro-otological tests and refined neuro-radiology is leading to the recognition of increasing numbers of small tumours, which has also improved operative results. Some are still confined to the porus acousticus, giving rise to no cerebellar or brain stem signs and no elevation of intracranial pressure; such tumours can sometimes be removed by a translabyrinthine route. When there are signs of encroachment on central structures or CSF pathways it is wise to explore the posterior fossa to facilitate dissection off the brain stem. In the case of really large tumours with critically raised pressure (and these are still a common occurrence), a two-stage procedure may be safest; first a posterior fossa decompression and intracapsular removal is effected, and at a later date micro-dissection is employed to complete the removal.

FURTHER READING

Dix, M. R. (1969). Modern tests of vestibular function with special reference to their value in clinical practice. *British Medical Journal* **3**, 317–323.

Drake, C. G. (1967). Surgical removal of acoustic neuroma with preservation or reconstitution of the facial nerve. *Journal of Neurosurgery*, **27**, 459–464.

Drake, C. G. (1967). Total removal of large acoustic neuromas. *Journal of Neurosurgery*, **27**, 554–561.

Edwards, C. H. and Paterson, J. H. (1951). A review of the symptoms and signs of acoustic neurofibromata. *Brain*, **74**, 144–190.

Horrax, G., Olivecrona, H., Pennybacker, J., Cairns, H. and Northfield, D. W. C. (1950). Symposium on the results of operations on acoustic neuromas. *Journal of Neurology, Neurosurgery and Psychiatry*, **13**, 268–279.

House. W. F. (1968). Monograph II: acoustic neuroma. *Archives of Otolaryngology*, **88**, 576–715.

Pool, J. L. (1966). Suboccipital surgery for acoustic neuromas: advantages and disadvantages. *Journal of Neurosurgery*, **24**, 483–492.

Rand, R. W. and Kurze, T. L. (1965). Facial nerve preservation by posterior fossa transmeatal microdissection in total removal of acoustic tumours. *Journal of Neurology, Neurosurgery and Psychiatry*, **28**, 311–316.

Shepherd, R. H. and Wadia, N. H. (1956). Some observations on atypical features in acoustic neuroma. *Brain*, **79**, 282–318.

Symposium (1969). Technique of acoustic neuroma survey. *Archives of Otolaryngology*, **89**, 326–340.

Symposium (1969). Early diagnosis of acoustic neuromas. *Archives of Otolaryngology*, **89**, 302–318.

Symposium (1973) Cerebellopontine angle tumours—diagnosis and survey. In: *Advances in Neurosurgery*. Eds. Schurmann, Brock, Reulen, Voth. Springer-Verlag, Berlin.

Metastatic tumours

PATHOLOGY

In the brain itself these tumours arise by hæmatogenous spread through the arterial system or the valveless vertebral veins. They comprise the majority of intracranial secondary neoplasms, and make up 20–30% of all brain tumours recorded by pathologists, but only 5% of surgical series. Almost one in five of all cancer deaths has intracranial metastases at autopsy, a fifth of these being diffuse carcinomatosis. Three quarters of those affected have major cerebral symptoms. Carcinoma of the bronchus is the commonest source of origin, a quarter of patients dying with this growth having brain metastases at autopsy; in a third the intracranial deposit is solitary although this is seldom the only secondary in the whole body. Breast cancer and hypernephroma, and less commonly carcinoma of the gut and malignant melanoma, also metastasise to the brain, sometimes producing symptoms years after the removal of the primary growth. In some 15% the primary site is never discovered.

Blood-borne metastases form discrete tumours in the cerebral or cerebellar hemisphere; most supratentorial deposits are around the posterior end of the Sylvian fissure, in the region of supply of the terminal branches of the middle cerebral artery. Solitary tumours are normally firm and well-circumscribed though there may be widespread œdema causing greater pressure effects than would be expected from the size of the tumour itself. Although the bulk of the mass is firm and may at first resemble a meningioma the centre is frequently soft and necrotic; thick creamy fluid aspirated from this is easily mistaken for pus. On smears a metastasis may be distinguished from a glioblastoma only with difficulty; less often it looks like a sarcomatous meningioma. On the other hand it may be possible to recognise the type of carcinoma, even to hazard a guess as to the site of the primary.

Invasion of the dura, usually of the skull base, is a less common form of secondary intracranial neoplasia. Ordinarily the underlying bone is first affected with later spread to the dura. *Bone involvement* may be by blood stream spread (carcinoma breast or stomach, multiple myeloma) or by the direct extension of regional carcinoma (naso-pharynx, paranasal air sinuses, middle ear; rodent ulcer or epithelioma of scalp). A dural carpet is formed which may spread over a wide area and become hæmorrhagic; clinically this is reflected in progressive multiple cranial nerve palsies without raised pressure; plain X-rays may reveal erosion of the skull. Dural deposits *without bone change* occur in reticulosis (Hodgkin's disease) and leukemia but are rarely the result of distant carcinoma.

Carcinomatosis of the meninges is a different entity arising from the dissemination of cancer cells in the subarachnoid space from a small deposit under the ventricular ependyma, in the choroid plexus or in the subpial part of the cerebral cortex. Although the arachnoid is infiltrated it looks only faintly opaque, or even quite normal to the naked eye. Cells may be recognised in the CSF.

CLINICAL

Carcinoma quite commonly declares itself first by intracranial invasion, sometimes at a stage when exhaustive investigation reveals no evidence of the primary tumour. Carcinoma of the bronchus by blood spread, and of the naso-pharynx by direct extension, are the tumours which most often behave in this deceptive way. Apart from this type of presentation patients with known primary malignancies, already treated or not, sometimes call for neurosurgical aid if intracranial extension is causing distressing symptoms.

Cerebral metastases usually give a short history of well-circumscribed focal signs, paralysis or focal epilepsy confined to one limb, and raised pressure. **Cerebellar** deposits cause distressing vertigo, vomiting and ataxia, usually with severe headache from internal hydrocephalus. Although a rapid course is the rule, intermittent symptoms may occur over a period of months. Sometimes clinical evidence of more than one tumour is found, and this is always suggestive of metastatic disease.

Congenital tumours

Teratomas contain multiple tissues foreign to the part in which they arise. Most develop in the *pineal* region, but there is controversy about whether tumours here are mostly teratomas of a kind or originate in adult tissue—pinealomas, pinealocytomas, etc. Some are frankly teratomatous with epithelial elements and smooth muscle; others are more uniform, resembling seminoma of testis, and may disseminate through the CSF and to the lungs. Many tumours here certainly are gliomas, ependymomas being the commonest type.

These tumours usually grow to a large size before detection. A hæmorrhagic and polycystic mass expands bilaterally above the tentorium, and presses below on the dorsal midbrain. All produce internal hydrocephalus, often with dilated pupils and impaired upward gaze with ptosis due to midbrain pressure. Many of the dubious tumours discussed above occur in young boys; a number of these patients develop precocious puberty which was at one time ascribed to endocrine activity in the tumour, but is probably due to involvement of the tuber cinereum by tumour which has seeded across the third ventricle.

Cholesteatoma (pearly tumours, epidermoids) consist of epithelial debris accumulating inside a thin capsule lined with flattened cells to form white glistening flakes of material resembling mother-of-pearl.

Most occur in the basal subarachnoid cisterns, usually near the sella but sometimes in the cerebello-pontine angle. Typical neighbourhood symptoms are produced but with a very long history. The capsule penetrates into every nook and cranny making complete removal impossible, although the tumour is non-invasive. Occasional cholesteatomas are related to the lateral ventricles, sometimes wholly intraventricular. These *intradural tumours* can be diagnosed by air studies, the air being dispersed through a sponge or lattice-work of tumour (fig. 41). They are also associated with aseptic or chemical meningitis after operation, pleocytosis and pyrexia persisting intermittently for months. Although reports of organisms isolated from these tumours at operation may explain the meningitis, it is difficult after numerous lumbar punctures to exclude secondary infection when frank bacterial meningitis does develop.

Diploic epidermoids cause a lump on the skull and may indent the brain; erosion of the vault with a scalloped, dense margin is diagnostic. Another bony site is the *petrous temporal* where a circular erosion, obvious on X-ray, gives rise to slowly progressive facial palsy. Although some patients have had previous ear disease this seems to be an entity distinct from infective cholesteatoma found with active otitis media. Early evacuation of this intra-petrous non-infective cholesteatoma through the middle fossa, using an extradural approach, like that used for trigeminal root section, may save the facial nerve from total destruction.

Dermoids also result from defective ectodermal closure, but the capsule includes dermal elements and the contents sebaceous material, hairs and oily fluid. *Pericranial* dermoids erode the bone near the anterior fontanelle in children. *Orbital* dermoids grow slowly from the lateral roof causing painless proptosis and bone erosion.

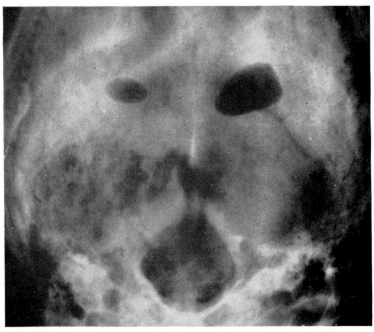

Lumbar encephalogram has filled interstices of tumour with air to give a fluffy appearance; clean air shadows are seen in the ventricles and cisterns.

Fig. 41 Cholesteatoma in cerebello-pontine angle

Posterior fossa dermoids are both more dangerous and more variable in their presentation. All are in the midline; those which are wholly extradural have a skin sinus leading to a dimple just above the external occipital protuberance; often there is a subcutaneous lump in addition. Intradural cysts in the fourth ventricle may occasionally extend through the foramen to cause spinal compression. A sinus to the surface will predispose to recurrent meningitis or a posterior fossa abscess; without a sinus the cysts may cause internal hydrocephalus with cerebellar signs of varying degree. Careful study of the back of the head may reveal the sinus, and the X-rays may show a circular defect in the inner table when there is an extradural cyst. The channel of a sinus may be seen as a fine groove in the bone.

Cordoma (chordoma) arises in notochordal remnants in the basis-phenoid or basiocciput to form a malignant and locally invasive tumour, which begins therefore in the midline. Extensive bone destruction follows with the spread of tumour into the dura, paranasal air sinuses and ear. Clinical progression is very slow and may be intermittent; parasellar syndromes are more common than posterior fossa symptoms, usually without increased pressure. Dense calcification often occurs, and although the tumour may be in part myxomatous it can be rock hard and cannot be removed completely.

FURTHER READING

Kamrin, R. P., Potanos, J. N. and Pool, J. L. (1964). An evaluation of the diagnosis and treatment of chordoma. *Journal of Neurology, Neurosurgery and Psychiatry*, **27**, 157–165.

Logue, V. and Till, K. (1952). Posterior fossa dermoid cysts with special reference to intracranial infection. *Journal of Neurology, Neurosurgery and Psychiatry*, **15**, 1–12.

Poppen, J. L. and Marino, R. (1968) Pinealomas and tumours of the posterior portion of the third ventricle. *Journal of Neurosurgery*, **28**, 357–364.

Tytus, J. S. and Pennybacker, J (1956). Pearly tumours in relation to the central nervous system. *Journal of Neurosurgery and Psychiatry*, **19**, 241–259.

Orbital tumours

The bony orbit is formed above by the floor of the anterior fossa, and the postero-lateral orbital wall is the sphenoidal wing. This is also the anterior wall of the middle fossa, and is perforated by the optic foramen and the superior orbital fissure. Neurosurgeons are concerned with orbital disease because this has often spread from, or is liable to spread to, the intracranial cavity. Surgical exploration of the orbit for tumour may call for simultaneous exposure of the anterior or middle cranial fossæ.

Orbital tumours are uncommon, but the main symptoms they cause are not; whenever proptosis or visual disturbance is found an orbital mass must be considered in the differential diagnosis.

PATHOLOGY

A wide variety of tumours have been reported in the orbit but only the most frequent will be mentioned. They arise in one of three situations:

1. **The optic nerve and its sheath** is most often affected by a *piloid glioma* (astrocytoma). This tumour is almost confined to children, many of whom have von Recklinghausen's syndrome (p. 155). It begins some 10 mm. behind the globe, and the enlargement of the optic nerve may cause expansion of the bony optic foramen which can be detected on plain X-rays. Spread backwards may result in involvement of the chiasm and the opposite optic nerve, or of the third ventricle with subsequent

hydrocephalus. Such spread is not inevitable, however, and this tumour can be very indolent; it may show little or no obvious progression for many years, wither without any treatment, or after only incomplete removal.

Meningioma of the sheath is much less common and occurs in adults. It is liable to cause pain and œdema in addition to proptosis and visual loss which are the usual symptoms common to it and glioma.

Retinoblastoma is a highly malignant familial glioma, occurring under the age of 4 years, often affecting both eyes and (exceptional among gliomas) metastasising to lymph nodes and distant organs.

2. **Other orbital tissues** may become tumorous and the commonest condition of all to cause proptosis is the *orbital granuloma* (pseudotumour) which affects all the orbital contents. This is an unexplained condition in which the orbital fat, muscles and adventitia of vessels are infiltrated with lymph cells and plasma cells; spread of low-grade infection from neighbouring air sinuses has been suggested as a cause but is unproven. The affected tissues are firm and swollen, and local masses may be felt both through the intact skin and when the orbit is opened surgically. This is a self-limiting process and its importance is the closeness with which it resembles true tumour clinically, which usually leads to orbital exploration.

Lachrymal gland tumours mostly resemble mixed salivary gland tumours and tend to recur locally, sometimes years after excision. Both *angiomas and lymphangiomas* occur and give rise to proptosis which may vary spontaneously or may be temporarily aggravated by the patient bending forwards and reduced by pressure on the globe.

3. **The bony orbital walls** may be affected by tumours which project partly into the orbit and partly either externally or into the surrounding cavities of the sinuses or cranium. Simple tumours include *dermoid cyst*, which often causes a palpable swelling at the outer upper angle of the orbit and a translucency on X-ray; *mucocæle* of the sinus, usually frontal, which is often associated with chronic or recurrent infection; *meningioma* of the sphenoidal wing, which gives rise to long-standing proptosis and visual loss, sometimes with a temporal swelling: and *osteoma* of the sinuses, usually frontal, which may also grow intracranially and breach the dura giving rise to rhinorrhœa or spontaneous ærocele. *Malignant* tumours may be primary, most often carcinoma of the ethmoid, or secondary, from distant carcinoma, sarcoma or melanoma.

CLINICAL

Proptosis is the most constant feature, and the globe may also be displaced downwards or laterally, occasionally upwards. In doubtful instances the eyes should be viewed from above; an exophthalmometer allows the amount of the protrusion (relative to the normal eye) to be measured and progression can then be assessed. *Intermittent* proptosis suggests a vascular, infective or granulomatous condition, whilst if the protrusion is *pulsatile* there is either an arteriovenous fistula (in the orbit or a carotico-cavernous fistula (p. 261)). Marked *œdema* of the lids and conjunctiva suggests either endocrine exophthalmos, carotico-cavernous fistula or orbital granuloma.

Visual failure is gradual and may not be noticed until the eye is totally blind. Because of the visual loss diplopia may never be complained of although the visual axes of the two eyes are far from parallel.

Ocular movements are surprisingly well preserved even when the globe is markedly displaced; if there is marked ophthalmoplegia either endocrine exophthalmos or a lesion in the cavernous sinus should be suspected.

Anteriorly placed tumours (lachrymal gland or dermoids) may be **palpable.** The fundus is affected only by tumours on the nerve and sheath, and **optic atrophy** is more common than **unilateral papillœdema.**

INVESTIGATION

Measurement of the degree of protrusion, and taking serial clinical photographs, are the best ways of documenting the progress of the condition, and assessing the result of treatment. Plain X-rays are always important, including views to show the air sinuses, the skull and the optic foraminæ. Thyroid function must be tested, and the possibility of a primary tumour elsewhere in the body excluded as far as seems reasonable. Carotid angiography may show up a vascular lesion within the orbit itself, a carotico-cavernous fistula or an intracranial tumour. Orbitograms, made by injecting air or iodine-containing contrast into the orbital tissues, may be useful in experienced hands.

TREATMENT

Few orbital tumours can be diagnosed without surgical exploration. The aim is to make this as limited as possible in the first place. Some tumours are easily removed, some call for a major orbito-cranial approach, whilst other conditions are either inoperable or do not call for surgical measures beyond a biopsy to establish the diagnosis (e.g. the common orbital granuloma). Most tumours can be biopsied, and some removed, through a lateral approach. An incision is made in the eyebrow (which is not shaved) and the superolateral angle of the bony margin turned back as a small flap. It is optic nerve gliomas which most often call for a frontal flap and opening of the orbit at the same time, in order to section the nerve behind the posterior margin of the tumour, if possible, to prevent backward extension. However, the indolent course of this tumour in many cases has led to controversy as to whether such drastic treatment is necessary or indeed justified. Certainly the globe need not be sacrificed, even though the nerve is sectioned and the eye left sightless, because this tumour rarely extends forwards to the globe.

Endocrine exophthalmos

Not only does this form an important differential diagnosis when orbital tumour is under discussion, but it may call for neurosurgical intervention in its own right. The physio-pathology cannot be fully discussed here. The link with overt thyroid disease may not be obvious; thyrotoxicosis may accompany the condition or have been treated months or years before, but some patients have no disturbance of thyroid function even when this is tested by modern isotope techniques.

Women are twice as frequently affected as men. Both eyes are usually involved, but there may be a delay of up to six months before the second eye is affected. Œdema and ophthalmoplegia are obvious, much more so than for a similar degree of proptosis due to tumour. Although the condition is commonly self-limiting, malignant cases occur in which vision is threatened by progressive protrusion and corneal ulceration. It is these cases that are sometimes sent to the neurosurgeon for decompression of the orbit.

Both this measure and such other treatment as is available are purely empirical. Correction of thyroid disorder by drugs or thyroidectomy may improve the condition or make it worse, or it may arise only when the treatment for thyrotoxicosis has been completed. Deep X-rays to the orbital tissues may be of value. Decompression does nothing to remove the cause, but may help to break the vicious circle of progressive œdema. As long as this involved a major frontal craniotomy (Naffziger's operation) the method was naturally looked on as a last resort, but several less drastic methods have been introduced in recent years. All involve a direct operation on the lateral wall of the orbit, with the removal of the orbital roof and lateral wall; the patient is left with a pulsating eye but this is not very noticeable nor subjectively troublesome. The method mentioned for approaching orbital tumours has proved successful and leaves an acceptable cosmetic scar. This relatively minor procedure can be considered for even mild cases, if symptoms are persistent and other measures are failing to afford relief.

FURTHER READING

Brain, W. R. (1959). Pathogenesis and treatment of endocrine exophthalmos *Lancet*, i, 109–115.
Foster, J. (1955). The diagnosis and treatment of orbital tumours. *Annals of the Royal College of Surgeons of England*, **17**, 114–129.
Hamby, W. B (1964). Pterional approach to the orbits for decompression or tumour removal. *Journal of Neurosurgery* **21**, 15–18.
Jelinick, E. H. (1969). The orbital pseudotumour syndrome and its differentiation from endocrine exophthalmos. *Brain*, **92**, 35–58.

Suspected tumour recurrence

Once a patient has had a brain tumour he and his medical advisers are always alert to the possibility of recurrence. Almost any symptom, but especially headache or vomiting, however trivial, is apt to raise suspicion and the decision must be made whether to re-investigate or not. Apart from irrelevant conditions, from influenza to hypertension, there are a number of intracranial events remotely related to the original operation which may mimic recurrence. Although most have been described already they may conveniently be listed together here.

1. **Radionecrosis** is characterised by the sudden onset of focal signs, frequently remote from the exact site of the previous tumour, without raised pressure as a rule, and often resolving spontaneously. This explanation should not be accepted for incidents occurring less than a year after treatment, and five years or more is the common interval.

2. **Obstructive hydrocephalus** due to post-operative adhesions may affect any part of the ventricular system. Reaction to the blood spilt at operation, or to low grade post-operative infection, may lead to an adhesive arachnoiditis in the posterior fossa or at the tentorial hiatus, which causes a block at the outlet of the fourth ventricle or at the cisterna ambiens resulting in total hydrocephalus. Occasionally the block is higher in the ventricular system with dilatation of one lateral ventricle or of only one temporal horn. A ventriculocisternostomy tube can become blocked and raised pressure recur; although reactions to rubber tubes are unusual a few patients develop a dense fibrous reaction to that part of the tube which is under the scalp; immediate recovery follows the replacement of the blocked tube by a new one of silicone. Third ventriculostomy is notorious for blocking off and is probably not worth trying to revise; some alternative drainage should be provided. Ventricular shunts, originally devised for treating infantile hydro-cephalus (p. 321), are effective in adults and probably offer the best solution to obstructive hydrocephalus which is unsuitable for ventri-culocisternostomy or in which this has proved unsuccessful. Once a ventriculo-caval shunt has been made, however, it is impossible to investigate the patient by air studies if a relapse should occur, because of the risk of air embolism; there is no such problem in re-investigating the patient with Torkildsen tubes in place or after ventriculo-peritoneal shunt.

3. **Hypopituitary crises** (p. 153) have characteristics which should lead to early recognition, and the site of the original tumour will suggest the likelihood of this explanation for coma or collapse.

4. **Infection** may take the form of meningitis, usually in patients who have had a CFS leak, and this may first develop years after operation. An abscess in the tumour cavity more often declares itself within a few months as a recurrence of raised pressure and focal signs, too soon to be likely to be due to tumour regrowth.

5. **Local brain atrophy** can occur in areas adjacent to the site of tumour removal. The ventricle may dilate into an atrophic area to form a porencephalic cyst; or such a cyst can develop in relation to the subarachnoid space and indent the ventricle, with which it does not

communicate. Local degenerative changes may be accelerated by vascular insufficiency, as arterial disease develops with advancing age; if a patient becomes arteriosclerotic, the area of brain surrounding the operation site, which has existed on a precarious blood supply for years, may be deprived more severely than the rest of the brain and focal signs and symptoms may then recur.

6. **Epilepsy** may occasionally be overlooked as a cause of relapse. A series of unwitnessed convulsions can leave a patient in post-epileptic stupor for hours or days, during which tumour recurrence may be suspected. Intoxication with epanutin causes ataxia and nystagmus which may mistakenly suggest intracranial mischief. Whether the development or recurrence of epilepsy itself should be taken as evidence of tumour recurrence is doubtful, but the sudden appearance of insistent focal epilepsy in a patient who has previously had a convexity or para-sagittal meningioma is certainly suspicious. In general, however, patients can rightly be reassured that the occurrence of epilepsy does not mean renewed tumour activity.

7. **A second intracranial tumour,** developing in a patient who has already had one removed, will naturally first be regarded as a recurrence. This possibility must be considered when the original tumour was a *metastasis*: or a *neurofibroma*, especially if this latter was in a patient with generalised von Recklinghausen's disease or a family history of this. *Meningiomas* are occasionally multiple, whilst most "recurrences" of cerebellar *hæmangioblastomas* are probably second tumours, again most often in patients with a family history. *Gliomas* which spread through CSF pathways (medulloblastoma, ependymoma and intra-ventricular astrocytoma), may recur at sites distant from the original mass.

8. **Recurrence of the original tumour** may be readily recognised because the symptoms and signs often closely resemble those which characterised the first illness. This is by no means the rule, however, and the issue may be further clouded by the absence of signs of raised pressure; not only are the fundi normal but the decompression often remains indrawn even when it has not become so firm as to be unyield-ing. Air studies are confusing when there has been previous surgery and angiography is a more reliable method of investigation if tumour circulation can be demonstrated. Shift of midline structures is difficult to interpret when there is a decompression, and perhaps also local atrophy, ventricular dilatation or a porencephalic cyst. Both angio-graphy and ventriculography may be required, as only air will show that a distortion of vessels on the angiogram is in fact due to a cyst or distorted ventricle rather than regrowth of tumour.

FURTHER READING (*Tumours in general*)

Dastui, D. K. and Lolitha, V. S. (1960). Pathological analysis of intracranial space-occupying lesions in 1000 cases. *Journal of Neurological Sciences*, **11**, 501–535.

Editorial (1968). Surgical treatment of intracranial tumours. *British Medical Journal*, **1**, 531–532.

Krayenbuhl, H., Maspes, P. E. and Sweet, W. H. (1965). *Progress in Neurological Surgery* 1 Karger, New York and Basel.

Krayenbuhl, H., Maspes, P. E. and Sweet, W. H. (1968). *Progress in Neurological Surgery* 2. Karger, New York and Basel.

Low, N. L., Correll, J. W. and Hammill, J. F. (1965). Tumours of the cerebral hemispheres in children. *Archives of Neurology*, **13**, 547–554.

Matson, D. D. (1969). *Neurosurgery of infancy and childhood.* Thomas, Springfield.

Russell, D. and Rubenstein, L. J. (1963). *The pathology of tumours of the nervous system.* 2nd edition. Arnold, London.

OTHER REFERENCES

CHAPTER 10

Intracranial Infection

Intracranial abscess

Meningitis

Encephalitis

Osteomyelitis of skull

Specific infections

Intracranial abscess

ORIGIN

Ear disease is the commonest source. In the present antibiotic era acute mastoiditis is liable to be treated without surgical drainage, and although survived may be followed by chronic disease and intracranial complications. Bronchiectasis and empyema are now rare causes, but now that patients with cyanotic heart disease survive longer they are liable to develop brain abscesses.

Chronic suppurative otitis media accounts for more than half of all cases. Infective cholesteatoma erodes the tegmen tympani allowing infection to spread upwards into the middle of the temporal lobe; or it destroys the bone of Trautman's triangle behind the middle ear, causing an abscess in the anterolateral segment of the cerebellar hemisphere. Temporal abscesses are twice as common as cerebellar; occasional patients have both. Chronic ear infection may be relatively silent, with minimal discharge, only occasional pain and gradual deafness. Neither inspection of the infected ear, nor study of X-rays of the petrous temporal bone, enable a reliable prediction to be made as to whether a particular infected ear is potentially dangerous. When acute otitis is promptly and properly treated so that chronic infection becomes unusual, and chronically infected ears with cholesteatoma, when they occur, are dealt with by early radical mastoidectomy otogenic intracranial abscesses should become a rarity.

Infection probably spreads by infective thrombosis in small veins traversing the diploe to join venous sinuses, so that suppuration can occur within the brain without involving the superficial planes. On the contrary extensive extradural collections of pus are frequently found in the course of performing mastoidectomy, even when there has been no reason to suspect an intracranial complication; the dura is remarkably resistant to infection.

Acute frontal sinusitis, like mastoiditis, now commonly responds to antibiotics without requiring surgical drainage; when frontal osteitis develops the risk of a frontal lobe abscess and subdural abscess is high. Less often extradural pus collects, usually when there is chronic infection of the sinus.

Hæmatogenous abscesses, due to blood stream spread from a distant focus, occur in the distribution of the middle cerebral artery, either posterior frontal or temporo-parietal. Cyanotic congenital heart disease now accounts for the majority, usually without an overt focus of infection elsewhere. Infection probably begins in small cerebral infarcts, arising from a combination of hypoxia and thrombosis, secondary to polycythæmia.

Trauma, either accidental or operative, accounts for most of the remaining cases. Infective material may be carried directly into the cranial cavity, as in a penetrating injury, or superficial infection in scalp or bone may spread secondarily. Dural tears affecting the air sinuses or middle ear provide another route.

A number of abscesses occur for which **no obvious cause** is found, and the presumption is that these are due to blood spread from primary foci too insignificant to have been noticed on their own account.

INTRACRANIAL PATHOLOGY

Subdural abscess most often arises from acute sinusitis but may be otogenic. Pus spreads back over the convexity of the cerebral hemisphere, and also collects beside the falx on the medial surface of the brain. From here it may reach the opposite side and the superior surface of the tentorium; and it can then gain access to the posterior fossa through the tentorial hiatus. Eventually there is widespread pus producing a plethora of neurological signs, probably due to infective thrombosis in small vessels.

Parenchymal brain abscess usually goes through a stage of diffuse suppurative encephalitis before liquefaction in the centre leads to a discrete collection of pus. A capsule then begins to form which eventually becomes quite tough and thick. Traumatic and hæmatogenous abscesses tend to become multilocular; if one loculus is sealed off from the main one, "recurrence" may arise from persistence of this loculus after the other has been drained. Untreated abscesses prove fatal either by causing acute brain compression (and can do so in the early encephalitic stage when brain œdema may be widespread) or by later rupturing into the ventricle or the subarachnoid space.

BACTERIOLOGY

Because most infections are from the ear Gram-negative organisms are common, often more than one type with B. proteus predominant. Sinus infections are frequently streptococcal (hæmolytic, viridans, anærobic) or pneumococcal. Subdural abscess is almost always streptococcal whether coming from sinus or ear. Metastatic abscesses vary according to source, those from lung infections often having a mixed growth like otogenic abscesses. Traumatic infections are usually due to staphylococcus pyogenes. Quite a number of abscesses are sterile by the time they are drained (at least no organisms can be grown), probably because so many patients have had prolonged antibiotic treatment for their primary infection.

CLINICAL

Brain abscess

This is a less dramatic complication, at least in its early stages, than is often imagined; and this is particularly true since antibiotics have been available. Eventually a picture of advancing brain compression with focal signs develops, but the diagnosis should be made before this. Suspicion should be roused whenever signs of intracranial mischief appear against the background of an infection known to predispose to brain abscess.

Otogenic abscess usually follows an acute recrudescence of infection in a chronically infected ear. A great deal of local pain in and around the ear gives way to headache, perhaps with some drowsiness and mild confusion. Not uncommonly this is taken to be part of an acute mastoiditis, and brain abscess is only recognised a week or so after mastoidectomy when post-operative recovery is unexpectedly slow, and pyrexia and toxicity persist. In most such instances intracranial complications were probably already present when the mastoid was dealt with, rather than having developed as the result of this operation.

Temporal lobe abscess does not produce florid CNS signs. Epilepsy and hemiplegia are quite unusual, whilst the most constant sign, an upper quadrantic homonymous hemianopia, is almost never complained of by the patient. It will be detected only by the clinician who specifically looks for it. On the left side mild dysphasia may occur, but if the patient is ill and pyrexial is readily mistaken for confusion or delirium. Papillœdema may develop but pressure can rise so rapidly with an abscess that there is not time for the fundi to become swollen.

Cerebellar abscess is more obvious because nystagmus, slow to the affected side, is almost constant, and some degree of ataxia usual; papillœdema may develop because of some degree of hydrocephalus.

Sinusitic abscess follows frontal osteitis which is associated with an œdematous swelling above the eye. Headache and pyrexia are accompanied by vomiting and some confusion. Epilepsy is very common, but marked hemiplegia is unusual (unless there is also subdural pus).

Abscesses of **hæmatogenous** origin are often more insidious, and there is seldom any recent acute infection to draw attention to the likelihood of intracranial mischief. A patient may be surprisingly well with 50 ml. of pus in the middle of the hemisphere, apyrexial and with no neurological signs detectable. However, some degree of hemiparesis is common, as these abscesses occur in the middle cerebral distribution, and epilepsy may develop.

Subdural abscess

Surface pus produces more profound disturbance of function than an abscess in the brain itself because cortical thrombophlebitis and arteritis develop with resulting ischæmic lesions. Following sinusitis, headache and toxicity persist and there is epilepsy; this commonly begins as focal motor attacks which may progress to status. Hemiplegia or dysphasia suddenly develop, often following a bout of fits. The picture is of a gravely ill patient in danger both from spreading infection and persisting epilepsy.

INVESTIGATIONS

These should be carried out in a neurosurgical unit and if the clinical condition is at all suspicious of intracranial complications the patient should be transferred because an emergency burr hole may be necessary.

Lumbar puncture is justified only if meningitis is strongly suspected. An abscess is a rapidly developing mass lesion, and intracranial pressure may become dangerously high before papillœdema is evident, and the risk of precipitating brain shifts is considerable. In any event, apart from excluding meningitis, examination of the CSF is not crucial, because it is occasionally completely normal. Often the protein is raised to 60–100 mg., and there are about 100 cells, either polymorphs or lymphocytes or both.

The EEG can be most useful in the recognition and localisation of parenchymal brain abscesses above the tentorium. A slow wave (delta) focus develops at less than one cycle per second, which is slower than is commonly seen with other disorders. Frequently it is sharply focal, with phase reversals between adjacent electrode pairs sharing a common placement indicating the site of the abscess. Experience and patience are required to change the electrode positions time and again until the exact site of maximal electrical abnormality is determined. Meningitis and surface suppuration give only non-specific and generalised abnormalities.

Isotope scanning is increasingly advocated as the investigation of choice for suspected supratentorial abscess, and if a reliable scan can be arranged as an emergency it should be done; but once an abscess is suspected no more than a few hours delay in establishing the diagnosis is acceptable.

EMI scanning is the most useful single investigation, because it can show not only displacement of the lateral ventricles, due to a supratentorial abscess and dilatation from one in the posterior fossa, but will usually locate the abscess directly as an area of reduced density. (Fig 42).

Carotid angiography is the safest radiological method available for *supratentorial* suppuration in the absence of EMI scanning. In many otogenic and sinusitic cases, however, it is unnecessary because the presence of an abscess is obvious from the clinical picture, whilst its site is so constant (temporal or frontal) that a burr hole can be correctly placed with some confidence (fig. 43). If shift is seen on angiography it is not possible to distinguish between diffuse suppurative encephalitis, œdema and actual pus as the cause of the displacement.

The clinical appearance of a *cerebellar* abscess is usually diagnostic, and again a burr hole can be made in the right place, having regard to the side of the affected ear and the lateralisation of the signs. If there is doubt **myodil ventriculography** is the investigation of choice. Air injections are liable to aggravate the condition of these patients with rapidly developing brain compression (either above or below the tentorium), but on occasions there may be no alternative. This most often occurs when a hæmatogenous abscess is suspected but cannot be localised by other means.

Subdural abscess is diagnosed clinically, by the rapid onset of hemiplegia and focal epilepsy. The thin film of pus may produce no displacement on contrast studies; or bilateral collections may balance each other. A burr hole must be made without delay in the area which is suspected from the distribution of the signs.

Other intracranial complications of infection must be considered as alternatives to abscess. *Meningitis* is diagnosed by lumbar puncture. Before accepting *otitic hydrocephalus* (p. 50) as an explanation for papillœdema undisplaced third and fourth ventricles should be seen on myodil ventriculography. *Cortical thrombophlebitis* is suspected when focal epilepsy and paralysis develop in a patient who remains remarkably well; however, a subdural abscess should always be excluded by burr hole.

TREATMENT

Whatever plane suppuration affects the basis of management is the same: the establishment of local drainage, the administration of local and systemic antibiotics and the treatment of the primary focus of infection. Active mastoid or sinus disease should be treated surgically as soon as the abscess is under control, usually about a week after it is first aspirated; otherwise re-infection or new extension may develop.

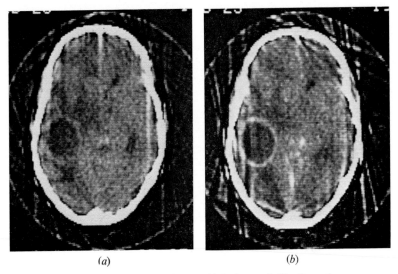

(a)   (b)

FIG. 42 Left temporal lobe abscess, (a) before and (b) after enhancement with Conray.

Methods of providing local drainage differ according to the type of abscess, but both parenchymal and subdural suppuration call for the utmost urgency. Once an abscess is diagnosed a burr hole should be made without delay. Compression can advance very rapidly with an acute lesion of this kind, and cerebellar abscess in particular is liable to produce sudden apnœa from medullary failure.

TREATMENT OF BRAIN ABSCESS

Burr hole aspiration

Most abscesses can be managed in this way. It is safer to make a clean burr hole than to attempt drainage through an existing incision (e.g. a mastoid wound) which could introduce fresh infection or allow brain to herniate.

A blunt brain cannula is introduced and will normally be held up by the capsule, the thickness and toughness of which can be estimated. It is unwise to empty a big abscess completely at first: collapse of the capsule may provoke hæmorrhage or block off the needle so that the cavity cannot be identified with certainty before injecting antibiotic and contrast medium. Because it is so important to make this injection the first time an abscess is tapped, it is a wise precaution to have the solution ready in a syringe before attempting aspiration.

As small a quantity as possible should be injected into the abscess cavity in order to gain the maximum decompressive benefit from

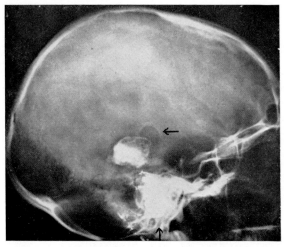

(a) Abscess cavity outlined by baruim and containing some air from recent aspiration through a burr hole (←). Radio-opaque BIPP pack (↑) from recent mastoidectomy is superimposed on the density of the petrous bone.

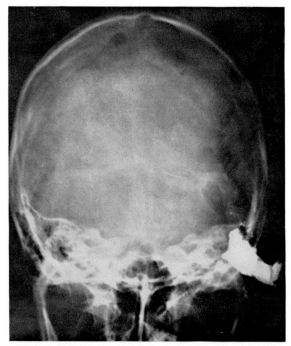

(b) Only the tegmen tympani separates the abscess cavity (large air bubble) from the middle ear (BIPP pack).

FIG. 43 Otogenic temporal lobe abscess

aspiration; 1–2 ml. of micropaque barium will enable skull X-rays after injection to show the site and size of the abscess (fig. 43). Frequently some air will be seen in the cavity, and by taking prone and supine films the full extent of the abscess can be judged. Pyograms are repeated every few days and aspiration is repeated if the outline becomes larger or smoother on the pyogram, or if the clinical condition deteriorates. Most abscesses require two or three taps, but some become crenated and shrivelled after the first tap and can be safely left. It is, however, always wise before discharging the patient to exclude an undiscovered, active loculus by air encephalography; the finding of normal lumbar CSF is also reassuring.

Early excision and decompression

Multilocular hæmatogenous and traumatic abscesses, from which often only small amounts of pus can be aspirated, are unsuitable for treatment by the above method. Excision under antibiotic cover is the only safe treatment. Occasionally an otogenic cerebellar abscess (less often a temporal) yields very little pus, yet compression is acute with a tight brain; perhaps it is still in the stage of diffuse infection prior to the formation of pus in quantity, or it is multilocular with the needle draining only one cavity. In such circumstances it is unsafe to rely on the removal of a small amount of pus, and an immediate decompression must be done. Sometimes when the dura is opened after the bone removal the brain overlying the abscess pouts out and bursts, releasing a mixture of necrotic and œdematous brain together with small amounts of pus. When this occurs the cavity must be sucked clean and irrigated with a dilute solution of penicillin (2,000 units per ml.); both meningitis and wound infection are quite unusual after such a procedure.

When no pus at all can be aspirated, yet the brain is tight, it may be advisable to perform a decompression, above or below the tentorium, and repeat the attempt to aspirate pus after a few days.

Late excision

The aspiration method of treating abscesses was introduced as a temporary measure prior to excision of the abscess, but very often the response is so satisfactory that excision is never needed. However, there is some evidence that excision of a shrivelled frontal abscess may reduce the risk of subsequent epilepsy, in spite of the brain scar which such an operation must inevitably leave. Sometimes the cavity will not collapse, perhaps because the capsule is too thick and rigid, or it repeatedly fills out again; in such circumstances excision is essential.

TREATMENT OF SUBDURAL ABSCESS

This space is difficult to drain efficiently. **Multiple burr holes** are needed because tight brain plugs off each one so that it deals with only a limited area; at least three holes should be made on each side, one of which is parasagittal in order to reach pus collecting alongside the falx. As when evacuating a subdural hæmatoma, the brain is depressed with a blunt instrument to allow pus to escape. When as much as possible has been sucked and irrigated away a fine rubber catheter (Jacques 3 or 4) is stitched in place, the burr hole incision being stitched up round it, and six-hourly irrigation with 5 cc. of weak penicillin (2,000 u. per ml.) instituted. If progress is satisfactory these tubes can be removed after 3 or 4 days. Massive doses of systemic antibiotics must be given in addition to intrathecal injections. Because the organism is usually a streptococcus, which is always sensitive, the response is normally satisfactory, but there remain the dangers of loculated collections of pus, and of intractable epilepsy. Further burr holes will be needed if progress is arrested or new signs develop; satisfactory drainage may be effected only by turning a large bone flap. This may be required at the outset, as a decompression, if the brain is very tight.

Extradural abscess is usually discovered when infected bone is removed, and the excision of the affected bone is all that is required to prevent re-collection, providing the primary condition is adequately treated.

MORTALITY AND SEQUELAE

Since antibiotics the mortality has fallen from about 50% to around 10%. Early recurrences are almost certainly due to untreated loculi rather than recrudescence of infection. Recovery is usually satisfactory after brain abscess, but subdural abscess may leave residual hemiplegia or dysphasia; occasionally ataxia persists after cerebellar abscess. Epilepsy is the most troublesome sequel, and follows in a third to a half of all abscesses above the tentorium; this risk is greater after frontal than after temporal lobe abscess and is common also after subdural suppuration.

Meningitis

The neurosurgeon has many interests in meningitis. He must be ready to recognise it when it mimics intracranial tumour or abscess or subarachnoid hæmorrhage; to deal with post-operative meningitis; to treat the primary lesions underlying secondary and recurrent pyogenic meningitis; and to manage certain complications of meningitis.

CLASSIFICATION

Pyogenic meningitis

This is of most surgical interest, and is often secondary to another condition such as a *local abscess*, either intracranial or in the mastoid or air sinuses. Meningitis may precede or follow intracranial abscess, but the two sometimes develop together when infection spreads from ear or sinus disease. Organisms may spread *by the blood stream* from a more distant focus such as pneumonia or a boil.

Recurrent pyogenic meningitis always raises suspicion of a dural defect, either *traumatic* following anterior fossa or petrous fracture (p. 253) or due to a *congenital sinus*, an inconspicuous skin hole over a spinal or posterior fossa dermoid, or due to one of the causes of *spontaneous* (i.e. *non-traumatic*) *rhinorrhœa* or *otorrhœa*. These include osteoma or mucocœle of the air sinuses which erode locally; chronic hydrocephalus from any cause (p. 308); radiation hypophysectomy with simultaneous destruction of bone and dura over the sphenoidal sinus and the diaphragma sellæ; and infective cholesteatomatous erosion of the petrous and overlying middle or posterior fossa dura.

Post-operative meningitis can develop after any neurosurgical procedure. Probably all wounds are bacteriologically contaminated when they are closed, but the body can deal with this in most cases. After prolonged procedures (>4 hours) contamination begins to be more serious, whilst excessive blood clot or necrotic tissue, which have no power to resist active invasion, also predispose to infection. A particular threat exists when operation is followed by a CSF leak, either directly through the wound after the dura of the posterior fossa has been left open and intracranial pressure remains high, or as rhinorrhœa after operation on pituitary or basal anterior fossa tumours. Nasal polypectomy and mastoidectomy may occasionally cause dural damage and lead to meningitis.

The commonest **organism** (taking all cases of pyogenic meningitis) is still the *meningococcus*, which causes a disease entity that is readily recognisable and largely confined to children. *Pneumococcal* infection results from otitis media, dural defects in the anterior fossa and from pneumonia. *Staphylococcal* meningitis commonly comes from a skin focus, and may be confined to the spinal meninges, sometimes as a complication of lumbar epidural abscess. *Streptococci* invade the meninges secondary to subdural abscess, usually the result of spread from sinusitis. *Hæmophilus influenzæ* infection is largely confined to children under 4, and the ear is the commonest primary source. *B. coli* causes meningitis in the early weeks of infancy, probably due to blood stream spread from the bowel. *Mixed infections*, frequently including Gram negative organisms and saprophytes of low virulence, characterise post-operative and otogenic infections; B. proteus, pyocycaneous, micrococci and staphylococcus albus are among those most often found.

Antibiotics are so commonly given for the preceding infection or for the preliminary symptoms of the meningitis that no organisms can be cultured from almost a quarter of patients with frankly turbid CSF teeming with polymorphs.

Primary specific meningitis

These are lymphocytic as a rule, less dramatic in onset and often more benign in outcome than pyogenic infections. **Viral** causes are many including *polio-encephalitis* due to a variety of polio-like viruses which may be cultured from CSF or bowel; meningitis may be the sole sign of infection in non-paralytic cases during an epidemic of polio. *Benign lymphocytic choriomeningitis* is characterised by a high cell count in CSF (up to 3000), but the patient is not as ill as would be expected if the infection were pyogenic or tuberculous.

Tuberculous meningitis (TBM) is an important condition to recognise since the results of treatment, if begun early enough, are good. When it complicates frank miliary infection or Pott's disease of the spine the diagnosis is obvious, but most often it develops as an insidious illness. Culture of CSF for tubercle bacilli is essential in every case of lymphocytic or chronic meningitis.

Aseptic meningitis

This term is sometimes applied when a CSF pleocytosis, usually lymphocytic, is associated with a sterile culture. The possibility of this being due to TBM, or to partly controlled pyogenic infection, must always be considered carefully because these are treatable conditions. Most of those previously regarded as suffering from **primary** aseptic meningitis probably had some kind of virus infection.

Secondary aseptic meningitis is largely overlapped by the term "chemical" meningitis. Any foreign material introduced into the CSF pathways is liable to provoke a meningeal reaction which at times may be clinically obvious with meningism, pyrexia and pleocytosis. Air or positive-contrast medium injected for radiological purposes, intrathecal antibiotics, blood and necrotic tissue after operation, all may give rise to a sterile meningitis which must be distinguished from true infection.

DIAGNOSIS

Meningitis is not always obvious. **Infantile** cases show few typical signs, but this diagnosis must be suspected whenever a child is drowsy and irritable for no obvious cause, or an infection responds poorly or relapses, or unexplained convulsions occur. **TBM** in both children and adults is insidious in onset; personality change, vomiting, constipation and headache make up the common complaints, none of which by itself might arouse suspicion of meningitis.

Pyogenic meningitis may strike so suddenly that coma supervenes within hours; but if infection is confined to the spinal meninges the CSF may be purulent without either disturbance of consciousness or even headache. Mild, aborted or arrested cases are common now that antibiotics are so freely given, and the possibility must be considered whenever an infection in the neighbourhood of the meninges unaccountably lingers or relapses.

Because of this inconsistency in clinical appearance, and the importance of instituting early treatment, lumbar puncture must be performed without delay whenever there is any possibility of meningitis. It provides the exception to the caution counselled against lumbar puncture after head injury and during the management of brain abscess. If there is concern about the risks on account of raised pressure a burr hole must be made first, and it will then be available for intraventricular therapy if needed. Not only is lumbar puncture required to diagnose meningitis, but it must be repeated to assess progress.

The pressure is usually raised, and the fluid, if containing more than 1,000 white cells per ml., is turbid. Pyogenic infection leads to high cell counts. It is less easy when there are only a few hundred lymphocytes, such as occur in TBM, to distinguish between a meningeal reaction to an intracranial abscess and low-grade meningitis. The CSF sugar is abnormally low in meningitis, especially in TBM in which the chlorides are also low. A very high protein suggests either an abscess or a CSF block. An immediate Gram smear must be made, and cultures put up under ærobic, anærobic and microærophilic conditions. Tubercle bacilli must be looked for in the smear of the centrifuged fluid—it may be a long time before even one bacillus is seen but this one is enough to clinch the diagnosis.

Although laboratory tests are essential for choosing the appropriate antibiotic, and for following progress, treatment must be started without waiting for bacteriological confirmation if the fluid is frankly turbid. Better treat an aseptic meningitis unnecessarily than reduce the chances of recovery from pyogenic or tuberculous meningitis by delaying treatment; hours may count in an acutely developing pyogenic case which deserves similar priority to a surgical emergency.

TREATMENT

Success depends on achieving a sufficient concentration of the correct antibiotic in the CSF, on treating any primary focus of infection, and on recognising and treating complications such as subdural effusions, spinal block and hydrocephalus.

Some antibiotics reach satisfactory levels in the CSF after systemic administration, particularly if high doses are given (e.g. 10–20 megaunits daily intravenously of penicillin). CSF levels are often higher than expected from experiments on normal tissues because the blood-brain barrier is altered by inflammation. However, intrathecal treatment should be started immediately in most pyogenic cases but can usually be discontinued once a satisfactory response is obtained. Provided solutions are properly prepared and buffered there is no danger from intrathecal antibiotics in the appropriate dosage—but this should be carefully checked. Commonly used are crystalline penicillin 20,000 units in 5 ml., or a vial of neonatal ampiclox (50 mg. ampicillin + 25 mg. cloxacillin).

The initial choice of antibotic must rest on the probability of a particular organism being responsible for the infection, having regard to the primary site incriminated. When there are no leads penicillin intrathecally and systemically, with the addition of sulphadimidine by mouth, probably provide the best cover with the least risk. If infection is serious, as judged by convulsions or coma and very turbid fluid, sulphonamide is best given by intravenous drip (6 gms. dissolved in the first litre of saline, and thereafter 4 gms., giving 2·5 litres in 24 hours). Levels of sulpha in CSF must be checked and should reach 12–15 mg./100 ml., although these may be achieved only at the price of some toxicity: bluish lips from sulphahæmoglobinæmia, mild confusion, abdominal distension with paralytic ileus and, rarely, crystalluria and hæmaturia. Ileus may necessistate the reduction of dosage.

Tuberculous meningitis calls for long term treatment with antituberculous drugs.

If meningitis due to a sensitive organism is being properly treated, the response should be rapid and unequivocal. Although clinical improvement is encouraging the only reliable **index of response** is the cell count in the CSF. If for some reason intrathecal treatment is not employed, repeated punctures must still be done, and immediate reports obtained on the fluid so that treatment can be modified as required. Meningitis can no more be treated safely without daily laboratory service than can diabetic coma. The cell count in pyogenic cases should fall from thousands to hundreds within 48 hours; should it fail to do so, or rise again after an initial reduction, treatment must be reviewed. A different antibiotic may be indicated by *in vitro* sensitivity tests, but these must not be taken as absolute criteria because many cases have been cured by high dosage of drugs to which resistance has been demonstrated.

Persisting or recurring pleocytosis does not always call for change of antibiotic; it may be that the primary condition requires treatment or that complications have developed. In a few cases it seems that prolonged therapy is irritating the meninges and maintaining a high cell count, and if the patient appears well by all other criteria it may be wise to stop all treatment and repeat the puncture after a few days.

Control of meningitis may depend on prompt **treatment of the primary condition.**

Profuse leakage of CSF may make it impossible to maintain an effective concentration of antibiotic in the CSF, and so call for early dural repair. A local source of infection, commonly mastoid disease or a brain abscess, may keep meningitis active by continually reinfecting the subarachnoid space, and this also calls for early surgery. Even if the meningitis is satisfactorily controlled without difficulty, surgery for any of these conditions should be delayed for only a week or so after recovery. No patient should go home with untreated mastoid disease or a dural defect after an attack of meningitis; he may decide not to come back for an operation, or defer it until a further and fatal attack of meningitis makes it too late.

COMPLICATIONS

Subdural effusions frequently complicate meningitis in children under the age of 4, and poor response to treatment or a bulging fontanelle call for a subdural tap. The fluid is yellow with a high protein content, but is rarely infected and does not become purulent. Its effect seems to be mechanical, like that of an infantile subdural hæmatoma and it requires the same treatment.

Spinal block, though characteristic of TBM, may occur with any organism if treatment is inadequate and partly controlled infection persists. Exudate accumulates in the basal cisterns and the spinal subarachnoid space and prevents intrathecal antibiotics from diffusing; this further diminishes the effectiveness of treatment. A block is suspected if lumbar puncture pressure becomes low while the protein level rises out of proportion to the cells. In the early stages, with active meningitis, a few days of treatment by the intraventricular route frequently controls the infection and the block may then resolve.

Epilepsy is particularly liable to develop in young children, and the outlook is considerably worse when this occurs. Not only do fits tend to develop in the more severely affected cases, but there is a risk of status epilepticus with its own considerable mortality. All epilepsy must therefore be treated vigorously (p. 268).

Late sequelæ are unusual. Even after intense meningitis a complete recovery without any intellectual or physical impairment is the rule, because the brain is very resistant to infection from the surface. Danger arises chiefly from arteritis of superficial vessels causing infarction, the focal signs of which may persist. In the brain stem infarcts may be responsible for a fatal outcome. Late hydrocephalus may develop due to permanent adhesions obstructing the various narrows—aqueduct, outlet of fourth ventricle or the basal cisterns.

Encephalitis

Non-pyogenic encephalitis is a fairly common provisional diagnosis in patients admitted to a Neurosurgical Unit for investigation of acute illness. In over 40% this diagnosis proves to be mistaken and half of these patients prove to have intracranial conditions requiring surgery, such as abscess, tumour and hæmorrhage. Of those finally diagnosed as encephalitis the causative virus is identified or strongly suspected in less than a third, herpes simplex being by far the commonest. Many of those in which the diagnosis remains unconfirmed follow a mild course with complete recovery.

Herpes simplex

The severe and frequently fatal encephalitis which results from invasion of the brain by this virus takes two forms: a fulminating disseminated infection in young infants who also have generalised visceral involvement, and, in older children and adults, acute necrotising encephalitis (ANE). In this latter condition the temporal lobes may be selectively and asymmetrically affected, so that a local space-occupying lesion is closely simulated. It is these cases of ANE, and those of acute hæmorrhagic leuco-encephalitis, which most often reach surgical units for investigation. Most patients are dead within 10–14 days of the onset of symptoms, which is usually abrupt. Headache, confusion and pyrexia are constant and there is usually some degree of hemiparesis, dysphasia or epilepsy to indicate involvement of one hemisphere. In the CSF the protein is raised, there is lymphocytosis and sometimes blood; occasionally atypical and primitive inflammatory cells are found.

A diagnosis has to be reached rapidly not only because other surgical conditions must be excluded, but because it is now possible to treat herpes simplex encephalitis successfully providing the diagnosis is made before necrosis is too advanced. The EEG is always abnormal, showing generalised slowing together with multiple focal abnormalities. Contrast radiology may show swelling of one hemisphere, particularly affecting the temporal lobe, and associated with lateral shift. A firm diagnosis at this stage depends on brain biopsy which should be carried out without delay on the temporal lobe which appears from all the evidence to be most affected; in cases of doubt bilateral biposies should be obtained. In severe cases liquefied necrotic brain will be aspirated and may be mistaken for pus. Immediate examination of the smears will show inflammatory infiltration with large mononucleurs, lymphocytes and plasma cells; if any neurones are identified necrosis may be obvious. This is good enough evidence to begin treatment but some brain tissue should also be sent to a virology laboratory in special transport medium; positive culture may be obtained in 48 hours or so. Confirmation may also come later from a rising titre of herpes anti-body in the blood, based on specimens taken at an interval of 10 days. Virus particles may subsequently be demonstrated by electron microscopy of the biopsy specimen.

Treatment with anti-viral agents is undergoing controlled trial, but dramatic effects are not yet evident. Decompression by hypertonic solutions or by operation may be life-saving, because some fatal cases have shown tentorial pressure cones due to temporal lobe swelling; however, survivors may be severely disabled from the widespread brain damage.

Post-infectious encephalitis, occurring after the common viral diseases such as measles and mumps is probably an immunological type of response, causing demyelination. As a result recovery may be rapid and this may be accelerated or initiated by giving ACTH or cortico-steroids. Measles is also incriminated as one of the causes of **sub-acute sclerosing encephalitis**, a chronic condition causing severe dementia and involuntary movements in children. It is associated with a very char-acteristic EEG pattern, all channels showing slowing and flattening but with repeated stereotyped high voltage complexes. Biopsy will confirm the diagnosis.

Osteomyelitis of the skull

This most often results from the local spread of infection from the middle ear or frontal sinus. It gives rise to no particular clinical features distinct from those associated with infection in these sites.

Osteomyelitis of the vault may develop after trauma, either accidental or operative. The scalp may become infected first and the bone is secondarily involved. More often the wound heals by first intention but then a swelling develops followed by a discharging sinus in the line of the wound. The discharge of rather watery pus persists and granu-lations form round the mouth of the sinus; a probe leads directly on to bare bone. The patient remains well and the sinus may heal for short periods, only to break down again. For several weeks X-rays show no abnormality but eventually irregular rarefaction appears, perhaps with areas of dense bone where sequestra have formed.

Treatment consists of removing the affected bone; until this is done local and systemic antibiotics are of little avail. Post-operative osteo-myelitis is seldom cured by nibbling the bone immediately under the sinus; it is best to remove the whole bone flap, which will usually be found irregularly eroded on its deep surface over a wide area (fig. 29). Granulations cover the dura which itself is almost never breached. Once the bone flap is removed the wound usually heals quickly and the infection does not recur. The bone may be preserved in the deep freezing compartment of a refrigerator after it has been cleaned of granulations and sterilised, either by boiling or exposing to irradiation. Each of these procedures kills the bone by denaturing the proteins, but the flap may still be replaced after 3 to 6 months and will form a frame-work for the body to build up a new segment of skull.

Occasionally osteomyelitis of the vault arises after closed trauma, from blood-borne organisms infecting a pericranial hæmatoma. A tender boggy swelling then forms, known as "Pott's puffy tumour". When a very wide area of the skull is involved it may not seem desirable to attempt to remove it completely; the contour of the skull may be preserved and the infection controlled if numerous burr holes are made, perhaps ten or twenty, to allow drainage of extradural pus. If the external table is more extensively involved it may be nibbled away between the burr holes, leaving open diploe.

Specific infection of the nervous system

Tuberculoma is the least rare of these, but in Great Britain is very much less common than in countries such as Spain and South America where it forms one of the common intracranial masses. Frank tuberculous infection elsewhere is unusual, and most cases are investigated and treated as tumours, the diagnosis being made at operation or by the pathologist. The cerebellar hemisphere is the commonest site. Many become inactive and calcify, but others terminate by producing TBM. Excision is now much safer than previously when post-operative meningitis kept the mortality at almost 50%.

Hydatid cysts in the brain present as neoplasms. In areas where the disease is common hydatid may be suspected if there are chest shadows in addition. Excision requires special care to avoid rupturing the cyst and spilling scolices which start fresh daughter cysts.

FURTHER READING

Adams, J. H. and Jennett, W. B. (1967). Acute necrotising encephalitis: a problem in diagnosis. *Journal of Neurology, Neurosurgery and Psychiatry*, **30**, 248–260.

Alphen, H. A. M. and Dreissen, J. J. R. (1976). Brain abscess and subdural empyema —factors influencing mortality and results of various surgical techniques. *Journal of Neurology, Neurosurgery and Psychiatry*. **39**, 481–490.

Beeden, A. G., Marsen, C. D., Meadows, J. C. and Michael, W. F. (1969). Intracranial complications of middle ear disease and mastoid surgery. *Journal of Neurological Sciences*, **9**, 261–272.

Beller, A. J., Sahar, A. and Praiss, I. (1973). Brain abscess—review of 89 cases over 30 years. *Journal of Neurology, Neurosurgery and Psychiatry*, **36**, 757–768.

Donald, G. and McKendrick, W. (1968). The treatment of pyogenic meningitis. *Journal of Neurology, Neurosurergy and Psychiatry*, **31**, 528–530.

Fallon, R. J. (1972). Bacterial infections of the central nervous system. In: *Scientific Foundations of Neurology*. pp. 451–459. Eds. Critchley, O'Leary and Jennett. Heinemann, London.

Garfield, J. (1969). Management of supratentorial intracranial abscess: a review of 200 cases. *British Medical Journal*, **2**, 7–11.

Martin, G. (1973). Non-otogenic cerebral abscess. *Journal of Neurology, Neurosurgery and Psychiatry*, **36**, 607–610.

Miller, J. D. and Ross, C. A. C. (1968). Encephalitis—a four year survey. *Lancet*, **i**, 1121–1126.

Ommaya, A. K., Di Chiro, G., Baldwin, M. and Pennybacker, J. B. (1968). Nontraumatic cerebrospinal fluid rhinorrhoea. *Journal of Neurology, Neurosurgery, and Psychiatry*, **31**, 214–225.

Price, D. J. E. and Sleigh, J. D. (1970). Control of infection due to Klebsiella aerogenes in a neurosurgical unit by the withdrawal of all antibiotics. *Lancet*, **ii**, 1213–1215.

Raimondi, A. J., Matsumoto, S. and Miller, R. A. (1965). Brain abscess in children with congenital heart disease. *Journal of Neurosurgery*, **23**, 588–595.

Tutton, G. K. (1953). Cerebral abscess—the present position. *Annals of the Royal College of Surgeons of England*, **13**, 281–311.

Wright, R. L. and Ballantine, H. T. (1967). Management of brain abscesses in children and adolescents. *American Journal of Diseases of Children*, **114**, 113–122.

CHAPTER 11

Surgery for Vascular Lesions

Subarachnoid hæmorrhage

Intracranial aneurysms

Angioma

Primary intracranial hæmorrhage

Occlusive cerebro-vascular disease

In a significant number of patients suffering from cerebrovascular accident or stroke, radiological investigations can indicate the underlying lesion, which may be suitable for surgical treatment. These include many patients with subarachnoid haemorrhage, due to aneurysm or angioma; some with primary intracerebral haemorrhage; and a few with ischæmic strokes—in effect the young patients who have stenosis of the cervical carotid artery. Radiology has taught that clinical criteria are unreliable in distinguishing between even the broadest categories of strokes.

These categories can be readily identified on a pathological basis as follows:

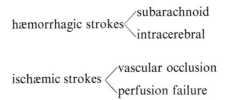

Hæmorrhagic strokes usually cause headache, and often clouding of consciousness or even coma, at the onset; ischæmic strokes are frequently painless and, if due to local vascular occlusion, cause focal signs related to the deprived area—a blind eye, a weak arm or dysphasia. Swelling of a large infarct may lead to headache and depression of consciousness after 24 hours or so, due to raised intracranial pressure and mid-brain shift and distortion.

HÆMORRHAGIC STROKES

Subarachnoid Hæmorrhage

Pathology

Most fatal cases of subarachnoid hæmorrhage prove to be due to ruptured aneurysm. But angiography fails to reveal any abnormality in some 30–40% of patients; most of these recover and have no further hæmorrhage; and the cause of hæmorrhage in such cases remains unknown. Aneurysm is the most frequent discoverable cause, although it accounts for only 40–50% of all cases. The next commonest cause is arteriovenous malformation; a few cases are due to intracranial tumours of various kinds, and, rarely, to blood dyscrasias.

Clinical

There is seldom an obvious precipitating cause of rupture, which is as likely to happen during relaxation as at the height of physical activity. The onset is usually sudden. When there is a considerable escape of blood from a large tear consciousness is rapidly lost. Recovery of consciousness may be quite rapid or the patient may remain deeply comatose; he may die within minutes or hours. Smaller leaks give less dramatic symptoms, severe headache being the most usual complaint. This is almost always followed within minutes or hours by vomiting, and later by neck stiffness. Meningitis may be suspected and result in admission to a fever hospital. Consciousness is often clouded but the illness may be so mild as to be mistaken for influenza or migraine. When a patient has a major hæmorrhage careful enquiry often reveals a minor incident in the recent past suggestive of, but not diagnosed as, subarachnoid hæmorrhage. In patients who remain ambulant lumbago and sciatica may develop due to the irritant effect of blood which has settled in the lumbar cul-de-sac of the subarachnoid space.

Headache is usual but not invariable. Commonly it comes on suddenly, and is either generalised or felt in the back of the neck, but occasionally it begins in one area and rapidly spreads. Pain limited to one eye suggests an ipilateral carotid aneurysm. **Vomiting** is almost invariable. **Neck stiffness** is also usual but may not appear until the second or third day and occasionally not at all; photophabia commonly develops sooner. Confirmation of the diagnosis rests on **lumbar puncture** though blood does not always appear in the lumbar fluid immediately. When CSF is very heavily bloodstained there may be doubt as to whether a blood vessel rather than the theca has been punctured by the needle; no matter how heavy the contamination blood in CSF does not clot. Red cells normally disappear in 9 days, but may go sooner after a small bleed. Xanthochromia of the CSF appears in 24 hours, sometimes sooner, and persists for a week or more, enabling a retrospective diagnosis to be made. This is important evidence in favour of a genuine hæmorrhage as against accidental contamination with blood. It should invariably be looked for either by centrifuging the fluid or allowing it to settle.

Clinical grades were proposed by Botterell as a means of indicating the overall state of the patient with recent subarachnoid hæmorrhage, particularly in regard to assessing suitability for surgery; Hunt and Hess have amended Botterell's system—and although neither is wholly satisfactory each is quite widely used both practically and in reporting results of surgery for ruptured aneurysm.

Focal CNS signs are not always a reliable indicator of the site or even the side of the lesion responsible especially when the hæmorrhage has been severe. Minor signs, such as an extensor plantar response, are of little value, and even hemiplegia may result from an intracerebral hæmatoma extending far from the ruptured vessel. Vascular spasm, embolism and thrombosis can develop in cerebral vessels remote from the lesion and give rise to bizarre and misleading signs. However, a marked hemiplegia with only a moderate hæmorrhage frequently proves to be due to a middle cerebral aneurysm. Isolated third nerve palsy associated with mild hæmorrhage is usually due to an aneurysm on the posterior communicating artery, but after severe hæmorrhage from any lesion brain shift can cause a tentorial cone and secondary third nerve palsy.

Management

Because of the possibility of finding an operable lesion such as an aneurysm or arteriovenous malformation, angiography is now always advised once the patient has recovered sufficiently to be likely to be fit for surgery. Because the risk of a second rupture from an aneurysm is so high in the first two weeks this investigation should then be carried out as soon as possible. Techniques employed are discussed in relation to ruptured aneurysm.

Prognosis

This depends entirely on the causative lesion. The mortality quoted for "subarachnoid hæmorrhage" proves often in reality to be that of ruptured aneurysm. As some 30–40% of cases of subarachnoid hæmorrhage have a negative angiogram and most of these survive the overall mortality of subarachnoid hæmorrhage is appreciably lower than that quoted for ruptured aneurysm.

Intracranial aneurysms

ÆTIOLOGY

The majority of saccular aneurysms are referred to as *congenital* in contrast to the less common fusiform *arteriosclerotic* dilatations, and the rare *mycotic* aneurysms associated with inflammatory lesions such as subacute bacterial endocarditis and polyarteritis nodosa. But it is only the predisposition to form aneurysms at the main junctions of the circle of Willis that appears to be developmentally determined, and aneurysms are rarely found in the course of post-mortems in children.

Deficiencies in the muscle coat of the main cerebral vessels tend to occur at junctions because the muscle of the main trunk and of the branch are separately developed and may fail to join. Other structural peculiarities of the normal cerebral vessels are the poorly developed media, compared with other arteries of similar size, and the concentration of all the elastic elements in the internal elastic lamina where they can be destroyed by a single patch of degeneration. Development of aneurysms is therefore related to many factors, including congenital and acquired weakness in the artery wall, together with the stresses imposed by local hæmodynamics and surges of systemic hypertension—either physiological or pathological.

These **anatomical anomalies** are the inheritance of the whole population, yet less than 1% develop aneurysms. Other factors must play a part, the most obvious being arterial degeneration and systemic hypertension. These exert their influence over a period of time, and angiograms repeated after an interval of years have shown that tiny vascular bulges can develop into fully formed aneurysms.

Arteriosclerosis in the circle of Willis appears in an increasing proportion of the population after the age of 20. In one series of ruptured aneurysms the incidence of severe coronary atheroma was much higher than in a control group of similar age, suggesting that these patients were prone to premature arterial degeneration.

Hypertension might be expected to accentuate any vascular weakness; patients with coarctation of the aorta, who have high arterial pressure in the carotico-vertebral system are liable to develop ruptured cerebral aneurysms at an unusually early age. But hypertension is certainly not a necessary causative factor either for the development or for the rupture of aneurysms; only half the cases in a recent large series had a pressure of more than 160/90 mm. Hg. Readings taken soon after rupture may be high, due to the hæmorrhage, which may also cause temporary abnormalities in the ECG (suggestive of myocardial ischæmia). This combination may be mistakenly regarded as supporting a diagnosis of hypertensive heart disease; it is due to sympathetic discharge and release of catecholamines.

Anomalous development of the circle of Willis is more frequent in patients with aneurysms; it may cause unusual strain on certain parts of the system, and may account for the occasional occurrence of bilaterally symmetrical aneurysms.

SITE

The majority of aneurysms occur in a few constant situations on the circle of Willis and most are on the anterior half of the circle (fig. 42). About a third of those that rupture are on the **anterior communicating** or proximal anterior cerebral artery; they may derive their blood supply from either or both internal carotids and are so situated that rupture may occur into either frontal lobe. **Middle cerebral** artery aneurysms are rather less common, and usually occur at the trifurcation, about 2 cm. lateral to its origin from the internal carotid. In women the aneurysm sometimes develops on a more proximal branch, and so lies among the perforating arteries. The **internal carotid** is itself the site of a similar proportion of aneurysms. Three main groups occur: at the origin of the posterior communicating artery (so-called **posterior communicating artery** aneurysms), at the terminal bifurcation, and in the cavernous sinus. **Pericallosal** artery aneurysms do occur, but are unusual. Half the posterior fossa aneurysms are on the **basilar** artery, most often at the terminal bifurcation into posterior cerebral arteries; some are on the **vertebral artery** or on its last branch, the **posterior**

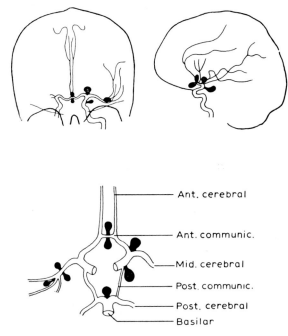

FIG. 44 Common sites for aneurysms

inferior cerebellar artery, and these may go undetected if both vertebral arteries are not seen on angiograms. Fusiform arteriosclerotic dilatation of the basilar is commoner than a saccular aneurysm.

About 10–15% of patients have more than one aneurysm, sometimes symmetrically disposed. The first aneurysm displayed by angiography may not therefore be the only one, nor necessarily the one which has ruptured.

NATURAL HISTORY

Most aneurysms **grow larger** with time: serial angiograms leave no doubt about this. Adhesions develop, to neighbouring structures, to other arteries, and to the brain in which the aneurysm can become so buried that no part remains in the subarachnoid space. Secondary dilatations may develop and patchy thrombosis lays down layers of clot; the irregular lumen which still fills with circulating blood, and which is all an angiogram can show, then represents only a fraction of the whole sac and bears little relation to its external shape.

Aneurysms usually become clinically obvious only when intra-cerebral or subarachnoid **rupture** occurs, but occasionally the sac is large enough to produce local pressure effects. Most aneurysms above the cavernous sinus eventually rupture, most often when they are about the size of a pea; if they become larger without rupture, stagnant blood near the edge of the sac may thrombose and reinforce the wall. The fundus gives way in most instances, the neck very seldom. If the aneurysm is buried in the brain the hæmorrhage will be intracerebral although blood may later reach the subarachnoid space via the ventricular system.

Intracerebral hæmatoma frequently follows rupture of a middle cerebral or anterior communicating artery aneurysm. Either frontal or temporal lobe hæmatomas may rupture into the ventricle, and the distension of the third and fourth ventricles probably contributes to the coma, mutism and hyperpyrexia which occur in some cases.

Cerebral infarction commonly develops after rupture of an aneurysm, and is invariably discovered in fatal cases. Large areas of cerebral cortex supplied by main vessels may be affected; but it is probably the involvement of the basal ganglia and hypothalamus, supplied by the perforating vessels, which proves fatal.

Infarction results from a combination of factors: local arterial *spasm* resulting from mechanical irritation of vessels by subarachnoid blood, or by vasoactive substances released locally; vascular *occlusion* from without, by an expanding aneurysm, or by clot; and *embolism* from thrombi formed during the period of vascular stasis caused by the two preceding factors.

Hydrocephalus, probably to impaired CFS absorption, sometimes develops soon after subarrachnoid hæmorrhage—and the clinical state may improve after shunting.

Intracavernous aneurysms are protected as they enlarge by the dural walls of the cavernous sinus, and consequently they rarely rupture. Occasionally, when still small, one does burst into the cavernous sinus giving rise to a caroticocavernous (arteriovenous) fistula, similar to that produced by trauma (p. 261).

SYNDROME DUE TO UNRUPTURED ANEURYSM

Local neurological dysfunction from distortion of neighbouring structures by the sac is largely limited to aneurysms of the internal carotid. Those which arise within the **cavernous sinus** are most common in middle-aged women; the usual complaint is of pain, and later sensory loss, in one or more divisions of the trigeminal nerve, together with ocular palsies (3, 4, 6 cranial nerves). Although symptoms characteristically begin or increase suddenly the onset can be insidious, exactly resembling a tumour; erosion of the clinoid processes seen on X-ray may be indistinguishable from changes produced by a sellar or parasellar tumour.

Aneurysms at the bifurcation of the **internal carotid** artery are often directed forwards. They may then produce symptoms resembling a pituitary tumour with visual failure, field defects and optic atrophy. Endocrine deficiency is unusual, but the sella may be eroded on X-ray.

Aneurysms arising at the point of origin of the **posterior communicating artery** are usually directed backwards and may cause pressure on the trunk of the third nerve. This leads to varying degrees of oculomotor palsy (dilated pupil, external strabismus and ptosis) sometimes accompanied by supraorbital pain but without trigeminal sensory loss.

ANGIOGRAPHY

Most recurrent hæmorrhages occur in the first fortnight, and the longer angiography is delayed the greater the chance of a second hæmorrhage, for which nothing can be done as long as the primary lesion is unidentified. Any risk of aggravating the patient's condition by angiography is outweighed by the danger of remaining in ignorance of the site and nature of the underlying pathology.

Angiograms should be performed as soon as it is clear that the patient will survive the initial hæmorrhage, provided he is not mute and akinetic and therefore unlikely to survive an operation. If he is unfit for surgery there is little to be gained from angiography, although the possibility that an intracerebral hæmatoma may be in part accounting for the clinical state should be considered; an EMI scan would be the safest way to exclude this. Should a large clot be discovered and evacuated the patient's condition may so improve that it becomes possible to consider operating on his aneurysm.

Bilateral carotid angiography should be done in most cases because even if an aneurysm is discovered on the first side injected, and is thought likely to be the source of hæmorrhage, the treatment may be influenced by information gained about the opposite carotid system. Multiple aneurysms may be found (fig. 47), and if one is inoperable it may be less justifiable to take considerable risks in the attempt to cure any of the others. On the other hand if one aneurysm is amenable to treatment only by common carotid ligation then some alternative must be sought for any aneurysms on the other side. Bilateral angiography will also reveal the relative contribution of blood flow from each carotid to an anterior communicating aneurysm (fig. 45); this may determine the operative approach. Visualisation of the whole circle of Willis is probably best achieved by femoral cathetisation, and selective injection of the separate neck vessels.

Apart from revealing the source of bleeding angiography sometimes shows an intracranial *hæmatoma*, usually intracerebral, which may require evacuation even though definitive surgery for the aneurysm is

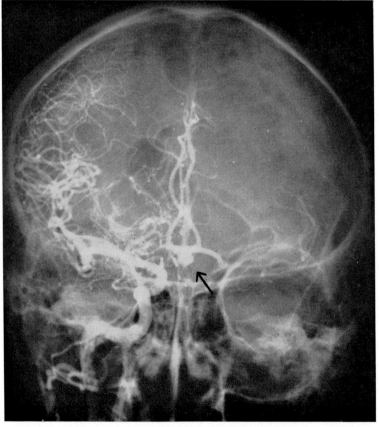

FIG. 45 Anterior communicating artery aneurysm
Sac projects downwards from an unusually large parent artery.

to be delayed. Vascular *spasm* may be recognised, irregular narrowing of the vessels in relation to the bleeding aneurysm (figs. 46, 47). If this spasm is associated with a clinical state which makes surgery doubtful it certainly strengthens the case for delaying operation. When more than one aneurysm is found the one which has bled may be recognised by the location of spasm and hæmatoma in the vicinity of one of them; localised EMI scan abnormalities may also provide evidence.

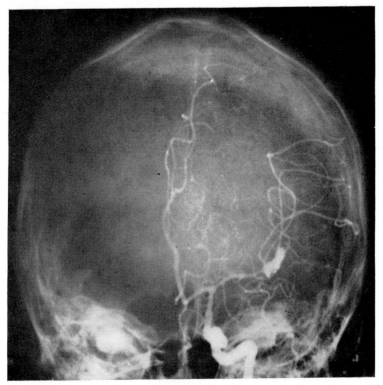

FIG. 46 Middle cerebral aneurysm with hæmatoma and spasm

Lateral displacement of anterior cerebral and upward displacement of middle cerebral indicate temporal lobe hæmatoma. Narrowing (spasm) of terminal carotid segment and horizontal part of anterior and middle cerebral arteries; distal anterior cerebral is of normal calibre.

Vertebral angiography is less likely to disclose an operable aneurysm. It should be considered in the presence of:

(i) Local symptoms and signs suggestive of a posterior fossa lesion—vertigo, nystagmus, cerebellar signs and lower cranial nerve palsies.

(ii) Multiple aneurysms shown on the carotid system—if there are still more on the vertebral system it may be judged pointless to treat any of them.

(iii) When carotid angiograms under the age of 50 either shown no aneurysm, or only an aneurysm without definite clinical or radiological evidence that it has recently ruptured.

(iv) Posteriorly situated angioma in the cerebral hemisphere, particularly if the posterior cerebral artery does not fill; there may be

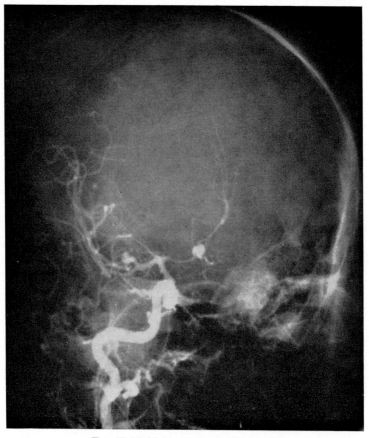

FIG. 47 Multiple aneurysms with spasm

Aneurysms on middle cerebral artery and anterior communicating artery. Marked narrowing of anterior cerebral artery from just distal to its origin.

a large contribution from the vertebral system and the lesion prove much more extensive than it appeared on the carotid angiogram.

CONSERVATIVE TREATMENT

The chances of surviving a severe hæmorrhage are now much greater than previously because the problems associated with the nursing of comatose patients are much more clearly understood. Beyond the conservation of life two positive measures may be taken in the hope of reducing the risk of early recurrent hæmorrhage. One is the reduction of an unduly high blood pressure by drugs, but this carries the risk of precipitating infarction which is already a hazard in view of vascular spasm and hæmatoma. The other is the use of anti-fibrinolytic agents, in the hope of firming up the clot which has presumably stopped the initial hæmorrhage. These do not take effect for 3–5 days, and their effect is probably not long-lasting.

In the event of operative treatment not being undertaken it is usual to keep the patient in bed for six or eight weeks in the hope that this will reduce the liability of blood pressure and so of further rupture. Once this period is over, however, it is important to encourage the patient to resume a normal life and not to impose restrictions when so little is known about the factors which precipitate rupture of an aneurysm. Pregnancy appears to increase the risk of recurrent hæmorrhage but this seldom occurs in labour. In the event of a patient with an aneurysm becoming pregnant or a pregnant patient developing subarachnoid hæmorrhage, a normal delivery at term should be suggested unless there are undue difficulties from an obstetrical viewpoint.

The **prognosis** of ruptured aneurysm without operation is of course important to know in order to assess the value of operation and yet accurate statistics are difficult to assemble. The only carefully controlled series come from neurosurgical units and these imply that the patient has survived the initial hæmorrhage sufficiently long to be transferred for investigation, and that angiograms have been completed and have shown an aneurysm. Some 20% of such patients die of the initial hæmorrhage and 40% die of a recurrent hæmorrhage within the first eight weeks. What remains unknown is how many other patients may have died at home, or at the first hospital to which they were admitted, before investigation; and how many may subsequently die of a late recurrent hæmorrhage. Some 10 or 15% of patients remain disabled, most commonly due to hemisphere disorders (hemiplegia or dysphasia) or epilepsy.

SURGICAL MEASURES FOR RUPTURED ANEURYSM

(1) Occlusion of neck of aneurysm.
(2) Reinforcement of sac.
(3) Ligation of one feeding vessel.
(4) Trapping by occlusion of feeding vessel on both sides.
(5) Induction of thrombosis in sac.

Occlusion of the neck

At present the best chance of a permanent cure appears to lie in isolating the aneurysm from its parent vessel either with a clip or by ligature. For an aneurysm neck to be safely clipped its neck should be reasonably narrow and accessible without the sacrifice of either vital brain tissue or other vessels in the vicinity. It is often difficult to decide from the angiographic appearances whether an aneurysm is suitable for clipping, and only exploration can resolve the matter. The dissection of a recently ruptured aneurysm from surrounding vessels, and from brain which is swollen and friable as a result of hæmorrhage, demands considerable skill. The morbidity and mortality of the operation diminish as the interval since the last subarachnoid hæmorrhage increases; operations in the first three days are especially hazardous. Not only may the aneurysm rupture during dissection and cause embarrassing bleeding, which may be controlled only by sacrificing important vessels, but chemical factors related to recent rupture appear to have an adverse effect locally. Permanent hemiplegia or mental changes due to frontal lobe damage can result from "successful" clipping in these circumstances, or the patient may die from hypo-thalamic damage.

Aneurysms on the anterior part of the circle are usually approached subfrontally; the carotid is identified lateral to the optic nerve, and the dissection carried medially or laterally as required, retracting the frontal and temporal lobes. The hazards of operation in the acute stage have been reduced by various techniques—controlled respiration, hypo-tension and, more recently, the use of the operating microscope. The last has been hailed as a major advance in the operative management of aneurysms, and there is no doubt that dissection of aneurysm and vital adjacent vessels and control of hæmorrhage can be done more precisely and with less need for retraction—especially if spinal drainage is also used. The bipolar coagulator and the use of sharp micro-dissection reduces the likelihood of thrombosis in adjacent vessels. Not only mortality but also morbidity may be reduced. It may be that the availability of the microscope will lead to operations being per-formed on aneurysms which would previously have been considered inoperable—and this may keep up the mortality and morbidity rate.

A month or so after rupture operation is both easier and safer but by then the risk of a recurrent hæmorrhage is also lessening; the benefits of delay must be weighed against this risk. Whenever operation is undertaken the risks vary with the site of the aneurysm. *Anterior com-municating* aneurysms are the most dangerous because they are tech-nically difficult to approach, and serious effects may ensue if the anterior cerebral arteries or their perforating branches are damaged; permanent personality changes may be the price of occlusion. Those at the tri-furcation of the *middle cerebral* are so intimately adherent to the branches that clipping is sometimes impossible without sacrifice of a branch and the risk of hemiplegia, and on the left of dysphasia. *Posterior communicating* aneurysms probably carry the least operative risk when they lie in a favourable situation.

Reinforcement of the sac

When dissection of an aneurysm reveals an anatomical arrangement which will not permit clipping, either because the sac is sessile or the branches inextricable, an attempt may be made to reinforce the wall. The sac can be wrapped with muscle, or terylene gauze or fibrin foam, or a combination of these agents. It is also possible to apply a rapidly solidifying polymer to the aneurysm which becomes closely invested with a non-yielding covering.

Proximal ligation

If dissection of the sac is thought too hazardous the main supplying vessel may be occluded proximally.

Clipping of the anterior cerebral for anterior communicating aneurysms is a comparatively simple operation, though there are risks of mental sequelæ the extent of which it is impossible to predict.

Carotid ligation in the neck is most effective for aneurysms arising directly from the internal carotid, and is the only treatment possible for sessile sacs arising from the terminal bifurcation. It is often used as an alternative to clipping for posterior communicating artery aneurysms, and as an alternative to trapping for aneurysms in the cavernous sinus.

The rationale is that the immediate risk of rupture is reduced because of the diminished pressure in the vessels above the ligature. A cure may even be effected by precipitating thrombosis in the aneurysm where blood becomes relatively stagnant due to the reduced pressure. Angiography has shown that aneurysms do sometimes disappear after ligation, and there is a marked reduction in the number of late hæmorrhages. Local pressure signs (third nerve palsy from posterior communicating aneurysm) often resolve quite soon after ligation. Usually the *common* carotid is ligated; this is probably less effective than tying the *internal* but the risk of hemiplegia is also smaller.

The *mortality and morbidity* of this simple operation result from depriving one hemisphere of an adequate blood supply. Hemiplegia is often delayed in onset, and this limits the value of trial ligation under local anæsthesia as a means of detecting those at risk. Isotope studies of cerebral blood flow (p. 74) have greatly extended understanding of intolerance of ligation, and can enable patients who are suceptible to be identified and permanent ligation avoided. These studies indicate that other measures of **tolerance** are unreliable—the EEG, evidence of angiographic cross-circulation and jugular venous oxygen during trial occlusion. Percutaneous compression of the carotid will identify those patients who are most sensitive to ligation; if the patient develops focal signs or impairment of consciousness during 5 minutes compression then it is unnecessary to proceed to more sophisticated tests. Occasionally tolerance increases as time passes since the rupture of the aneurysm, and it may be worthwhile repeating tests of tolerance after an interval.

Patients are less tolerant within 7 days of a bleed, and if they are less than Grade I.

The patient is kept flat in bed to minimise the risk of postural hypotension precipitating cerebral ischæmia in the first two or three days after operation and the blood pressure is recorded regularly and any fall promptly treated.

Trapping

Aneurysms in certain situations lend themselves to trapping, that is ligation of the artery of supply on both the proximal and distal side. Those most frequently treated in this way are aneurysms in the cavernous sinus, including the carotico-cavernous arteriovenous fistula; a clip is placed on the internal carotid artery immediately above the anterior clinoid and on the vessel in the neck just above the bifurcation.

SURGICAL RESULTS

The efficacy of surgery for ruptured aneurysm is judged by comparing survival rates after operations with those following conservative treatment. Prevention of a fatal recurrent hæmorrhage is the primary object of surgery, and as 80% of such recurrences occur within the first eight weeks a relatively short follow-up will give significant information, although the possibility of late recurrence must not be overlooked. A survivor at six months with his aneurysm clipped is obviously in a better situation than the patient who has naturally survived for that long but who still has an aneurysmal sac at risk.

Matching of comparable surgical and medical series needs to take account of many factors; it is because of these and the complex inter-relationships between them that so much difficulty has been experienced in assessing the exact value of surgery. Three categories of patient are commonly recognised:

(a) Patients in immediate danger of dying from the hæmorrhage which has led to admission to hospital. Whatever the site or other factors the poor outlook for these patients is almost certainly not improved by any form of operative surgery.

(b) Patients who are recovering from the most recent hæmorrhage and are seen within eight weeks of it; these patients are at risk from a recurrence and it is this group which the surgeon claims to help; they are discussed in greater detail below.

(c) Patients seen more than eight weeks after subarachnoid hæmorrhage, having completely recovered, and those in whom an unruptured aneurysm has been discovered. Such patients are in no immediate danger and the risk of future rupture is difficult to assess. Therefore any procedure attempted for these patients must have a low mortality and morbidity if it is to match the natural prognosis, or improve upon it. On the other hand operations in this quiescent stage are both easier and safer than in the first few weeks after rupture, and the mortality is probably less than 2% either for craniotomy or carotid ligation in these circumstances.

The factors influencing the risk of surgery in category (b) cases can be set out thus:

FACTORS AFFECTING THE RISK OF ANEURYSM SURGERY

Patient	Aneurysm	Hæmorrhage	Brain damage
Age	Site	Number of incidents	Conscious state
Sex	Side	Interval since last	Focal signs
Blood pressure	Size	Hæmatoma	Grade
Arteriopathy	Shape	Spasm	

Because there are so many variables generalisations about surgical results are of limited value, but with this proviso some overall figures may be given. Probably the most important variable is the site of the aneurysm and it is really valid to discuss only one type of aneurysm at a time; thus, **posterior communicating** artery aneurysm tends to cause very little brain damage on rupture (apart from third nerve palsy), and the results of surgery, whether by clipping or by carotid ligation, are definitely superior to those of conservative management (less than 10% mortality at six months compared with over 30% without operation). **Middle cerebral** aneurysms not infrequently cause hemiplegia (with or without dysphasia), and whether or not surgery is employed a proportion will retain some permanent disability; mortality is improved by surgery from about 30–40% to 15–25%. **Anterior communicating** aneurysms when they rupture commonly cause brain damage in the distribution of the perforating arteries supplying deep posterior frontal structures; this is often manifested by prolonged stupor followed by some degree of dementia which may be permanent, and operation tends to aggravate such damage; results are poor in patients already showing signs of persisting damage before operation, whilst some patients who are quite well before surgery suffer such damage as a result of operation. These aneurysms are technically the most difficult to deal with surgically, and unless all the factors are favourable many surgeons are reluctant to operate although the conservative mortality for "operable" cases is over 40% in six months.

Vascular spasm is believed by many to make the likelihood of post-operative infarction greater whatever the site of the aneurysm and surgery is frequently postponed until the spasm has passed off; this is in accord with the finding that the longer the interval since the rupture the lower the operative risk. But every day's delay runs the risk of a recurrent hæmorrhage; the lower surgical mortality of delayed operation must always be balanced by the number of deaths which will have occurred whilst awaiting surgery. The best guide to the patient's having reached the stage when operation can reasonably be undertaken is the conscious level; if he is still markedly confused or stuporose operation should be postponed, unless it is considered that the continuance of this state is due to a compressing hæmatoma. In that case it may be wise to evacuate the clot, without directly attacking the aneurysm, which is dealt with some days later when the patient's condition has improved. Focal signs (hemiplegia or third nerve palsy) are no reason for deferring operation if the patient is alert. The only place to make these day to day assessments is a neurosurgical unit, and only there can compression by hæmatoma be dealt with; every patient should therefore be transferred to a surgical unit for investigation and assessment once it is clear that the initial hæmorrhage will be survived, and provided there is no other factor which would absolutely contra-indicate surgery should an operable lesion be discovered.

Angioma
(angiomatous malformation, arteriovenous aneurysm)

These collections of abnormal vessels increase in size with time although they are not true tumours, but congenital malformations. One of a small tangle of abnormal capillaries ruptures to form a tiny arterio-venous fistula, and the veins then progressively enlarge as arterial blood fills them. In time the resistance in quite large vessels in the angioma may be less than that offered by normal arteries in the surrounding brain; not only does the angioma enlarge but the brain may be deprived of an adequate blood supply and chronic ischæmia develop.

Most angiomas (90%) occur in the cerebral hemispheres, the majority in the parietal or occipital lobes. About half reach the cortical surface, but may do so only on the medial aspect of the hemisphere. The Sturge–Weber syndrome is a rare form consisting of a capillary angioma confined to the meninges in association with a superficial angiomatous malformation (port-wine nævus of skin or bucconasal mucosa, or uveal or conjuctival angioma). The cerebral cortex underlying the meningeal abnormality may suffer gliosis and calcification, which may be detected radiologically. Angiomas sometimes affect the brain stem and cerebellum.

Most of these lesions eventually rupture and *hæmorrhage*, either intracerebral or subarachnoid, is the initial symptom in more than a third; they account for only 10% of subarachnoid bleeds. The immediate and ultimate outlook is considerably better than for ruptured aneurysm, and even after repeated hæmorrhage many patients with angioma have little disability. Large malformations seem less likely to bleed recurrently than small ones. *Epilepsy* is the initial symptom in a quarter of the cases, and by the time the diagnosis is made half the patients have had one or more fits, which are usually focal; because angiomas are commonly situated in the posterior part of the hemisphere these are often sensory. *Migrainous headaches* occur in less than a fifth of cases and are not always relieved by removal of the angioma; a family history of migraine is common in patients with angioma, even in those who do not themselves suffer from headache. *Dementia* and slowly progressive *hemiplegia* are late developments due to ischæmia from diversion of blood into the angioma. Giant aneurysms of the vein of Galen occur in neonates and can cause heart failure.

A cranial *bruit* of a continuous to-and-fro type may be heard in about a quarter of cases and sometimes the patient is aware of this. Intracranial *calcification* is seen in a quarter of cases and a plain skull film should be done before seeking confirmation of the diagnosis from angiography.

Angiography shows the abnormal vessels which fill earlier than the normal arteries in the rest of the brain (fig. 46). By the time the normal brain capillaries are filled contrast is already seen in the veins draining the angioma. This rapid circulation is also a feature of some glioblastomas and confusion may arise between these two lesions angiographically. Some angiomas are so tiny that they may easily be overlooked if an early enough film is not taken, and in cases of doubt a second series should be done. The vertebral artery often contributes substantially (through the posterior cerebral artery) to angiomas in the posterior half of the hemisphere; if only a carotid angiogram is done a lesion may appear deceptively small and easy to remove.

Accurate information about long-term **prognosis** is scanty because these lesions have only been recognised in life since angiography became available. Certainly some patients live long with little disability, and this is a comfort for those with massive angiomas beyond the scope of operative treatment; but the threat of rupture remains, and if operation is possible it should be done.

Excision is the method of choice, but is applicable only for circumscribed hemisphere lesions well away from the motor area of the cortex and other vital areas.

Ligation of the main feeding vessels has been employed most often for an angioma exposed at operation and impossible to excise. It is doubtful if lesions become any smaller after this procedure, or if the risk of recurrent hæmorrhage and epilepsy is much reduced. **Radiotherapy** likewise excites controversy, but circumscribed lesions (in surgically inaccessible sites) to which effective dosage can safely be directed have been shown by serial angiography to disappear. The effect of radiation is only gradual and may not be complete for years.

Cerebral hæmorrhage

Most patients suffering primary cerebral hæmorrhage are hypertensives between the ages of 50 and 70. The hæmorrhage occurs in the region of the basal ganglia, and causes hemiplegia associated with coma and

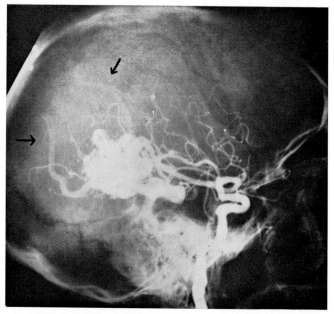

(*a*) Arterial phase—contrast already filling two large draining veins.

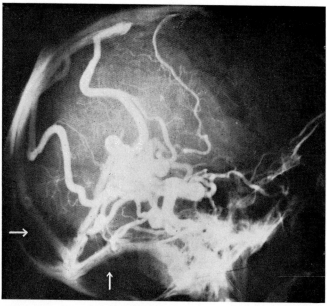

(*b*) Capillary phase—contrast already in huge draining veins and in sagittal (→), straight and transverse (↑) sinuses.

Fig. 48 Arteriovenous malformation (angioma), showing rapid circulation

bloody CSF. Given modern nursing care about 50% of such patients survive, but two thirds of them remain disabled due to persisting hemiplegia. Surgery has nothing to offer such patients, who are suffering from the effects of the initial brain damage caused by the hæmorrhage; cerebral compression is not an important element and there is not the threat of recurrence associated with ruptured aneurysm or angioma.

Sometimes, however, the hæmorrhage is more superficially placed and this produces rather a different clinical syndrome. The hæmorrhage is normally parietal in situation and, because of its superficial situation, has been termed **spontaneous subcortical hæmatoma.** All ages can be affected, including children, and hypertension is a feature of only a few. Prodromal headaches precede the acute illness for weeks or months in half the cases. Sudden headache is followed by hemiplegia, but consciousness is only seriously impaired as a secondary development; in other cases the illness may be limited to sudden confusion without any hemiplegia. Some patients deny headache and a few prove to have clear CSF on lumbar puncture. EMI scan is the ideal investigation. Angiography may show lateral displacement of the arteries but, as the lesion is often very posteriorly placed, no shift may be shown by this investigation or by echoencephalography; in such cases only ventriculography will locate the lesion. Surgical evacuation is better carried out through a trephine opening than a burr hole, and recovery is often very satisfactory. Naturally there are patients who do not fall clearly into either of these groups, and it may be difficult to decide whether to investigate or not.

Cerebellar hæmorrhage occasionally takes this sub-acute form and it may then closely resemble metastatic tumour. The history of rapidly developing headache and posterior fossa signs may be associated with stiff neck and the discovery of blood-stained or xanthochromic CSF. Evacuation of the clot usually relieves the symptoms and is followed by good recovery.

FURTHER READING

Allcock, J. M. and Drake, C. G. (1965). Ruptured intracranial aneurysms—the role of arterial spasm. *Journal of Neurosurgery*, **22,** 21–29.

Amacher, A. L., Allcock, J. M. and Drake, C. G. (1972). Cerebral angiomas: the sequelæ of surgical treatment. *Journal of Neurosurgery*, **37,** 571–575.

Amacher, A. L. and Shillito, J. (1973). Syndromes and surgical treatment of aneurysms of the great vein of Galen. *Journal of Neurosurgery*, **39,** 89–98.

Crompton, M. R. (1966). The comparative pathology of cerebral aneurysms. *Brain*, **89,** 789–796.

Crompton, M. R. (1966). The pathogenesis of cerebral aneurysms. *Brain*, **89,** 797–814.

Drake, C. G. (1968). Further experience with surgical treatment of aneurysms of the basilar artery. *Journal of Neurosurgery*, **29,** 372–392.

Farrar, J. K. (1975). Chronic cerebral arterial spasm: the role of intracranial pressure *Journal of Neurosurgery*, **42,** 408–417.

Fein, J. M., Flor, W. J., Cohan, S. L. and Parkhurst, J. (1974). Sequential changes of vascular ultrastructure in experimental cerebral vasospasm. *Journal of Neurosurgery*, **41**, 49–58.

Heilbrun, M. P., Olesen, J. and Lassen, N. A. (1971). Regional cerebral blood flow studied in subarachnoid hæmorrhage. *Journal of Neurosurgery*, **37**, 36–44.

Hockley, A. (1975). Proximal occlusion of the anterior cerebral artery for anterior communicating aneurysm. *Journal of Neurosurgery*, **43**, 406–431.

Hollin, S. A. and Decker, R. E. (1973). Effectiveness of microsurgery for intracranial aneurysms. *Journal of Neurosurgery*, **39**, 690–693.

Hosobuchi, Y. (1975). Electrothombosis of carotid cavernous fistula. *Journal of Neurosurgery*, **42**, 76–85.

Jennett, B., Miller, J. D., and Harper, A. M. (1976). *Effect of Carotid Artery Surgery on Cerebral Blood Flow*. Exerpta Medica. Amsterdam, London, New York.

Krayenbuhl, H. A., Yasargil, M. G., Flamm, E. S. and Tew, J. M. (1972). Microsurgical treatment of intracranial saccular aneurysms. *Journal of Neurosurgery*, **37**, 678–686.

Leech, P. J., Miller, J. D., Fitch, W. and Barker J. (1974). Cerebral blood flow, internal carotid artery pressure, and the EEG as a guide to the safety of carotid ligation. *Journal of Neurology Psychiat.*, **37**, 854.

Locksley, H. (1966). Natural history of subarachnoid hæmorrhage, intracranial aneurysm and arteriovenous malformation. *Journal of Neurosurgery*, **25**, 321–369.

Logue, V., Durward, M., Pratt, R. T. C., Piercy, M. and Nixon, W. L. B. (1968). The quality of survival after rupture of an anterior cerebral aneurysm. *British Journal of Psychiatry*, **114**, 137–160.

McKissock, W., Richardson, A. and Taylor, J. (1961). Primary intracerebral hæmorrhage. *Lancet*, **ii**, 221–226.

McKissock, W., Richardson, A. and Walsh, L. (1960). Posterior communicating aneurysms. *Lancet*, **i**, 1203–1206.

McKissock, W., Richardson, A. and Walsh, L. (1962). Middle cerebral aneurysms. *Lancet*, **ii**, 407–428.

Millikan, C. H. (1975). Cerebral vasospasm and ruptured intracranial aneurysm. *Archives of Neurology*, **32**, 433.

Mount, L. A. and Anturas, T. (1975). Results of treatment of intracranial aneurysms by wrapping and coating. *Journal of Neurosurgery*, **42**, 189–193.

Mullan, S. (1974). Experiences with surgical thrombosis of intracranial berry aneurysms and carotid cavernous fistulas. *Journal of Neurosurgery*, **41**, 657–670.

Nishioka, H. (1966). Evaluation of the conservative management of ruptured intracranial aneurysms. *Journal of Neurosurgery*, **25**, 574–592.

Paillas, Jean, E. and Alliez, B. (1973). Surgical Treatment of spontaneous intracerebral hæmorrhage. Immediate and long-term results in 250 cases. *Journal of Neurosurgery*, **39**, 145–151.

Paterson, J. H. and McKissock, W. (1956). A clinical survey of intracranial angiomas, with special reference to their mode of progression and surgical treatment. *Brain*, **79**, 233–266.

Perret, G. and Nishioka, H. (1966). Arteriovenous malformations: and analysis of 545 cases. *Journal of Neurosurgery*, **25**, 467–490.

Pool, J. L. (1972). Bifrontal craniotomy for anterior communicating artery aneurysms. *Journal of Neurosurgery*, **36**, 212–220.

Potter, J. M. (1955). Angiomatous malformations of the brain; their nature and prognosis. *Annals of the Royal College of Surgeons of England*, **16**, 227–243.

Robinson, J. L., Hall, C. S. and Sedzimir, Carol, B. (1974). Arterial venous malformation aneaurysms and pregnancy. *Journal of Neurosurgery*, **41**, 63–70.

Skultety, F. M. and Nishioka, H. (1966). Report of the co-operative study of intracranial aneurysms and subarachnoid hæmorrhage. *Journal of Neurosurgery*, **25**, 660–704.

Sonntag, V. K. H. and Stein, B. M. (1974). Arteriopathic complications during treatment of subarachnoid hæmorrhage with epsilon-aminocaproic acid. *Journal of Neurosurgery*, **40**, 480–485.

Troupp, H. and Bjorkesten, G. A. (1971). Results of controlled trial of late surgical versus conservative treatment of intracranial arterial aneurysms. *Journal of Neurosurgery*, **35**, 20–24.

Wilkins, R. H., Alexander, J. A. and Odom, G. L. (1968). Intracranial arterial spasm: a clinical analysis. *Journal of Neurosurgery*, **29**, 121–134.

Yasargil, M. G., Yonekawa, Y., Zumstein, B. and Stahl, H.-J. (1973). Hydrocephalus following spontaneous subarachnoid hæmorrhage. *Journal of Neurosurgery*, **37**, 474–479.

ISCHÆMIC STROKES

Occlusive cerebro-vascular disease

Angiography has revealed that cerebral ischæmia is twice as often due to extracranial as to intracranial vascular occlusion; some patients have vascular lesions in both sites. It is possible now, to carry out reconstructive surgery on the extracranial (neck) vessels and this is quite widely practised for patients with threatened cerebral ischæmia. The role of surgery is prophylactic and operation cannot revive infarcted brain tissue; however, the inclusion in some series of patients already hemiplegic makes it difficult to define clearly the value of this type of surgery. The following account emphasises the neck vessels because at present it is only these which are accessible to surgery; development of micro-surgical techniques makes it possible for intracranial vessels to be similarly reconstructed but definite evidence that this procedure is clinically beneficial is still awaited.

PHYSIOPATHOLOGY

Severe disease of the neck vessels can be completely symptomless because of the efficiency of the anatomical and physiological arrangements in the circle of Willis for ensuring an adequate blood supply to the brain under even adverse circumstances. The resting total cerebral blood flow is significantly reduced only when each of the four neck vessels is 90% obstructed, or three of the four are completely blocked, but the reserve is obviously diminished before this stage is reached. Although such severe disease is rarely found, half the patients with one carotid completely blocked do have at least one of the remaining three trunks affected to some degree. Although it is local defects in perfusion rather than alterations in total blood flow which produce symptoms, the potential total flow, or vascular reserve, is certainly important for establishing collateral circulation if further occlusions develop in extracranial or intracranial vessels. The chief contribution of surgery may be to improve this available reserve rather than to re-establish local blood flow directly.

Many factors other than occlusion of main vessels are of importance in determining whether or when ischæmia will develop and how extensive or long-lasting it will be. Among these are the collateral channels available in an individual patient, variations in systemic blood pressure, vasospasm, alterations in blood viscosity, sludging in capillaries and the formation of platelet microemboli. These latter are most likely responsible for repeated transitory symptoms associated with occlusion of intracranial vessels, such as intermittent monocular blindness.

This multiplicity of factors influencing the cerebral circulation accounts in part for the difficulty of correlating clinical, angiographic and pathological findings in these patients. The inexact use of various terms contributes further to the confusion. *Stenosis* implies narrowing only, *occlusion* a complete block, while *thrombosis* describes a pathological state which may sometimes be the cause of an occlusion but is more often a consequence of obstruction. *Ischæmia* refers to inadequate perfusion of an area of brain with functional failure; only if it is sufficiently severe and prolonged does *infarction* develop. *Carotico-vertebral insufficiency* is a useful term for symptomatic extracranial obstructive vascular disease, and emphasises that the state of the quartet of neck vessels as a whole is more important than the condition of any one of them alone.

ÆTIOLOGY

Atheroma is the usual cause of stenosis, and commonly affects the first two centimetres of the internal carotid artery above the bifurcation of the common carotid. *Thrombosis* may complete the block, or develop only secondarily when atheromatous occlusion becomes total. In either event it frequently spreads up the whole length of the internal carotid to its first intracranial branch (the ophthalmic). *Macro-embolism*, associated with auricular fibrillation, is much less common than formerly, but *micro-embolism* from an atheromatous plaque or a thrombus in a narrowed internal carotid may occlude cerebral vessels, often temporarily.

Trauma is an occasional cause of carotid thrombosis; this may be added to underlying atheroma, but can also develop in young individuals with healthy arteries. Up to two days after closed injury to the neck, or after head injury without overt neck injury, hemiplegia and impaired consciousness can develop. Most cases will rightly be suspected first of having an intracranial hæmatoma, and it is usually wise to make burr holes before assuming that the carotid thrombosis is responsible. Rarely local *infection* may induce thrombosis, and so may involvement by local *carcinoma* in the neck.

Oral contraceptives have recently been suspected of precipitating arterial thrombosis in the cerebral circulation, but an association has not been statistically established. What the controversy has emphasised is that spontaneous occlusions both of the cervical internal carotid and of the middle cerebral artery are not uncommon under the age of 40, and even under 30. Moreover *pregnancy* considerably increases the risk of intracranial arterial thrombosis, and the mortality is significantly greater than in non-pregnant females or males of similar age. Post-mortem in such cases usually reveals primary thrombosis without atheroma. Before angiography was available many such cases were ascribed to intracranial venous thrombosis, but this now appears to be a rather unusual occurrence.

CLINICAL SYNDROMES

Obstruction of the *carotid* has claimed most clinical attention because since angiography has been available carotid disease has frequently been recognised, and because almost all surgical endeavours have been directed to this artery. The *vertebral* is less often examined radiologically and is less accessible surgically.

Carotid occlusion can produce a wide variety of symptoms and of modes of onset, all of them manifestations of ischæmia of one cerebral hemisphere. Hemiplegia may be so severe and sudden as to suggest cerebral hæmorrhage; or it may develop rapidly but remain incomplete, resembling the classical picture of cerebral thrombosis; or it may be so gradual and progressive that an intracranial tumour is suspected. All these types of stroke imply infarction and are therefore unlikely to be benefited by surgery. Of more interest to the surgeon is the patient who suffers *transient ischæmic attacks*. These temporary strokes may last a few minutes or a few hours, but recovery is complete; a limb may be weak or merely numb or there may be dysphasia. Occasionally transient blindness in one eye occurs, and the eye affected is ipsilateral to the affected carotid, whilst any signs referable to the cerebral hemisphere are of course contralateral. Micro-emboli are commonly held responsible for these transitory attacks, and such have been observed passing across the retinal vessels during the course of episodes.

Vertebro-basilar occlusions cause episodes of vertigo, tinnitus and ataxia due to brain stem ischæmia; the syndrome of the posterior inferior cerebellar artery is most often a reflection of more proximal block, in a main vessel.

Physical signs related to the neck vessels, as distinct from those related to failure of cerebral function, are unreliable. A carotid **bruit** may be heard when there is stenosis (but not with occlusion), though this may be mimicked by a bruit transmitted from the thyroid or aortic arch and branches. **Ophthalmodynanometry** as a means of detecting occlusion (but not stenosis) depends on measuring the pressure which must be applied to the globe to obliterate the retinal circulation, as observed with an ophthalmoscope. The two sides are compared and a marked difference is taken to indicate carotid occlusion on that side. Clearly the method takes no account of the extent to which collaterals have opened up, and there may be no significant difference between the two sides once compensation is adequate or if there is bilateral stenosis. As a preliminary test and in skilled hands it has some value but a diagnosis should not be based on this alone.

INVESTIGATION

Clinical diagnosis is clearly difficult. It is much less easy to distinguish with certainty between cerebral hæmorrhage, thrombosis and embolism than was formerly thought; indeed it is often impossible on clinical grounds to decide whether the primary disturbance is intracranial or extracranial. It is as unwise to try to decide the cause of hæmoptysis without a chest X-ray as to attempt to guess the cause of stroke without visualising the brain or its vessels.

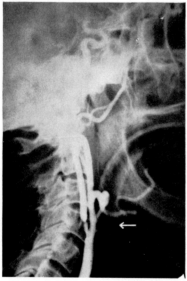 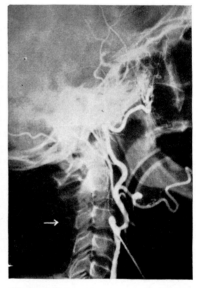

(a) Stenosis—segment of narrowing of internal carotid immediately above its origin.

(b) Occlusion—a stump of internal carotid remains above the bifurcation.

FIG. 49 Carotid disease in the neck

Note low site of puncture and inclusion of the bifurcation of the common carotid artery on the film.

Isotope scanning will often show increased uptake around an infarct and an improving appearance on repeated investigation would be in favour of a vascular lesion rather than a tumour. **Echo-encephalography** may show a shift of midline structures and if this is discovered within a few hours of onset then hæmorrhage is much more likely than infarct; however, massive infarcts can cause a great deal of shift once there has been time for the swelling to develop (see fig. 50).

EMI scan will distinguish between infarct and hæmorrhage, and it is the most reliable way to determine the cause of a persisting focal deficit. In the patient with transient attacks it will likely be normal, and only angiography will show whether there is an ulcerated plaque in the cervical carotid, or stenosis or occlusion.

Angiography is the only method at present available for establishing the diagnosis; care must be taken to make a low puncture in the common carotid and to include the neck down to the needle point on the film (fig. 49). If a complete occlusion is found no information will be available as to how far up the vessel the block extends. An intracranial occlusion may be found (fig. 50).

If surgery is contemplated the other three extracranial arteries must also be demonstrated. Direct puncture of these possibly diseased vessels is to be avoided because of the risk of precipitating even a temporary occlusion in one of the still patent vessels. An aortogram (injection into the arch after retrograde catheterisation via the femoral or subclavian artery) enables the origins of all four vessels to be visualised without inflicting any local trauma, but satisfactory films of the intracranial circulation are not usually produced. Many of these patients are investigated initially as suspected brain tumours, the symptoms not being particularly suggestive of vascular disease; the intracranial distribution of the patent carotid artery ought therefore to be visualised to exclude other disease. If the left carotid is occluded the right may be filled (together with the vertebral) by subclavian injection, but the left carotid can only be satisfactorily examined by direct puncture in the neck. The alternative is to exclude an intracranial mass lesion by air studies, once a carotid occlusion has been shown, and rely on an aortogram to demonstrate the remaining vessels in the neck.

TREATMENT

Cerebrovascular disease could be treated only expectantly until anticoagulants became available and surgical clearance of obstructed neck arteries became possible; more recently aspirin has been used to present platelet aggregation.

Anticoagulants carry the risk of precipitating fatal intracerebral hæmorrhage. The risk is greatest when they are given in error to cases with hæmorrhagic lesions. But the distinction between hæmorrhage and occlusion is not always clear; both develop against a similar background of hypertension and carotico-vertebral disease, and begin with symptoms of local ischæmia. In any event an ischæmic infarct may become hæmorrhagic under the influence of anticoagulants, and their use for established cerebral ischæmia has been largely abandoned. However, these drugs may effectively stop transient ischæmic attacks when these are occurring frequently; even though micro-embolism is

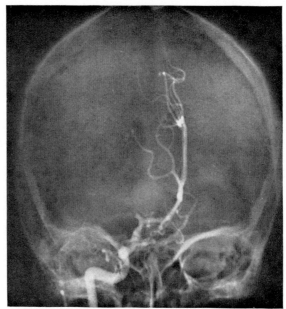

(*a*) Main artery blocked immediately beyond its origin. Massive displacement of anterior cerebral branches due to swelling of the hemisphere containing a large infarct.

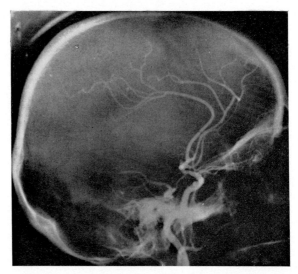

(*b*) Complete absence of vessels in middle cerebral territory. Posterior cerebral artery displaced downwards by transtentorial hernia.

FIG. 50 Middle cerebral artery occlusion (post-partum)

thereby prevented the atheromatous process in the carotid may progress and eventually lead to complete occlusion.

The question of **operation** arises when carotid stenosis has been demonstrated angiographically and the patient is not yet hemiplegic. This will most commonly be when the patient has suffered one or more temporary strokes. Three distinct aims may be achieved as a result of surgery. The most important is the *prevention of complete occlusion of* the artery. It is of course well known that occlusion of a single carotid vessel may be tolerated without any symptoms whatever and there are even cases with bilateral occlusion which are symptomless. However, in the background of atheromatous disease there is usually affection of several vessels both extracranial and intracranial and the total circulation must be considered. Surgery for a narrowed carotid is more urgently needed if the opposite carotid is also narrowed or occluded, or if the vertebrals or basilar are also affected. Secondly, surgery may *remove a source of micro-emboli*, although, as indicated, anti-coagulants may control this particular phenomenon fairly satisfactorily. The third, and most dubious, outcome of surgery is the *improvement of the circulation* to the brain; experiments suggest that narrowing is not important until the last 10% of the lumen is encroached on, but that is when all other vessels are normal. Radioactive blood flow measurements (p. 74) carried out immediately before and after endarterectomy show no significant difference in most instances; but the reserve of the cerebral circulation may be improved, as revealed by a greater response to increasing $PaCO_2$ after operation.

Surgery is therefore prophylactic and there is probably no case for emergency disobliteration of the carotid apart from the exceptional circumstances when this occurs in the environs of a surgical unit and operation can be carried out within a matter of hours. A bypass may be put in place whilst endarterectomy is completed and a saphenous vein patch is usually employed in order to prevent stenosis developing as a result of suturing the arterial incision. Anticoagulants need only be given during the course of the operation. In the event of the circulation being extremely critical the operation may be made safer by hypothermia, or even by hyperbaric oxygen.

FURTHER READING

Adams, J. H. (1967). Patterns of cerebral infarction: some comments on their topography and pathogenesis. *Scottish Medical Journal*, **12**, 339–348.

Battacharji, S. K., Hutchinson, E. C. and McCall, A. J. (1967). Stenosis and occlusion of vessels in cerebral infarction. *British Medical Journal*, **3**, 270–274.

Cross, J. N., Castro, P. O. and Jennett, W. B. (1968). Cerebral strokes associated with pregnancy and the puerperium. *British Medical Journal*, **3**, 214–218.

Gillespie, J. A. (1969). Extracranial cerebrovascular disease and its management. Butterworths, London.

Jennett, W. B. (1967). Ischæmic carotid strokes. *Scottish Medical Journal*, **12**, 368–376.

McDowall, D. G. (1970). Cerebral circulation. *International Anaesthesiology Clinics* 7. Little, Brown. Boston.

Marshall, J. (1966). The management of occlusion and stenosis of the internal carotid artery. *Neurology* (Minneapolis) **16,** 1087–1093.

Meyer, J. S., Lechner, H. and Eichorn, O. (1969). *Research on the cerebral circulation.* Thomas, Springfield.

Yates, P. O. and Hutchinson, E. C. (1961). Cerebral infarction: the role of stenosis of the extracranial cerebral arteries. *H.M.S.O. Spec. Rep. Ser. Med. Res. Coun. No.* 300, London.

III: Head Injuries

CHAPTER 12

Pathology and Natural History of Head Injury

Mechanism of injury

Scalp and skull injury

Impact brain damage

Secondary events and their consequences

Findings in fatal cases

Outcome in survivors

Assessment of severity

MECHANISM OF INJURY

Most head injuries in civilian life are *blunt* injuries caused either by the moving head striking a static surface, usually the road, or by the head being struck by a moving object. The damage suffered by the brain depends on the rapid deceleration when the moving head comes abruptly to rest on the road or the acceleration imparted when the stationary head is struck. This causes diffuse brain damage which is usually accompanied by loss of consciousness, at least for a brief period. Quite different are *penetrating injuries*, which may be due to low velocity agents (sharp objects falling or fallen against, or used as weapons of assault), or to high velocity ballistic missiles. At close range the latter may cause extensive damage, but if the missile is nearly spent the effect is to produce only local damage, like that due to the low velocity agents. With only local brain damage consciousness is often not lost at all. Whilst penetrating injuries are always open, not all acceleration-deceleration injuries are closed, because the basal dura may be torn (see page 261). The traditional classification into closed and open injuries is therefore less fundamental than that based on the mechanism of brain damage.

Scalp and Skull Injuries

It is brain damage that matters in a head injury and fatal brain damage can occur without a blemish on the scalp or any fracture of the skull. Scalp injury and skull fracture may, however, be important as evidence that the head has suffered violence, it may also indicate the sites where brain damage is likely to be accentuated, and may raise the possibility that the injury is an open one (page 257), or that intracranial haematoma may develop (page 247).

Brain Damage

The brain is highly incompressible but easily deformed, and experiments with models suggest that shearing strains due to rotational acceleration do most damage; the brain moves within the skull and the stresses are felt most acutely at interfaces between structures of different density, such as between grey and white matter. Direct damage also results from the brain impinging on the free edges of the falx cerebri, tentorium and sphenoidal wing; local damage occurs under a depressed fracture, and sometimes under the intact skull opposite to where a blow was applied (contre-coup lesion). In all sites damage may fall directly on nervous structures, on blood vessels or on both.

In addition to this impact damage there may be secondary brain damage due to subsequent events occurring intracranially or extra-cranially or both. Whilst these processes may be initiated within minutes of impact, their effects may not appear until hours or days after injury; when they develop quickly it may be difficult to distinguish clinically between the effects of impact and secondary brain damage.

Impact Damage

Contusion and laceration are the two obvious naked-eye brain injuries and, until the discovery of the microscopical lesions described below, were thought to be the most important. Yet the frequent disparity between their severity and distribution, and the clinical state of the patient, had long made it obvious that the whole story of brain injury did not lie in these coarse lesions. Contusions are most frequent on the summits of gyri, which bear the brunt of the impact against the skull during injury. The pia is usually torn, leading to subarachnoid haemorrhage, and sometimes to acute subdural and intracerebral haematoma. These lesions are most obvious in the tips of the temporal lobes and the inferior surface of the frontal lobes.

Concussion used to be regarded as a functional condition unaccompanied by structural changes and associated with rapid recovery. It is now known that even in these mild cases microscopic damage, chiefly to nerve fibres, occurs in many areas of the brain; this probably accounts for the observation that concussional injuries are cumulative (e.g. in boxing), and may have a more marked effect in older patients who have less neuronal reserve. Similar but more severe and widespread shearing lesions of nerve fibres in the brain stem and subcortical regions account for more severe cases of concussion—which cause prolonged unconsciousness. The most severely affected are those patients, usually young and without a skull fracture, who survive for weeks or months in a vegetative state. When they die extensive demyelination of the cortico-spinal tracts in the brain stem and spinal cord may be identified by appropriate staining. In patients who die more rapidly, shearing lesions can be inferred by the presence of retraction balls or of microglial stars; and there are often small lacerations in the superior cerebellar peduncle and the corpus callosum after severe shearing injuries.

Having shown that even the mildest injuries are associated with brain damage, which differs in quantity rather than in kind from that in severe injuries, the term concussion has taken on a new meaning—because it may be mild or severe. It is commonly used to describe the diffuse damage, attended by loss of consciousness of varying duration, in distinction to the clinical evidence of focal brain damage in the cerebral hemisphere, in the brain stem/cerebellar systems or in the cranial nerves.

SECONDARY EVENTS

Intracranial

Haemorrhage on the surface or in the substance of the brain may appear to be a secondary development, but it seems likely that bleeding starts at the time of impact. Nonetheless there may be an interval of hours or days (or, in the case of chronic subdural haematoma, weeks) before the effects of haemorrhage are evident clinically.

Infection is a risk in all open injuries until they are surgically closed, and may take the form of meningitis or intracranial abscess—extradural, subdural or parenchymal.

Brain swelling may be due to oedema (page 6) or to engorgement (page 3) which is added to the petechial haemorrhages and contusions from the impact.

Extracranial

Hypoxia and **hypercapnia** may be due to associated chest injury or to pulmonary complications. Hypoxia may also arise due to depleted haemoglobin from blood loss, again usually from associated injuries. Systemic **hypotension** is likewise usually due to associated injury. Each of these phenomena may be aggravated by anaesthesia or by drugs causing respiratory depression. If there is respiratory obstruction not only may there be alteration in blood gases but **intrathoracic pressure** may rise; the net effect of all these events will be to cause engorgement of cerebral vessels with consequent rise in intracranial pressure.

Consequences of Secondary Events

More than one of the secondary events listed frequently occurs at the same time, and the interactions intracranially can be complex. Most of them result in a rise in intracranial pressure, with the possibility of brain shifts and herniae if gradients develop between one intracranial compartment and another (pp. 9, 51). Perfusion pressure may be eroded, both because of raised intracranial pressure and of lowered systemic arterial pressure; cerebral circulation may therefore be impaired, and the oxygenation of the brain may be further threatened if there is systemic hypoxia.

Findings in Fatal Cases

Half of fatal head injuries die before admission to hospital. What follows applies to deaths in hospital, in a third of which the patients have talked at some time after injury; this indicates that the impact injury was not overwhelming and that secondary events have presumably been largely responsible for the fatal outcome. About two thirds of hospital deaths occur within the first 24 hours after injury.

Overwhelming or irrecoverable primary brain injury is relatively rare, and care is needed not to accept too readily that a patient has sustained such an injury; modern resuscitative methods can revive deeply unconscious patients and some of these may make a good ultimate recovery.

Primary brain stem haemorrhage and contusion, or lacerations involving the hypothalamus, can reasonably be accepted as a cause of death. Assumptions about irrecoverable injuries are based only on cases examined post-mortem, and there is little information about the extent of the lesions in those who do survive.

The common findings in patients who die from their head injury, are a combination of impact injury and the consequences of secondary events. **Contusions** may be now be associated with a certain amount of local swelling, or there may be **widespread oedema** either throughout a lobe, throughout a hemisphere or throughout the brain. In young children widespread oedema like this is sometimes found with hardly any contusions at all. In about 90% of fatal head injuries there is pathological evidence of **raised intracranial pressure** (page 9); in about 75% there is an **intracranial haematoma.** Almost as common, but less obvious, is **ischaemic brain damage,** either distributed widely throughout the cortex and basal ganglia or, sometimes restricted to one major arterial territory. The pattern of this is suggestive of a perfusion failure in that it is often aggravated in the boundary zones of cortex and it seems likely that this contributes not only to death but maybe an important contributing factor in continuing morbidity in survivors.

Death ascribed to head injury may, however, be largely due to *associated injuries or extracranial complications.* Combined chest and head injuries are particularly lethal and pre-occupation with the head injury may distract attention from the need for treating shock, or even lead to other serious injuries being overlooked and thereby undertreated (see page 231). Fracture dislocations of the cervical spine are quite common in association with head injury but are easily overlooked and the death may be mistakenly ascribed to head injury. Extracranial complications which may develop after some time include fat embolism, gastrointestinal hæmorrhage and œsophageal perforation.

The mortality of head injury is a rather abstract concept, because the figure will differ considerably according to whether overall mortality or hospital mortality is being considered; and the case mortality in hospital will depend on the admission policy. For head injuries admitted to general hospitals it is usually quoted as less than 2%; but severe head injuries admitted to a special unit carry a mortality of about 50%. Unless severity of injury is clearly defined then comparison of mortality rates is unhelpful.

Outcome in Survivors

Mental sequelae consists of personality change, memory disorders and reduction in reasoning powers. The latter are often the least severely affected and it is personality change which is the most consistent and often the most damaging. This may be obvious only to relatives or close associates of the patient, and may easily be overlooked by the doctor unless he takes the trouble to see the relatives alone and to ask the right questions. The change may take the form of apathy or lack of drive or of disinhibition so that the patient becomes talkative and tactless. Whilst personality changes may be most distressing to those around the patient, it is defective recent memory which most handicaps the patient, particularly if he is a white-collar worker.

Hemisphere sequelae consist of sensori-motor hemiplegia, including hemianopia and dysphasia, which, however, usually recovers well. Epilepsy may also develop (see page 265). Children in particular may be left with ponto-cerebellar disorders—bilateral motor spasticity, ataxia and dysarthria.

Cranial nerve palsies may result from injury of the central connections, or the intracranial nerve trunks or of the extracranial course in the orbit or face; lesions in the last situation may occur without any head (= brain) injury at all. **Anosmia** is the commonest persisting complaint and occurs after almost 10% of head injuries; it may result from frontal fractures but is also frequent in mild injuries, and may then result from occipital blows. Recovery occurs only after mild injuries, usually within 3 months. Apart from loss of pleasure anosmia constitutes a hazard, because the warning smells of escaping gas or burning will not be appreciated. **Optic nerve injuries** usually occur in the optic canal, frequently without fracture and after only mild concussion; altitudinal field defects are found in incomplete lesions, and if recovery is to occur it begins in a few days. Lesions of the **oculomotor mechanism** (III, IV, VI) occur in 5% of injuries, most often due to secondary cerebral compression and tentorial herniation or to carotico-cavernous fistula; most primary injuries are due to orbital and superior orbital fissure damage. **Facial anæsthesia** is usually due to maxillary fracture involving the infra-orbital nerve. **Facial palsy** occurs quite commonly, with or without petrous fracture but usually associated with hæmotympanum. Paralysis may be delayed for a few days, and is then always temporary; most immediate palsies also recover.

The **eighth nerve** is probably the most commonly damaged of all, but neuro-otological tests may be required to discover milder degrees of trauma. *Vertigo* and nystagmus indicate vestibular nerve or end organ damage and these may persist for months after even a mild injury. Sudden movements of the head or putting it in certain positions, precipitate the sensation of movement and unsteadiness. *Nystagmus* may occur only in these positions, or may be revealed only by electro-nystagmography; caloric tests may reveal reduced labyrinthic function on one or both sides. *Deafness* may be due to damage of the conductive system (with hæmotympanum), of the end organ or of the nerve; neuro-otological tests will distinguish these and measure the amount of functional loss.

Assessment of Outcome

Whatever the actual sequelæ it is useful to evaluate the overall social outcome for the patient who has survived an episode of brain damage— whether due to head injury or any other lesion. The Glasgow Outcome Scale enables this to be done in a simple fashion. The **vegetative state** has already been described (page 23). **Severe disability** will usually be due to a combination of mental and physical disabilities, but includes some patients whose sole handicap is devastating dementia. Dependence implies an inability to get through a day without reliance on someone else—either for activities such as dressing, feeding or mobility; or because of a need for someone to organise the day. A patient who is independent for activity of daily living might therefore still be judged to be severely disabled in many instances. **Moderate disability** covers a wide range of handicaps, but such patients are able to cope on their own at home, to travel by public transport and to undertake work— albeit at a reduced level compared with their pre-traumatic capabilities. **Good recovery** does not imply complete recovery, but does indicate the capacity to undertake work and leisure activities similar to those previously possible. Return to work is a poor indicator of outcome; not only is it difficult to apply to housewives and children, but there are many disabled persons able to return to a particular type of work, whilst some find themselves unemployed although minimally disabled. Studies on disabled survivors have shown that mental disability contributes more significantly than does physical to the ultimate handicap; in fact everyone with marked physical handicap has some degree of mental disability, but there are many patients who make a good physical recovery who have marked mental disability. The combination of mental and physical disability makes the overall handicap more serious than might be expected from either of the problems alone; the mental disability interferes with the rehabilitation processes, with their family relationships and with the capability of adapting to disability.

It has long been held that recovery can continue for prolonged periods after severe head injury, even for years. However, objective serial testing now indicates that over two thirds of patients have reached their final outcome category on the Glasgow Scale within 3 months of injury, and that few change category after 6 months; those who are severely disabled at 3 months rarely make a good recovery. This is not to deny that some improvement occurs, but that it is seldom sufficient to change the outcome category; much of the very late "recovery" reported is probably due to social adaptation to a relatively fixed disability.

Glasgow Outcome Scale

Dead	—
Vegetative state	(sleep/wake but not sentient)
Severely disabled	(conscious but dependent)
Moderately disabled	(independent but disabled)
Good recovery	(may have minor sequelae)

Prediction of Outcome

It used to be regarded as fairly difficult to predict the ultimate outcome after injury, and reports of remarkable recoveries after severe injuries were frequent. If the input severity is critically assessed, and likewise the outcome, then it transpires that outcome can often be predicted with considerable accuracy within 24 hours of injury, and in most cases by the end of the first week. The basis of these predictions is probability statistics, using Bayesian methods, and computerised data processing of information from a large series of carefully studied patients; however, it is likely that much more simple predictive systems will emerge from these studies. The data on which these are based is clinical, without laboratory data.

Assessment of Severity of Injury

It is almost impossible to discuss head injury either in groups or in individual patients without reference to severity. Management, outcome and its prediction, the quantum of legal damages and so on, all these differ according to severity. Several indicators of severity are available, not all of which can be applied to every injury; but if reference is made to as many of these as possible a clear picture of severity will emerge. The two occasions when it is most important to have a readily understood way of describing severity is when the patient first presents to a doctor; and when the case is finally closed. Soon after injury the state of consciousness (page 19), and whether or not there is a skull fracture or neurological signs, provide the most useful guides.

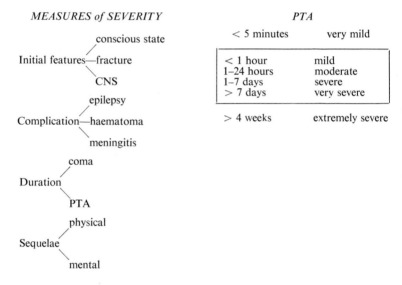

MEASURES of SEVERITY

Initial features	conscious state
	fracture
	CNS
Complication	epilepsy
	haematoma
	meningitis
Duration	coma
	PTA
Sequelae	physical
	mental

PTA

< 5 minutes	very mild
< 1 hour	mild
1–24 hours	moderate
1–7 days	severe
> 7 days	very severe
> 4 weeks	extremely severe

Once recovery has occurred the severity of the original diffuse brain damage is best judged by the duration of the coma; but that may be difficult to assess long after the occasion; notes made at the time of the initial admission may be unavailable or uninformative. Fortunately the patient carries with him the information required—which is the duration of the post-traumatic amnesia (PTA). This is defined as the lapse of time between the injury and the return of continuous memory. The capacity of the brain to store day to day memory appears to be one of the last functions to return after diffuse brain damage, and the end of PTA is always some time after the return of the ability to talk, to recognise relatives—which will commonly be judged to have been the end of coma. Sometimes there are isolated recollections of significant events in the early period after injury, such as an ambulance ride or having stitches put in the scalp; but the patient can usually recall that they then "went out again", before coming round and staying round. An assessment of PTA within these limits is therefore usually possible by direct questioning of the patient, without reference to written or remembered testimony from others. Within broad limits this is a good guide to severity and has been shown to correlate closely with outcome, whether this is assessed by mental, physical or social handicap.

FURTHER READING

Adams, J. H. (1975). The neuropathology of head injuries. In: *Handbook of Clinical Neurology*, **23**, p. 35. North Holland Publishing Company, Amsterdam.

Carlsson, C. A., Von Essen, C. and Lofgren, J. (1968). Factor affecting the clinical course of patients with severe head injuries. Part 1: Influence of biological factors. Part 2: Significance of post-traumatic coma. *Journal of Neurosurgery*, **29**, 242–251.

Caverness, W. F. and Walker, A. E. (eds.) (1966). *Head Injury*. Lippincott, Philadelphia.

Ciba Foundation Symposium 34 (1975). *Outcome after severe CNS damage*. Elsevier, Exerpta Medica, North Holland Publishing Company, Amsterdam.

Gurdjian, E. S. (ed.) (1975). Mechanistic, clinical and preventive correlations. In: *Impact Head Injury*. Thomas, Springfield.

Jennett, B., Teasdale, G., Braakman, R., Minderhoud, J. and Knill-Jones, R. P. (1976). Predicting outcome in individual patients after severe head injury. *Lancet*, **i**, 1031–1034.

Jennett, B. (1976). Resource allocation for the severe brain damaged. *Archives of Neurology*, Volume 33.

Jennett, B. and Bond, M. (1975). Assessment of outcome after severe brain damage. A practical scale. *Lancet*, **i**, 480–484.

Jennett, B. (1976). Assessment of the severity of head injury. *Journal of Neurology, Neurosurgery and Psychiatry*, **39**, 647.

Jennett, B. and Plum, F. (1972). Persistent vegetative state after brain damage. *Lancet*, **i**, 734–737.

Ommaya, A. K. and Gennarelli, T. A. (1973). Neural trauma: correlations between the biomechanics and pathophysiology of head injury. In: *Recent Progress in Neurological Surgery*. 275–285. Eds. K. Sano and S. Ishli, Exerpta Medica, Amsterdam.

Oppenheimer, D. (1968). Microscopic lesions: the brain following trauma. *Journal of Neurology, Neurosurgery and Psychiatry*, **31**, 299–306.

Overgaard, J., Hvid-Hansen, O., Land, Anne-Marie, Pedersen, K. K., Christensen, S., Haase, J., Hein, O. and Tweed, W. A. (1973). Prognosis after head injury based on early clinical examination. *Lancet*, **ii**, 631–636.

Reilly, P. I., Graham, D. I., Adams, J. H. and Jennett, B. (1975). Patients with head injury who talk and die. *Lancet*, **ii**, 375.

Strich, S. J. (1961). Shearing of nerve fibres as a cause of brain damage due to head injury. *Lancet*, **ii**, 443–448.

Symposium on Head Injuries (1966). *Clinical Neurosurgery* 12. William and Wilkins, Baltimore.

CHAPTER 13

Management of Uncomplicated Injuries

Is it a head injury?

Is there diffuse or focal brain damage?

Is the patient getting worse or better?

Is there a skull fracture?

Primary care of mild injuries

Initial care of unconscious patient
    Airway
    Fluid
    Observation
    Investigation

Care of continuing coma
    Nutrition
    Chest
    Pyrexia and infection

Recovery from coma

Less severely injured

MANAGEMENT OF UNCOMPLICATED INJURIES

Most head injuries are mild and whatever is done for them will make a good recovery. Yet all who are unconscious, no matter how briefly, run the risk of respiratory obstruction; and a few of the mildly injured will develop complications such as intracranial hæmatoma. Unconscious patients must be afforded the care proper for this state, and all head injured patients must be adequately observed in case complications developed and the brain suffers a second accident.

Is it a head injury, and only a head injury?

Doubt as to whether a head injury has in fact been sustained arises in two different situations; when a patient is known to have banged his head but appears to have fully recovered, and when an unconscious or confused patient is brought to hospital with no clear story of injury. In the first instance the question is whether there is evidence of the violence being sufficient to indicate the possibility of intracranial damage—and that evidence will usually be the presence of a skull fracture or of a brief period of post-traumatic amnesia. In the second case, when there is clearly brain dysfunction, the question is whether it is wholly or partly due to head injury. Patients who collapse due to a fit, due to a cerebrovascular accident or to alcoholic intoxication may readily sustain a head injury. Every effort must be made to find witnesses at the instant, but as long as there is doubt it is wise to regard the altered consciousness as due to head injury—because this is the condition that may need active intervention. It is known that the commonest reasons for delayed diagnosis of traumatic intracranial hæmatoma is a mistaken diagnosis of vascular accident or drunkenness.

A third of patients with a head injury have *another injury* in addition, usually a facial or upper limb fracture. A careful search should always be made for other injuries, particularly if surgical "shock" is marked because this is rarely due to head injury alone, unless there has been heavy blood loss from the scalp. The unconscious patient cannot complain and draw attention to his injuries, for which a positive search must be made; a swollen thigh may indicate a fractured femur, hæmaturia a fractured pelvis and surgical emphysema fractured ribs. Chest injuries are important because they tend to aggravate the effects of the head injury; abdominal injuries call for more urgent immediate treatment than most head injuries but are easily overlooked in an unconscious patient; the abdomen should always be examined, and bowel sounds listened for. Tyre marks or impression patterns of clothing on the yielding skin of the abdominal wall bespeak severe crushing, and warrant abdominal exploration for ruptured viscera. Injuries to the cervical spine can result from hyperextension strains secondary to frontal blows, and CNS damage here or in the brachial plexus can cause Horner's syndrome (with inequality of the pupils) or a paralysed arm. Flaccid paralysis of both legs is always suspicious of spinal injury, brain damage normally causing spasticity with extensor plantar responses. Facial fractures may be obvious or may be diagnosed on the skull X-rays; Towne's projection shows the ascending ramus of the mandible, a common fracture site.

Is there evidence of diffuse or focal brain damage?

Altered consciousness is the sign of diffuse brain damage. It is therfore useful to classify patients soon after injury according to whether or not they are talking; if so, whether they are orientated, and if they are whether they can remember the accident and everything since quite clearly. Even a brief period of amnesia indicates an episode of brain damage. If a patient is not talking then there is obviously diffuse brain dysfunction and what then matters is whether the level of unconsciousness is improving or worsening (vide infra).

Focal neurological signs indicate local damage, but only a minority of recently injured patients have any such signs. Dysphasia may be wrongly interpreted as mental confusion; hemiparesis may be overlooked if there are also limb injuries; cranial nerve palsies are important to detect early, particularly eye signs, because changes in these can be important evidence of progressive cerebral compression. The pupils should therefore be examined early, before the swelling of a black eye makes them difficult to see. If one pupil is already dilated, and the patient has not otherwise deteriorated this may be evidence of injury to the optic or the third nerve, or to traumatic mydriasis. Analysis of the pupil reaction on each side should enable the distinction to be made (fig. 12).

Is the patient getting worse or better?

Alterations in the **conscious level** are the most reliable evidence of change in the patient's intracranial state. It is vital to discover whether the level of consciousness has altered since the time of injury, and ambulance personnel, police and any other witnesses must be detained and questioned, or if not available actively sought; the information obtained, with as accurate an account as possible of the timing of events must be clearly recorded in the notes. Without such information a surgeon may feel bound to open the skull, unsure whether or not the present state represents deterioration due to developing compression or an initial severe injury. If the patient is not talking when first seen the question is whether he has ever talked since injury—in other words, has there been a lucid interval. Changes in the level of consciousness are most easily recorded on the coma scale described on page 19. This depends on evaluating simple responses to stimuli, and can be reliably used by relatively untrained personnel. If the patient is talking care should be taken to discover whether or not he is correctly orientated in time and place, will answer questions appropriately—and whether or not this represents improvement or worsening according to his previous state. It is here that alcohol may be a confusing factor. It seems that quite high levels are required (over 200 mg/100 ml. in the blood) before patients will become disoriented or unresponsive. Even if there is evidence of intoxication coma should never be ascribed wholly to alcohol if the level is below this.

If the **pupils** are known to have been equal and reacting at some stage after injury and have now become unequal then hæmatoma must be suspected on the side of the dilated unreacting pupil. If both pupils are fixed and dilated, and the state of the patient does not otherwise suggest that he is in the final stages of unrelieved cerebral compression or has sustained an overwhelming injury, other explanations should be sought—such as homatropine drops (instilled to facilitate ophthalmoscopy) or the recent occurrence of an epileptic fit. If the pupils have become small and fixed the possibility is that morphine may have been given or that the patient has sustained a pontine injury.

Alterations in vital functions such as rising blood pressure, slowing pulse and the development of periodic, sterterous breathing occur as late features of cerebral compression. Hyperpyrexia usually indicates upper brain stem injury. Rapid shallow respirations more likely to indicate hypoxia, fat embolism or other pulmonary complications than primary brain stem injury.

Increasing **hemiplegia,** perhaps associated with decerebrate or extensor posturing, usually indicates brain stem distortion due to an expanding hemisphere lesion; but these signs may have been present bilaterally from the beginning and would then bespeak severe primary diffuse damage.

Is there a skull fracture, and is it an open injury?

Overwhelming brain injury can occur without skull fracture, whilst many patients with linear vault fracture have no evidence of brain damage. This has led to a view that skull X-rays are unhelpful, therefore an unnecessary, investigation in the early stages after head injury. However, in the patient who appears to be only mildly injured, linear skull fracture may be the only evidence which justifies admission to hospital —over 80% of patients who subsequently develop intracranial hæmatoma have a skull fracture; it is therefore prudent to keep anyone with a fractured skull under observation. Again, only an X-ray of skull may indicate that an innocent scalp laceration is in fact overlying a compound depressed fracture of the vault; or that a black eye bespeaks a basal fracture of the anterior fossa. The prevention and early diagnosis of complications depends on anticipation; knowledge of the presence and site of the skull fracture can be invaluable in the early recognition of the two most important complications of mild injury—intracranial hæmatoma and infection.

Primary Care of Mild Injuries

1. Assessment of conscious level and CNS signs
2. Skull X-ray
3. Scalp suture
4. Continued observation

Whilst no-one would be likely to disagree with this list, views differ as to how continued observation is best arranged. Criteria for the admission of mild injuries to hospital will depend, *inter alia*, upon the availability of caring relatives and on whether there is ready access to short stay or to in-patient ward beds. Most hospitals would want to admit, at least for 24–48 hours, all patients with any degree of altered consciousness in the accident department and with neurological signs, severe headache or vomiting, and all patients with fractures of the skull even if fully conscious and otherwise well, Patients in whom the history is in doubt, or assessment is difficult (e.g. infants and drunks) should also be admitted. Views will differ about patients who have no skull fracture and who are now fully conscious, without signs or symptoms, but who have a brief amnesia for the period immediately following the accident. Traditionally it has been recommended that such patients be admitted, but in practice so few of them ever develop complications that it is doubtful whether this is a wise policy—unless beds and nurses are freely available. How long mildly injured patients who are admitted should remain in hospital for observation is difficult to say, because a few may develop complications only after a few days; it is certainly unwise to have a rigid policy based on an arbitrary period, rather than letting each case be considered on its merits; these may depend not only on the patient's clinical state but on what further observation is possible after discharge. These factors will also determine whether or not the patient is admitted in the first place, in the doubtful categories mentioned above. Modern reaction against the unnecessary admission of children to hospital, makes it entirely reasonable to instruct parents in the observation of their children in the first 24 hours or so after a mild injury and the same may go for adults with suitable relatives. They must be told to wake the patient regularly to discover whether his conscious state is still satisfactory and to report back to the hospital if there is any suggestion of abnormal behaviour, or has developed headache or vomiting or any other new complaint.

Initial care of the unconscious patient

Except for the small number with compound depressed fractures, or a profusely bleeding scalp, the only urgent care required for most head injuries is the maintenance of a clear airway. Once this is attended to management resolves itself into careful observation for signs of complications and general sustaining treatment until consciousness is fully regained.

THE AIRWAY

The airway must be kept clear from the moment the unconscious patient is picked up off the road, during the ambulance journey, in the accident room, whilst X-rays are taken and when being wheeled from one department to another. Every unconscious patient runs the risk of developing a blocked airway from swallowing the tongue or inhaling vomit or naso-pharyngeal secretions. Blood may collect in the mouth and throat from fractures of the nose or jaws or base of skull; salivary and mucous secretions may be stimulated by local damage or by central brain injury affecting the autonomic outflow. The stomach is often full (frequently of beer) and a massive vomit can occur at any moment with the risk of fatal aspiration. Some patients with relatively mild brain damage die of asphyxia before they ever reach hospital.

Methods of keeping clear

The simplest way to keep the airway clear is by the correct **positioning of the patient.** In the prone or semiprone position the jaw and tongue fall forward, and any potential aspirate in the mouth dribbles out rather than down into the trachea; if the feet are elevated safety is further increased and there need be no hesitation about having the head down after a head injury.

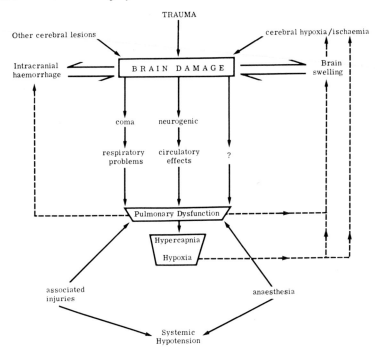

This alone must suffice for the roadside, but as soon as possible **mechanical suction** should be employed. This ought to be available in ambulances and casualty departments and also in a portable form to accompany patients along hospital corridors, in lifts and to the X-ray department. Severe injuries with hypersecretion of salivary and mucous glands, blood in the pharynx and some degree of pulmonary œdema may require suction every five or ten minutes (using soft rubber catheters with suction about 5–20 cm. water). A tube passed at this stage to aspirate the stomach will prevent a massive vomit occurring unexpectedly later.

If aspiration has already occurred, or if suction has to be repeated every few minutes, an **endotracheal tube** should be passed provided the patient is deep enough to tolerate it. This is also advisable if an operation is to be done (even under local anæsthesia) so that suction can easily be continued after the head is draped with towels. The cuff of the tube should be deflated for 5 minutes every two hours, but even so should not remain *in situ* much longer than 7 days because of the risk of laryngeal pressure necrosis; if the patient cannot then do without it a tracheostomy must be considered. Temporary intubation or **bronchoscopy** may deal satisfactorily with a particular incident of aspiration or the accumulation of secretions in the lower passages.

When these measures are not immediately successful or have to be repeated the question of **tracheostomy** arises. This should be considered whenever unconsciousness is prolonged. The majority of patients, however, regain their swallowing and cough reflexes within a few hours of injury and the danger of choking and the likelihood of aspiration pneumonia is greatly reduced, even though full consciousness is not regained for several days.

Indications for Tracheostomy

By excluding supratracheal obstructions a clear airway is assured and it becomes possible to remove abnormal secretions from the lower respiratory tract, minimising stasis and its sequelæ; the effort of breathing is lessened by reducing the dead space and increasing the effective tidal volume. The benefits are such that some recommend it for every patient unconscious for more than 12 or 24 hours, but this takes no account of the many patients (including most children) who can remain in coma for many days without presenting any difficulty with their airway or threatening to develop chest complications, providing they are skilfully nursed. When such nursing care is not readily available tracheostomy may rightly be recommended, because it certainly makes less demands on the nursing staff. However, tracheostomy is by no means free of risk itself; hæmorrhage, mediastinitis and blockage from drying secretions can all lead to death, whilst the stoma invariably becomes infected, often with resistant organisms which can spread through a whole ward. Children are particularly liable to develop crusting, and in any event derive less benefit mechanically from the procedure because of the relatively small diameter of the trachea.

Tracheostomy is indicated for unconscious patients after head injury, in the following circumstances:

1. Associated fractures of jaw or cervical spine which make endotracheal intubation and bronchoscopy unwise or impractical.

2. Major chest injury, or complications requiring prolonged mechanical ventilation.

3. Endotracheal tube already in place for several days in a patient unable to manage without it, yet likely to recover; children tolerate

endotracheal tubes for longer, and are more liable to complications from tracheostomy.

In this last category the indication for tracheostomy is only relative and the resources of the nursing staff and the way in which the individual patient is behaving must be considered. If constant suction is needed, or repeated obstructions develop, tracheostomy should be done without delay. Obviously it is more beneficial if done before chest complications are established. The operation is simple to perform, and if it has been properly carried out the stoma heals rapidly without leaving an unsightly scar.

Technique

Tracheostomy is very rarely required as an absolute emergency, in the casualty department or in the patient's bed. Immediate crises are best dealt with by an endotracheal tube which is left in place until tracheostomy can be done under proper conditions. Indeed it is always safer to have an endotracheal tube in place before operation, and to withdraw it as the tracheostomy tube is introduced. The operation can then be done without the venous congestion in the neck which is inevitable when there is partial respiratory obstruction. The one indispensable requirement is adequate suction without which it is unsafe to operate.

Local anæsthesia is used, and the neck is slightly extended over a sandbag placed between the shoulders. A transverse incision below the cricoid cartilage gives the best cosmetic result. The isthmus of the thyroid is divided and bleeding controlled before the anterior parts of the second and third rings of the trachea are excised with a solid scalpel (thin detachable blades may snap and be inhaled) to form a hole to fit the tube snugly. If the first ring is interfered with, stenosis is liable to develop. A sharp hook pulls the thyroid cartilage upwards and steadies the trachea whilst dilators are inserted; suction is applied immediately to prevent tracheal secretions from being inhaled deep into the lungs by the sudden inflow of air. Only then is the tube inserted, either a size 28–32 silver tube with its introducer or a cuffed rubber tube (James size 8–12); the latter allows mechanically assisted ventilation to be set up if necessary. In any event these tubes are probably easier to manage, and a recent type with a movable rubber flange enables an adjustment to be made according to the thickness of the soft tissues of the neck. The wound does not usually need stitching and should never be tightly closed as surgical emphysema may then develop.

To prevent crusting and tenacious sputum air should be delivered through the humidifier, at least for the first few days.

Fluid Requirements

Most of the patients who are admitted unconscious are sufficiently recovered within 24 hours to take fluids. Head injury alone is seldom associated with hypovolæmia. It is therefore unnecessary to institute intravenous fluid therapy in the first 12 hours—unless there are associated injuries which call for this. If unable to take oral fluids after 12 hours intravenous dextrose saline should be started (2L in 24 hours for an adult); if coma continues the aim should be to change to naso-gastric feeding as soon as possible.

Clinical Observation

Having made an initial assessment, and decided whether the intra-cranial condition is improving, static or deteriorating, it is essential to keep the situation under constant review, particularly in the first 24 hours—48 hours after injury. When a talking patient lapses into coma it is obvious that something is wrong; when the already un-conscious patient becomes worse the change is less striking and its recognition may be delayed unless regular monitoring of the conscious level, of focal neurological signs, and of vital signs is not instituted. It is in such cases that special investigations may prove useful.

INVESTIGATIONS

The majority of head injuries who reach hospital show steady clinical improvement and, in Europe at least, never reach neuro-surgeons or come within range of the special investigative techniques which are mostly confined to neurosurgical or neurological units. In North America neurosurgeons are more frequently involved at an early stage, and investigations are more widely used. Some of these (echoencepahlography and EMI scanning) are now becoming available in general hospitals, and may be used to determine which patients should be transferred to special units where more invasive techniques are available (angiography, exploratory burr holes, intracranial pressure monitoring). These various tests have already been described but it is intended here to review the role which they may play in the management of head injury.

Skull X-ray is essential, but in unconscious patients it is quite reasonably often deferred when the patient presents in the accident department. Even if it is not needed for initial diagnosis, or for a decision about an admission to hospital, it may be invaluable to know that there is a fracture in the location which would indicate the likeli-hood of a particular complication (e.g. basal fracture involving a dural tear or a posterior fossa fracture predicting an anomalously placed hæmatoma).

Echo-encephalography has proved unreliable in most centres but where one or two individuals devote care and attention to the technique it may prove useful. Only shift can be determined (page 72). If this develops afresh, or increases, there is clearly need for further investigation.

Isotope scanning and EEG are of very little help in the early stages after head injury, because abnormalities are apt to be widespread and focal accentuations difficult to detect; in any event it is the distinction between the primary and secondary intracranial events which these investigations are required to determine and that is not within the scope of these tests.

EMI scanning provides a reliable means of detecting intracranial hæmatomas in the first week or so after injury, when they usually show up as a dense area. Subdural collections sometimes have to be deduced from the presence of ventricular shift on the EMI scan, which will also show oedema, infarction and ventricular dilatation. After about two weeks extravasated blood approaches the density of normal brain and care is needed not to miss chronic subdural hæmatoma, which may not cause lateral ventricular shift if it is bilateral. When EMI scanning if readily available it therefore promises to alter attitudes to the early management of head injuries. Being free from the risks associated with angiography or ventriculography EMI scanning can be repeated. However, an anæsthetic is often required to ensure freedom from movement artefact in the confused patient. When scanning is used routinely it may sometimes disclose an intracranial hæmatoma in a patient in whom this complication is not suspected and whose state is stable or is improving. Surgical intervention may not be needed, and such patients are known to have made rapid and full recovery without removal of the hæmatoma—the absorption of which can be verified by repeat scanning.

Angiography is chiefly used to indicate brain shift, and the location of intracranial hæmatoma. However, it frequently fails to distinguish between the shift due to more or less generalised swelling in one side of the brain and the presence of a hæmatoma; moreover it is impractical to repeat it frequently. The same restrictions apply to **ventriculography.** Moreover, each of these investigations may aggravate the intracranial condition.

Exploratory burr holes may be the right way to investigate patient who is rapidly deteriorating and in whom there is some indication as to the likely cause and its location (see page 251). However, the policy of putting 4 or 6 burr holes in as a primary method of investigation of a deteriorating, or stable but comatose patient with head injury, is much less often used than previously as alternative investigative measures become available. The information gained by exploratory burr holes is limited, and even a surface hæmatoma may be missed if it is in an unusual situation, even quite close to one of the burr holes. Judgements about intracranial pressure and brain contusion based on burr hole exploration are of no value.

Intracranial pressure monitoring is becoming more widely used, and it is interesting to reflect that many of the signs sought during clinical monitoring of head injuries are those which are associated with lesions which also cause raised intracranial pressure. It is therefore logical to undertake direct measurement if this is possible. Various techniques are available (page 8) and the method used will depend on local conditions. A twist drill makes it possible to do this without exploratory burr holes or the use of an operating theatre. The ventricles may be small after head injury and difficult to enter, and in that event subdural or extradural recording may be adequate.

CARE OF CONTINUING COMA

Patients still in coma 24 hours after injury may well remain unconscious for several days, sometimes for a week or more. It then becomes important to take steps to prevent the complications of prolonged unconsciousness.

Nutrition

It is not enough to provide the theoretical requirements because it is difficult to estimate the fluid and metabolic demands of the brain damaged patient. Not only may he expend energy in hypertonic muscles or in hyperactivity in bed, unlike other sick people, but damage to the hypothalamic/pituitary region may cause specific metabolic disorders.

Water depletion can result from insufficient intake which can readily occur when a patient who is sufficiently co-operative to take sips but who is not given supplementary tube feeds. Even when the standard requirement of 2 litres in 24 hours is met dehydration can develop if there is unsuspected **diabetes insipidus** due to the head injury. The conscious patient would demand more fluid but with unconsciousness and incontinence the situation can rapidly get out of control. **Uraemia** can follow dehydration and may be exaggerated by too generous a diet, especially if proprietary protein concentrates are used too freely. **Altered salt excretion,** resulting in either salt-hoarding or losing syndromes, is a specific post-traumatic metabolic upset which may be accentuated by excessive salt intake (too much protein or intravenous saline) or inadequate intake (dextrose in water by gastric tube or intravenously).

The importance of all these complications is that they may cause increased drowsiness and vomiting, accounting for failure to improve and in some cases contributing to death. These disorders should be anticipated by careful attention to nutritional needs, and frequent checking of the blood electrolytes, urea and the urinary output.

Intravenous administration is unnecessary except when there is persistent ileus, and nothing is needed on the first day when the gut is often unreceptive in any event. After 24 hours an ounce of water should be given by naso-œsophageal tube every hour, and if this is retained the amount can be rapidly increased to a litre or more a day (in 250 ml. feeds). After two or three days a 2,000 calorie high protein diet must be introduced, gradually at first as diarrhœa may be precipitated. Either proprietary powders may be mixed or milk, eggs, sugar and vitamins are made up by a dietitian.

Chest

Depressed consciousness and bulbar palsy predispose to aspiration which may result in a small area of infected atelectasis, diffuse broncho-pneumonia or massive pulmonary collapse. In either event the pointer to the chest as the cause of pyrexia is an increased respiratory rate; there may be cough and pleural pain, and with massive collapse obvious dyspnoea and mediastinal shift. If these complications are anticipated they can often be prevented; when they do develop the treatment is to institute, or intensify, the prophylactic measures.

Position is critical. The patient should be a semiprone both to prevent the tongue from falling back and to stop secretions, food or vomit from passively entering the trachea. Passive breathing exercises by the physiotherapist are supplemented by two periods a day of postural drainage during which the foot of the bed is elevated and chest percussion performed; no harm comes from the head-down position which may indeed be maintained for most of the day, but the head should be up for half an hour after feeds. Suction is needed to remove nasopharyngeal secretions, and if the catheter is passed through the nose no co-operation is demanded of the patient and he cannot bite the tube, which should be passed far enough down to stimulate cough-ing. No fluids should be given by mouth unless a good swallowing and cough reflex is present. When a bulbar palsy is anticipated, it is wise to return the patient from the theatre with a naso-œsophagael tube in place, and remove it only when it is clear that the danger of choking has passed. Bronchoscopy may be needed for main bronchus obstructions, and should be availabe in the ward or dressing room with a minimum of preparation; it may be done repeatedly, though if this proves necessary tracheostomy is probably called for. This may be done prophylactically once it is obvious that a patient will remain unconscious for several days or a severe bulbar palsy had developed; indications and technique have been discussed (p. 236). Antibiotics for chest complications are less important in treatment than establishing mechanical drainage and ensuring re-expansion of the lung. If there has been a definite aspiration then it is proper to give a five-day course.

Pulmonary embolism complicates neurosurgical procedures on occasion, and may be mistaken for chest infection. Commonly occurring in the second week, in patients not specially predisposed to infection, a mild pyrexia due to the leg thrombosis may precede the chest symptoms by a few days; pleural pain, dyspnoea and small hæmoptysis suggest the diagnosis.

The value of chest X-rays in ill patients soon after injury (or operation) is sometimes debated. Films taken in bed are subject to such distortion that it is seldom that much information is gained. If there is a main bronchus block calling for bronchoscopy the area of limited air entry can usually be detected clinically; also the wedge-shaped shadow of pulmonary infarction does not develop until the clinical syndrome is obvious and treatment has already been instituted. When chest infection is recurrent or difficult to control, or the patient has a tracheostomy or a naso-œsophageal tube, it may be as well to have regular films lest an effusion or an abscess has developed. Soon after injury films can be helpful in detecting pneumothorax, lung contusion and collapse—and the response of these to therapy.

Pyrexia and Infection

The commonest cause of pyrexia is probably **chest infection**. However, high temperature developing within hours of injury may indicate a lesion affecting the hypothalamic temperature regulating centres. Heat-losing mechanisms are paralysed and the skin may be dry and even cool. It may be aggravated by the heat production associated with extensor rigidity or epileptic fits. Unless promptly controlled **central hyperpyrexia** itself can be damaging. An auxiliary temperature of 38·5°C is cause for removal of blankets, a fan by the bed and, in non-centrally heated wards, perhaps opening the window. These actions may have to be explained to relatives, who might otherwise regard them as possibly harmful to the patient. If there is no response, or the initial temperature is higher, tepid sponging is required; more effective still is sponging with Savlon (chlorhexidine) or alcohol or the application of icepacks. Chlorpromazine 25–50 mg. intramuscularly every 6 or 8 hours is useful for controlling hyperpyrexia because it prevents shivering, the body's principal mechanism for increasing temperature.

After a few days sudden pyrexia suggests **urinary infection** if the chest is not to blame. **Parotitis** rarely occurs with adequate nursing care but in the later stages when patients are recovering from coma and are being given solid food they may retain food in their mouths from one meal to the next unless carefully watched. Infection of a **scalp wound** may indicate the possibility of **intracranial suppuration** (abscess or meningitis). The latter may develop quite rapidly in a patient who was not hitherto suspected of having an open injury; pyrexia, stiff neck and further lowering of conscious level are the clues.

Septicaeima must also be considered, especially in patients with associated injuries or where intravenous therapy has been needed.

Other problems

Skin excoriation readily occurs in restless patients in wet beds, and pressure sores in the quietly comatose. The unconscious, immobile patients must be **turned in bed several times daily.** Paul's tubing strapped on the penis is a useful way of collecting the urine and helps to keep the bed dry; in women an indwelling catheter is the only effective method, but the possibility of urinary infection and its sequelæ must be remembered.

Corneal drying and abrasion is a danger in the unconscious patient who lies with his eyes wide open. The lids should be closed with thin strips of waterproof strapping applied by a responsible person who will make certain that the strapping cannot itself rub against the cornea. Parolene drops should be instilled four-hourly and watch kept for infection. Care is taken to avoid damage from bed linen and observers should not repeatedly elicit the corneal reflex as a guide to conscious level.

Recovery from coma

All but the mildest injuries pass through a stage of restless, disorganised behaviour before regaining normal consciousness. This comes earlier and is briefer after mild injuries, often confined to an hour or less as the senses return within 24 hours of the accident. But after severe injuries several days of unconsciousness may be followed by many more days of cerebral irritation during which, although anxiety about life is allayed, doubts are sometimes entertained by relatives about the patient's future sanity. The continual restlessness and noisiness which characterises this stage of recovery can be a great annoyance to other patients and to the nursing staff, the bed-clothes thrown off, feeders and urinals pitched on the floor, to the sound of swearing and shouting. When such disturbed behaviour is prolonged there may be administrative pressure to give strong sedatives, or to transfer the patient to a mental hospital. But complete recovery is usual and permanent dementia exceptional.

The physical activity associated with this state is not necessarily harmful to the patient; indeed he thereby exercises his lungs and limbs better than any physiotherapist could do for him. **Sedative drugs** should not therefore be given freely; not only is there a greater risk of chest complications if the patient lies quietly all day, but intracranial complications may be difficult to detect if the conscious level is artificially depressed. However, if this stage is not reached until several days after injury, when the danger of a rapidly developing hæmatoma has passed, it is reasonable to give a mild sedative at night. Chlorpromazine (25 mg. t.d.s.) may quieten the patient by day without seriously depressing either the conscious level or the respiratory centre. Sometimes sleep rhythm is reversed, the patient sleeping all day and lying awake all night. Pain from other injuries may call for analgesics, but narcotics must be avoided.

A sound-insulated cubicle meets the needs of this condition because the patient can then be allowed to come through the noisy stage without disturbance to others. Some physical restraint may be needed by way of wrist straps, particularly if there is an accessible open wound or an œsophageal tube which could be pulled up. Cot sides and wrist straps prevent most falls out of bed, but many such falls result from frustrated attempts to reach the toilet by patients dimly aware of their needs; **a full bladder** often contributes to agitation which may subside once it is emptied.

Another source of irritation is the **traumatic subarachnoid hæmorrhage** which probably accompanies most severe injuries but also occurs with relatively mild injuries; after these the patient may be sent home, only to return next day with severe headache, a stiff neck and photophobia.

As the patient begins to recover he often benefits from the company of other patients in an open ward; and he may be less disturbed at night than when shut up alone in a dark room.

THE LESS SEVERELY INJURED

Most patients have regained full consciousness within 24 hours of the accident, though they still call for sympathetic care if their recovery is to be as smooth and rapid as possible. A head injury is not only a bewildering experience in itself but is apt to have sinister associations. Both the patient and his relatives will be concerned to know whether the skull was fractured, whether there was concussion and to what extent the function of the brain will be affected in the future.

Headache is commonly complained of by the less severely injured as soon as they regain their senses. As long as it persists they should remain lying in bed. Aspirin or codeine tablets give as good relief as anything more elaborate without the risk of masking complications. There has been a welcome reaction against treating head injuries in a darkened room, with visitors and reading forbidden—measures which tended to emphasise the seriousness of the injury and gave ample opportunity to brood on it. Once the headache has subsided the patient should begin to sit up in bed, and if it is not brought on again by this he may begin to get up. Gradual return to normal activities is the secret of smooth recovery, but reappearance of headache is the sign to go back one stage and take it more slowly. Recurrence is almost inevitable if a patient is suddenly got up and sent home after a few days flat in bed. Each patient will take his recovery at a different speed, some slower because traumatic subarachnoid hæmorrhage gives prolonged headache, others because they are unnerved by the experience.

The final stage of recovery may be prolonged after even mild injuries. The patient finds his power of concentration poor, that he lacks confidence, and that noise, especially that of children, irritates him; he may become depressed or anxious because of these symptoms and begin again to complain of headache. This is described as pressure, heaviness or a band round the head, sometimes associated with dizziness and light-headedness. Not even previous pleasures are enjoyed; books bore him, television annoys him and libido is low. The remarkable consistency of the symptomatology of this **post-concussional syndrome** from one patient to another suggests an organic basis. Many of the symptoms may be related to 8th nerve damage, which has been found to be common after mild injuries (p. 226).

The wide variation in its severity, or perhaps rather in the significance which the patient gives it and the amount he complains about it, appear to depend more on the individual patient than on the severity of the injury. It is often most marked after apparently mild injuries, perhaps because less care and consideration are extended than after a severe injury, which earns sympathy from everyone. But a mild injury may be equally upsetting for a patient. After a severe injury he remains quite oblivious of all the events during the period of unconsciousness and cerebral irritation, which are so distressing to his relatives. For the patient the illness begins the day he comes out of his PTA, whether this is an hour or a week after injury. After severe concussion little is expected of him for some time, whilst the mildly injured man is expected to pull himself together in a few days. Moreover by the time the severely injured patient wakes up the unpleasant meningism of subarachnoid hæmorrhage has usually subsided and he may never remember suffering a severe headache.

How well and quickly a patient recovers depends also on confident and sympathetic handling in the acute stage, on properly graded resumption of normal activities, on the patient's personality and on the demands made on him by his domestic and occupational background. An understanding spouse, and an employer who will enable a man to regain his confidence by starting him half time in his old job quite soon after the accident, can make the difference between an illness lasting a month and a year. Waiting for legal settlement of compensation claims sometimes seems to retard recovery, for lawyers quite legitimately press the patient to recall in detail all his complaints, many of which the doctor is trying to minimise; symptoms sometimes resolve rapidly once a settlement is completed, even when it is unfavourable for the patient. Gronwall and Wrightson have recently shown that even patients so mildly injured as not to require overnight admission to hospital often show impaired information processing for two to three weeks. Post-traumatic symptoms are markedly reduced by simple but formal rehabilitation.

FURTHER READING

Editorial (1968). Severe head injures. *Lancet*, **i**, 514–516.
Galbraith, S., Blaiklock, C. T., Jennett, B. and Steven, J. L. (1976). The reliability of computerised transaxial tomography in diagnosing acute traumatic intra-cranial hæmatoma. *British Medical Journal*.

Lewin, W. (1968). Rehabilitation after head injury. *British Medical Journal,* **1,** 465–470.

London, P. S. (1967). Some observations on the course of events after severe injury of the head. *Annals of the Royal College of Surgeons of England,* **41,** 460–479.

McClelland, R. M. A. (1965). Complications of tracheostomy. *British Medical Journal,* **2,** 567–579.

Miller, J. D. (1974). Studies of intracranial pressure and volume in patients with head injury. *Journal of Neurosurgical Sciences,* **17,** 217.

Potter, J. M. (1968). The practical management of head injuries. 2nd edition. Lloyd-Luke, London.

Russell, W. R. and Smith. A (1961). Post-traumatic amnesia in closed head injury. *Archives of Neurology,* **5,** 4–17.

Symonds, C. (1962). Concussion and its sequelæ. *Lancet,* **i,** 1–5.

Walker, A. E., Caveness, W. F. and Critchley, M. (eds.) (1989). The late effects of head injury. Thomas, Springfield.

CHAPTER 14

Complications after head injury

Intracranial haematoma
    Extradural
    Acute intradural
    Chronic subdural (adult)
    Infantile subdural

Depressed fracture

Basal dural tears

Traumatic epilepsy

Fat embolism

Carotico-cavernous fisula

Intracranial Haematoma

Many fatal head injuries prove at autopsy to have an intracranial hæmatoma. Some have been recognised in life but too late to be treated effectively; some remain quite unsuspected and are revealed at autopsy. Some hæmatomas develop so rapidly, or in patients so remote from surgical care, that there is never a chance of saving their lives. This is the exception; many could be saved if the criteria for diagnosing intracranial hæmatoma were more widely known, and, when recognised, were more promptly heeded.

In mildly injured patients the possibility of a hæmatoma may not ever be considered; in patients unconscious from the beginning the commonest reasons for delayed recognition of hæmatoma is a mistaken diagnosis of either drunkenness or a stroke. This would happen less often if a fracture were more often sought, because most adults who develop traumatic intracranial hæmatoma have a skull fracture.

Extradural Haematoma

Classically this consists of a clot in the extradural space in the temporal region resulting from a tear of the middle meningeal artery; but a quarter of extradural hæmatomas are elsewhere, either frontal or parietal or in the posterior fossa. The source of the bleeding in these is probably diploic veins or venous sinuses or connections between these two other sites. Failure to locate and evacuate clots in these unusual situations, even when cerebral compression has been correctly diagnosed, accounts in part for the continuing mortality of operated cases; but delayed diagnosis is probably more important.

Clinical Features (temporal clot)

The initial injury is frequently mild, and in a quarter of patients is not followed by any amnesia; the majority have less than an hour's PTA. This complication is therefore liable to arise in those mildly injured patients most likely to be sent home from casualty departments. Four-fifths have a *skull fracture* which is usually obvious on X-ray; and if everyone with a fracture was kept under observation, no matter how well they seemed, the majority at risk from this complication would be safe. Deterioration of the conscious level is almost always a feature of a developing hæmatoma. When this follows recovery from an initial period of unconsciousness, or there was no initial unconsciousness, the patient is said to have had a "lucid interval".

But extradural hæmatoma can develop after more severe injuries without consciousness ever being regained, although a lowering of the level can still usually be detected if primary assessment and subsequent observation are meticulous. Indeed it is in the hope that no patient will succumb from this essentially remediable complication that so much stress is laid upon careful observation of all head injuries; many must be watched for the sake of the few, probably about 1% of head injuries admitted to hospital.

Increasing CNS signs due to hemisphere compression include hemi-paresis and, in those still able to co-operate, dysphasia; extensor rigidity in the limbs is a late sign, indicative of midbrain distortion from tentorial herniation.

Pupillary dilatation on the side of the clot is a reliable sign when it occurs; it does not usually develop until late, sometimes not at all—and occasionally the contralateral pupil dilates first. Too much dependence must not therefore be put on watching the pupils, but any inequality should be recorded; some temporary variation in pupil size (lasting only a few minutes) is not uncommon during recovery from a head injury, but progressive dilatation is always significant. The value of this observation depends on knowing that the pupils were not only equal but also normally reacting at an earlier stage after the injury. Pupillary signs may be invalidated if atropine drops have been instilled, or if morphine has been given, or if there has been an injury to the globe, the optic nerve or the third nerve.

In cases when compression has not been relieved in time **autonomic**

abnormalities due to brain stem compromise may develop. *Pulse slowing* (to<60 per min.) is a late inconstant sign, occurring in less than half the cases; often the pulse is rapid. *Blood pressure* commonly rises and *respiration* becomes deep and stertorous; later periodic rhythm may develop.

The location of the clot may be indicated by a **boggy scalp swelling** in the temporal region and this is characteristic when it occurs; and short of this there may be **scalp marks** in the temporal region or a **fracture** line crossing the middle meningeal groove.

Extradural hæmorrhage is usually an early complication of head injury, more than half coming to operation within 24 hours of injury, often within 6 hours. Sometimes pressure builds up less dramatically during the first week after injury; and a few cases may be discovered even later than this.

Unusual Sites

Parietal or frontal clots should be suspected if fracture involves these areas, but the clinical syndrome is usually similar to that caused by temporal hæmatoma. Exploratory burr holes are advisable if compression is rapidly advancing; but if there is time EMI scan or carotid angiography can be most helpful (fig. 53). The EMI scan is both more informative and more reliable. Contusional swelling can produce angiographic shift, but with good films and skilled interpretation this can usually be distinguished from surface hæmatoma.

Posterior fossa hæmatomas are usually associated with neck stiffness and vomiting, but there may be no definite signs of cerebellar disorder. Often there is marked contre-coup frontal contusion which confuses the clinical picture. An occipital fracture passing down to the foramen magnum is highly suggestive. Bleeding comes from the transverse sinus, and sometimes there is hæmatoma in both the parietal region and the posterior fossa.

Operation

The urgency with which this may have to be done is not always appreciated. The degree of urgency depends on how quickly the signs of cerebral compression have developed, and how far advanced these are. There may be circumstances when transferring the patient to a neurosurgical centre is out of the question, and an attempt must be made to relieve the pressure wherever the patient is and by whoever is available. The skull should be opened with any sort of drill or trephine in the hope that an extradural hæmatoma will be found. The initial hole may have to be nibbled to reveal the clot, or to allow enough of it to extrude to save the situation. Stopping the bleeding and completing the evacuation of the clot can be left until more help is at hand; either a neurosurgeon can travel out or the patient can be transferred in with the wound lightly packed with gauze.

With proper observation this kind of desperate situation should seldom arise; there should usually be time for transfer to a neuro-surgical unit. **Mannitol** may be useful in gaining time, even though its effect may last in these circumstances for only an hour or so; there-for it should always be given if the diagnosis of hæmatoma is seriously suspected, whilst arrangements are made for transfer.

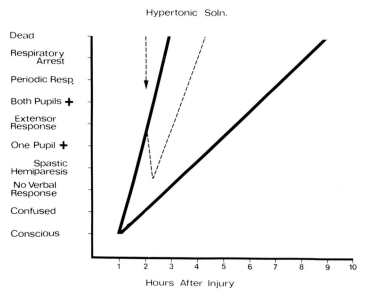

Time-sign graph to indicate different rates of clinical progression; note that hypertonic solutions provide only a temporary respite.

Fɪɢ. 51 Extradural hæmatoma

When time is available blood should be taken for **grouping and cross-matching** because, especially in children, the blood loss in the hæma-toma added to that lost during operation can be enough to demand immediate replacement. The whole head should usually be shaved because scalp marks and swellings can then be seen. Local anæsthesia will suffice, but if an anæsthetist can be summoned without delay it is preferable to have an endotracheal tube in situ; this makes for quieter and more efficient respiration, reducing cerebral congestion; and if the patient begins to wake up once the clot is released, an agent can be given to prevent restlessness whilst the wound is closed.

The first burr hole should be made in the region of the fracture, or under any boggy swelling or scalp mark; failing these guides it should be over the middle meningeal artery on the side of the dilated pupil, 2 inches above the zygoma and 2 inches behind the posterior margin of the orbital crest (fig. 52). Before obscuring the surface anatomy with drapes a second scratch should be made over the posterior branch of the middle meningeal artery, above and behind the ear, so placed that the two can be joined to form a small skin flap if necessary.

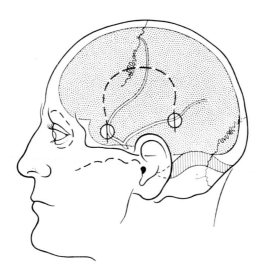

FIG. 52 Extradural hæmatoma

Burr holes are sited over the anterior and posterior branches of the middle meningeal artery; vertical skin incisions are made, so that a skin flap could be turned if necessary (dotted lines).

If the burr hole is correctly sited the clot will begin to extrude as soon as the bone is perforated. If none is seen the dura should be depressed with a blunt instrument (periosteal elevator) in the hope of seeing the edge of the clot. It is seldom possible to evacuate all the clot and secure bleeding points through a burr hole, and further access is gained either by nibbling away bone (which will leave a permanent skull defect) or by turning a small bone flap. Neurosurgeons usually prefer the latter, but no one should be deterred because they have not the instruments or do not wish to tackle the problem in this particular way. Diathermy coagulation is effective for arterial bleeding, bone wax for diploic bony oozing, and gelfoam for venous leakage. The wound need not be drained but if the dura is slow to come up to the surface it may be stitched up to muscle or periosteum.

If no clot is found a decision must be made whether to search for a clot elsewhere, to do an angiogram, or to accept some alternative diagnosis. If the brain is found slack it is probably safe to assume there is no large clot causing compression provided the patient has not recently had hypertonic solutions and is not being hyperventilated.

The surgeon must quite often expect to make exploratory burr holes and find no surface hæmatoma; indeed it has been said that if half the burr holes made in a hospital are not negative (for clot), then not enough burr holes are being made. An exploratory burr hole should be regarded not as an operation but as an investigation; once considered, it should be performed rather than discussed.

Children

Under the age of 15 extradural hæmatoma often follows a very trivial injury, with no loss of consciousness and no fracture. It tends to develop more slowly, many children coming to operation more than 24 hours after injury. Vomiting is a common complaint, and the blood loss into the hæmatoma may amount to a considerable fraction of the blood volume, causing exsanguination and shock.

Mortality and sequelae

Some 30% of injuries complicated by extradural hæmatoma are fatal, and few of these by reason of the primary brain damage. Most follow milder injuries from which a good recovery would have been expected if uncomplicated; death occurs either because the clot is not evacuated at all or is dealt with too late, after irreversible midbrain shifts and secondary midbrain damage has occurred. However good the accident service, and however alert those caring for head injuries, there will always be occasional cases of mild injuries which do not initially come to hospital, or come and are quite reasonably sent home again, only to develop rapid compression which cannot be dealt with in time.

Sometimes a clot is evacuated from an advanced case and the patient remains in coma, presumably due to midbrain damage, but survives for a few weeks. Timely evacuation normally leads to complete recovery though there is rarely some residual hemiparesis, and partial third nerve palsy sometimes persists. Epilepsy is liable to develop later in almost a third of the cases. If a craniectomy has been done the bone defect can be repaired later by cranioplasty if necessary.

Acute and Sub-acute Intradural Haematoma
(within 14 days of injury)

Intradural hæmatoma commonly occurs in association with severe injury, and there has usually been continuous alteration of consciousness since the injury. The brain is usually contused and lacerated, and the hæmatoma is often a mixture of subdural and intracerebral blood, associated with damaged brain. The source of the bleeding is usually the lacerated cortical vessels, but bleeding from veins bridging the subdural space between the cerebral cortex and the sagittal, transverse or sphenoparietal venous sinuses may contribute. Less commonly a pure subdural hæmatoma occurs without cortical laceration and it is these veins which are then the cause of the bleeding. Least common is a pure intracerebral hæmatoma; when it does occur the frontal lobe is most often affected.

The distinction between acute (first 48 hours) and sub-acute is not always clear-cut, nor is it invariably associated with one type or site of the hæmatoma. However, there is an obvious practical difference between the rapidly deteriorating patients with early intradural hæmatomas, associated with a high mortality and morbidity, and the more gradual and less dangerous type of hæmatoma which is diagnosed only several days after injury.

Acute intradural hæmatomas are most often due to the mixed intradural hæmatoma/contusion which most often affects the temporal lobe, and is sometimes bilateral; some surgeons term this condition a "burst temporal lobe". The patient has usually had impaired consciousness from the time of injury, but if the lesion is a pure subdural hæmatoma there may have been a lucid interval and the clinical picture may be indistinguishable from extradural hæmatoma; occasional patients have both hæmatomas. Deteriorating conscious level, epilepsy (often focal), unilateral pupil dilatation and contralateral heimiparesis are typical—but may not all occur. Diagnosis is by no means straight-forward—angiography may show evidence of temporal lobe swelling

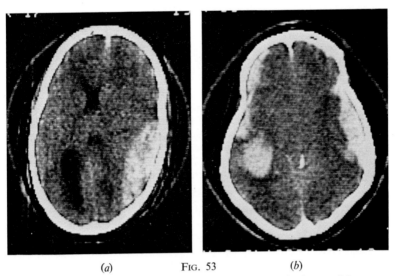

(a)   Fig. 53   (b)

(a) Extradural hæmatoma—note displacement of anterior horns of the ventricles and obliteration of much of the body of the ipsilateral ventricle.

(b) Bilateral acute subdural hæmatoma with left temporal intra-cerebral hæmatoma.

but this may as well reflect contusional swelling as hæmatoma; in practice there is usually both. The EMI scan will show not only shift but areas of hæmorrhage and oedema (fig. 53). Care is needed not to misinterpret the findings from this invaluable method of investigation or from angiography. When these are carried out consistently, rather than to confirm a suspected clot, a sizeable hæmatoma will be shown in some patients who are not deteriorating, and may even be improving. Radiological demonstration of an unexpected hæmatoma may result in patients being exposed to the hazards of unnecessary surgery, hazards which derive from the difficulty of distinguishing at operation between irretrievably damaged brain and contused brain which might recover; indiscriminate sucking away of damaged brain may therefore do more harm than good, in respect of ultimate disability. In many cases of course clinical deterioration is obvious and operation is clearly needed.

Exploration may begin with temporal burr holes, but it is almost always necessary to turn a flap (or to do an extensive craniectomy) in order to get adequate exposure to control bleeding from lacerated brain. In those who require operation in the first 48 hours after injury the mortality is high (c. 50%) and many survivors are disabled. Much of this is probably due to brain damage already sustained by the time the patients come to operation.

Subacute intradural haematomas (3–14 days after injury) are usually much less dramatic in appearance. Failure to improve, or to maintain improvement may be the first evidence; epilepsy occurring after the first 24 hours and before the end of the first week after injury quite often indicates this kind of hæmatoma. This is the period when the pure intracerebral hæmatoma is most often found, usually in the frontal lobe. The patient may even have been sent home after initial hospital admission for 24–48 hours observation before there is definite evidence of this complication.

After acute or subacute hæmatoma has been removed epilepsy frequently complicates the immediate post-operative period, and over a third of survivors develop late post-traumatic epilepsy. It is wise to prescribe anticonvulsants after intradural hæmatoma (page 269).

Chronic subdural hæmatoma (Adult)

Only half the patients with this type of hæmatoma admit to a head injury and then it has often been a very mild one. A few result from tumours, rupture of an aneurysm or angioma, or reduced coagulability of the blood from primary blood diseases or anticoagulant therapy. In some no cause is discovered; most of these are elderly and may have sustained a minor injury which they cannot remember.

The exact pathogenesis is still obscure, but an outer and inner membrane are formed which can be cleanly stripped from dura and arachnoid respectively. Solid clot may fill most of the space between these membranes, but more often there is a collection of fluid consisting of liquefied blood and CSF. Whether the hæmatoma slowly increases in size due to recurrent bleeding, or to the liquefied clot attracting CSF into the cavity by osmosis, is uncertain. Compression alone cannot account for the symptomatology because not only is the CSF pressure often low but at operation under local anæsthesia the hæmatoma may not be under pressure and the brain show no immediate tendency to re-expand once clot is removed. The most extreme examples of tentorial herniation and midbrain distortion are seen with chronic subdural hæmatoma, and many of the signs probably result from this.

Headache is the commonest complaint, and is apt to be more severe than with a brain tumour. In children it may be episodic and devastating, often interpreted as migraine. **Mental changes** can lead to admission to a mental hospital, the patient's condition being regarded as due to the effects of diffuse cerebrovascular disease or, even more vaguely, to ageing (two-thirds are over 50 years old). Drowsiness and apathy are the most usual features but confusion may be prominent; dysphasia, if not recognised for what it is, may accentuate the appearance of dementia. The patient may by this time be unable to give any account of an injury which may have been so trivial that his relatives know nothing of it. A characteristic feature is the variability of the conscious level, the patient unrousable at one time and a few hours later awake, talking and eating, only to relapse later.

Although signs of hemisphere dysfunction are common, they are often slight, perhaps restricted to reflex change and minimal weakness. Sometimes, due to severe shift, hemisphere signs are ipsilateral to the clot, and they must never be taken as reliable localising signs in this condition. Only a fifth have a dilated pupil. A much more common sign of tentorial coning is **bilateral loss of upward gaze with mild ptosis,** which may lead to the diagnosis of a pineal tumour. Papillœdema is not uncommon, and some patients are investigated as brain tumour suspects, the hæmatoma being discovered unexpectedly on angiography, or when burr holes are made for ventriculography. Epilepsy occurs in less than a tenth of cases.

X-rays rarely show a fracture, but displacement of a calcified pineal is quite often seen. **Lumbar puncture** may reveal normal CSF under normal or low pressure, but frequently the fluid is yellow and the protein level is raised. **EEG** is sometimes helpful, but suppressed activity overlying a clot is only occasionally seen. If **EMI** scanning is not available **angiography** is the investigation of choice because not only the location but also the size of the clot may be deduced if a good film of the capillary phase is available. Small posterior hæmatomas may show only on oblique views. **Echoencephalography** (fig. 20) may be deceptive when bilateral hæmatomas balance each other, and there is no displacement of midline structures.

Most **chronic** hæmatomas can be drained by making at least two **burr holes** and irrigating saline between them, but if the clot is solid a bone flap has to be turned. One hole should be in the parietal region and the other in the frontal or temporal area, according to where most hæmatoma seems to be located. Although less than a fifth of chronic subdurals are bilateral it is probably wise always to make one hole on the other side to confirm that there is not a second hæmatoma. The brain does not always re-expand immediately but unless the patient is in coma it can be left to come up slowly, encouraged by nursing him head down.

Failure to improve may be due to persisting **low pressure state** with the brain failing to re-expand. The head-down position and attention to general hydration may be enough to improve the condition, but failing this intrathecal saline may be tried.

Re-accumulation of a hæmatoma is unusual but some of the original fluid, missed at the first operation, may appear on the surface and be released either by introducing a brain cannula through one of the burr holes or by opening this formally in the operating theatre. Sometimes the patient, who is often old and arteriosclerotic, simply takes time to recover, and needs only to be protected from developing fresh complications such as chest infection, retention of urine or bedsores until he is restored to normal. The ultimate recovery is usually satisfactory, although a few do not regain entirely normal mental alertness and some develop epilepsy.

Infantile subdural hæmatoma

Subdural hæmatoma or effusion in the first two years of life forms a clear-cut entity, in regard to presentation and management. Most of these infants are under 6 months and less than half have any history of trauma (including birth injury); however, evidence of trauma elsewhere is not uncommon and this, with denial of injury by the parents, usually points to the "battered baby" syndrome. Vomiting and convulsions are the usual presenting symptoms, and a tense fontanelle with retinal hæmorrhages the most frequent signs; the latter are almost pathognomonic and occur in more than half the cases. Many of these infants are anæmic.

The diagnosis is confirmed, and the condition treated, by subdural taps, using a sharp needle inserted obliquely beneath the bone at the outer angle of the fontanelle. Both sides should always be tapped, but only 10 ml. removed from each side on the first occasion as bleeding may be started again and brain shifts aggravated if too sudden a decompression is performed. The fluid is usually yellow with a variable amount of blood, but always a high protein content (over 1 G.). Up to 1,500 white cells are commonly found, both polymorphs and lymphocytes, but this need not cause suspicion of infection. However, a small number of effusions do form as a complication of meningitis, particularly due to hæmophilus influenzæ.

Repeated tapping may show a diminishing amount of fluid and no further treatment is then required. More often the fluid keeps re-accumulating, and injection of air into the space shows the brain still depressed more than 1 cm. away from the skull. In that event membranes have formed on the dural surface (thick and vascular) and on the arachnoid surface (thin and transparent), and surgical intervention is required. The vogue for removing the inner membrane by craniotomy has given way to subdural shunting procedures, to peritoneal or pleural cavities; either no valve or a low pressure valve is used in this system.

Open Injuries

COMPOUND DEPRESSED FRACTURE

These occur from impact with sharp objects of low mass which impart little acceleration to the skull as a whole, and the brain damage is therefore localised. Because there is often little (or no) concussional damage unconsciousness is frequently lost only briefly or not at all, and unless there is obvious penetration of the skull it is possible to overlook this fracture and treat the patient as having only a simple scalp laceration. On the other hand the injury can look worse than it really is, because even when there is brain oozing out of the wound the

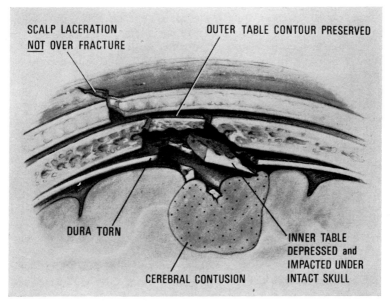

SCALP LACERATION NOT OVER FRACTURE

OUTER TABLE CONTOUR PRESERVED

DURA TORN

CEREBRAL CONTUSION

INNER TABLE DEPRESSED and IMPACTED UNDER INTACT SKULL

Fig. 54 Depressed fracture: to illustrate how diagnosis may be missed.

Note splitting of inner from outer table with only inner fragment depressed. Double density shadow (see fig. 55) produced by fragment driven under intact skull.

patient may be fully conscious; focal neurological signs will occur only if the fracture overlies the region of the central sulcus (fig. 20).

About 10% of diagnosed depressed fractures are closed (no scalp wound) and these are common in children. Even under a closed fracture the dura may be torn and the cortex lacerated. In compound fractures the dura is torn in half the cases; about half all depressed fractures are in children.

Diagnosis

Clinical examination may be misleading because the scalp laceration may not overlie the fracture; or an apparently intact outer table may conceal a depression of the inner table of the skull (fig. 54); X-ray is therefore usually necessary for the diagnosis. It is essential that two views at right angles be taken because depression is usually obvious on only one of them (fig. 55).

Treatment

The skin should be closed within 24 hours, but there is no immediate urgency provided the wound is cleaned, the surrounding hair shaved and local and systemic antibiotics given. Other factors may need to be considered before undertaking formal closure, such as the treatment of penetrating abdominal or chest injuries, or of shock due to associated injuries, which claim priority. If the fracture seems likely to involve one of the venous sinuses it may be wise not to attempt elevation; when this is essential, because of obvious contamination with marked depression, then plenty of cross-matched blood should be available before embarking on the operation.

The débridement required is the same as that employed for wounds elsewhere, the removal of devitalised tissue and foreign bodies and the provision of primary skin closure. Local anæsthesia may suffice, but first the mobility of the scalp should be tested, and any extensions of the existing scalp laceration which may be needed to allow closure should be marked; only then is local anæsthetic infiltrated.

The depth of depression of a fracture should not be judged from the degree of indentation of the outer table, because the inner table may be much more severely angulated. A burr hole is made beside the depression, and a periosteal elevator inserted; it may be possible to lever the depressed piece up but often it has to be teased out completely, taking care not to tear the dura if that is still intact. If it is already open any brain tissue which is badly bruised should be sucked away, and bleeding controlled by coagulation. Small dural tears can be sutured; larger ones are either left open or patched with a piece of pericranium. Providing the wound is clean and toilet has not been delayed, large pieces of bone can be replaced, making a loose jigsaw, and the pericranium stitched over to keep them in position. After applying topical antibiotics the scalp is sutured in two layers. If bone

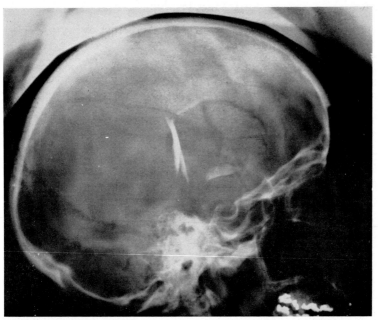

(*a*) Double density indicates depressed fragment, although angulation not directly seen.

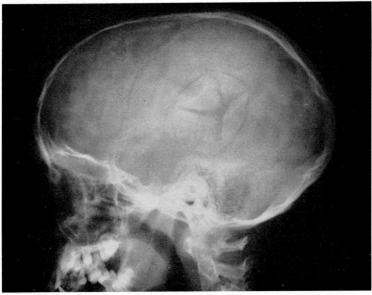

(*b*) Radiating and circumferential fracture lines (cartwheel) but no certain evidence of depression.

FIG. 55 Depressed fractures

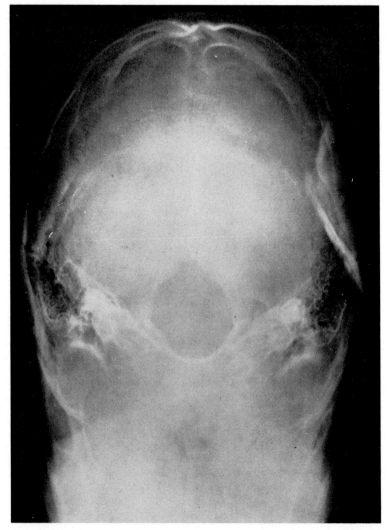

(c) Axial view of same skull as (b), showing marked depression.

FIG. 55 (continued)

has to be sacrificed and cranioplasty is considered necessary this should be carried out as a delayed procedure, never immediately because of the risk of infection.

Sequelae

Most patients make a rapid recovery if properly managed, and few suffer from persisting sequelæ. However, inadequate initial treatment, usually due to failure to recognise that there is a depressed fracture under a scalp laceration, may result in infection—meningitis and intracranial abscess may then cause death or disability. Involvement of the venous sinuses is another hazard because torrential hæmorrhage may result from dislodging a fragment at operation. A small proportion of patients develop an intracranial hæmatoma usually intracerebral, and this considerably increases the mortality and morbidity rate. Epilepsy is another complication; it occurs in the first week after injury in 10% of cases, and later than this in 15%. However, the incidence of late epilepsy after depressed fracture varies between 70% and less than 3% according to various contributory factors (see page 267).

Basal Dural Tears

Meningitis still causes death after head injuries yet the means are available in most cases both for preventing this complication and for treating it effectively should it develop.

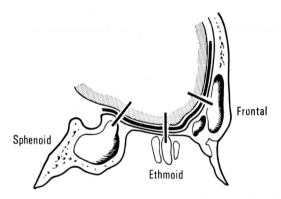

Fig. 56 Dural tears into air sinuses, associated with anterior fossa fractures.

A dural tear is presumed in the following circumstances:

(a) Proved CSF leak from nose or ear.
(b) Aerocele.
(c) Meningitis.
(d) Broad fracture line or elevated fragments involving roof of sinuses.

CSF Leak

Otorrhœa is usually profuse but short-lived and there is seldom any doubt about its nature. Once it stops the risk of infection is small unless the ear is already the site of chronic otitis media.

Rhinorrhœa is less obvious and even after careful observation there may be no certainty of a CSF leak. Injuries likely to cause rhinorrhœa often occur in association with facial and nasal fractures; the nose is filled with blood which exudes serum, and the damaged mucuos membrane of the sinuses secretes excessively, in each case simulating a CSF leak. If enough fluid can be collected to test for glucose its presence is diagnostic of CSF. Tracer substances may be introduced by lumbar puncture into the CSF, and then looked for in the nasal discharge. Rhinorrhœa may first appear several days after injury when blood clot filling the dural defect dissolves. More often rhinorrhœa noticed immediately after the accident dries up after a few days, probably because a plug of brain occupies the hole in the dura. Although this prevents CSF from continuing to leak it is no protection against ascending infection from the nose, and meningitis may develop many years after injury in patients who deny ever suffering from rhinorrhœa. Sometimes rhinorrhœa is reported by an observant nurse who finds a wet pillow in the morning; the recumbent patient may admit to a salty taste in his mouth due to CSF trickling directly down his throat; occasionally a leak first declares itself when the patient is placed prone for skull X-rays, and there is a sudden discharge of fluid. Late CSF rhinorrhœa may be simulated by allergic rhinitis or discharge from nasal polypi.

Meningitis

Infection may develop in the first few days while the patient is still unconscious; it is then difficult to detect and is rapidly fatal if not expeditiously treated. The suspicion of meningitis is the one indication for lumbar puncture after head injury, and it is an urgent one. Immediate treatment is needed. If turbid fluid is discovered intrathecal penicillin, 10,000 units in 5 ml., or a vial of neonatal ampiclox (50 mg. ampicillin +25 mg. cloxacillin) should be instilled without waiting for laboratory reports. Large doses of antibiotic must be given systemically (see p. 187). Even though the pneumococcus is the usual organism, and is always sensitive to penicillin, a delay of a few hours can still cost the patient his life.

Aerocele

Air may enter the cranium through a dural defect and collect in the subdural or subarachnoid space; it may gain access to the ventricles and produce a spontaneous ventriculogram. It may accumulate in the brain itself through a cerebral laceration, and a tension pneumocephalus develops—an unusual cause of brain compression after injury. A straight X-ray clinches the diagnosis in either case (fig. 57).

Fracture lines

The roof of the ethmoidal sinuses and the posterior wall of the frontal sinus are difficult to see clearly on routine skull X-rays, and stereoscopic

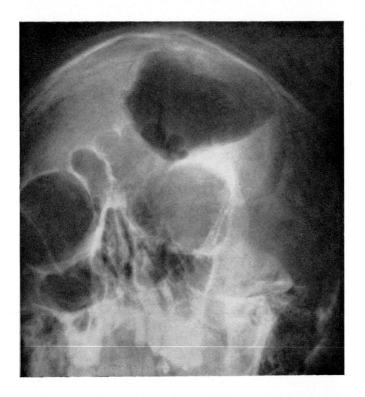

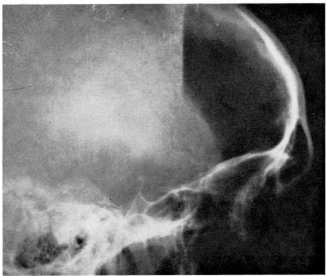

A fracture line runs into the frontal sinus.

FIG. 57 Traumatic aerocele

projections may help an expert to identify a fracture line. When a broad fracture line is seen in this area, or a chip of bone is cocked up towards the brain, a dural tear should be presumed; but X-rays can never make this diagnosis a certainty. Opacity of the sinuses suggests a fluid collection from a tear, but this may be due to blood from local external injury. Rhinorrhœa can occur without a fracture, probably due to avulsion of filaments of the olfactory nerve at the cribriform plate after a frontal or occipital injury.

Treatment of dural tear

There is some difference of opinion about the indications for repair of a dural tear, when the CSF leak dries up within a few days of injury. It it persists beyond a week, or there has been an aerocoele or an attack of meningitis, or there is radiological evidence of a broad fracture line, or an angulated spicule of bone in the roof of one of the air sinuses, then all surgeons would recommend exploration.

In the first few days after injury it may be impossible to diagnose a dural tear with confidence, unless there is an obvious CSF leak. It should be suspected in any patient with bilateral orbital hæmatoma or a fracture which involves the air sinuses; such patients, as well as those with a leak, should have prophylactic antibiotics. The careful stereoscopic films which are often required to visualise a fracture in the air sinuses cannot usually be carried out until the patient is sufficiently recovered to be fully co-operative in positioning his head for X-rays.

By the end of the first week, when X-ray examination has been completed, the rhinorrhœa has often stopped. The question is whether this is due to healing of the dural tear or to a plug of brain filling the dural defect. The latter case does not provide a bacterial barrier from the normal nasal commensals, and operation is best delayed until the scalp has healed and recovery is under way, usually 2–3 weeks after the accident. Fracture lines are the best guide to the site of the tear. If the fracture and rhinorrhoea are on the same side, then only that side need be explored. Bilateral rhinorrhœa does not always indicate two tears because a fracture of the bony septum may have put the two sides of the frontal sinus into communication. When no fractures are seen, or there is bilateral damage, it may be necessary to explore both sides through a coronal skin and bone flap. In an effort to avoid this an attempt may be made to recognise into which meatus of the nose the CSF is escaping and so deduce the origin of the leak, right or left and frontal, ethmoidal or sphenoidal. Anosmia is almost invariable with ethmoidal tears, whilst those into the sphenoid usually cause profuse and persistent rhinorrhœa. Occasionally rhinorrhœa results from a petrous fracture, the fluid running along the Eustachian tube to the nasopharynx. Petrous defects are usually on the floor of the middle fossa, and can be apprpached through a vertical skin incision and craniectomy, as in the exposure of the fifth trigeminal root (p. 352), or by a small temporal flap. Both here and in the frontal region intra-dural explorations are most reliable, because the small hernias of brain which are commonly found lead the surgeon to the dural defect.

Tears should be repaired with a fascial graft. For a small tear temporal fascia or periosteum is satisfactory, but fascia lata from the thigh is used to cover a large defect. Fascial patches need not be stitched in place, for they are kept in position by the pressure of the brain, and rapidly unite; some surgeons now use tissue glues.

Traumatic Epilepsy

Early Epilepsy (first week)

Early epilepsy is more common when the injury is more severe (i.e. associated with PTA 24 hours, depressed fracture or intracranial hæmatoma); but in children 5 years it may complicate a trivial injury. A fit may give rise to alarm, and it may cause a patient's conscious level to deteriorate temporarily; if the fit itself is not witnessed this may result in an immediate suspicion of intracranial complications. But although early epilepsy is commoner in patients with an intracranial hæmatoma it is never the only sign of this complication, and only about 2% of patients prove to be developing an extradural hæmatoma at the time of the first fit. Status epilepticus, which is commoner in children, is a hazard and calls for urgent treatment (p. 268). But the main significance of an early fit is that it increases the risk of future (late) epilepsy by a factor of 4 times. This risk applies to both children and adults, whether the injury has been mild or severe, and whether these have been repeated early fits or within 24 hours of injury. Focal motor attacks are common, and about 5% of hospitalised head injuries have one or more fits during the first week after injury. The first early fit occurred within 24 hours of injury in half the cases, and in half of these it was within the first hour. Two thirds of these patients had more than one seizure in the first week, and in more than half the seizures were focal. Epilepsy occurs 30 times more often in the first week than in any of the next 7 weeks (fig. 58); this and various other features indicate that first week epilepsy is a distinct entity.

Late Epilepsy (more than a week after injury)

This occurs in about 5% of non-missile injuries and is of importance because it tends to persist and may constitute a considerable disability in a patient who has otherwise made a good recovery. About half of those who will develop late epilepsy have had their first fit within a year of injury, but this is delayed for more than 4 years in about a quarter of cases. Prediction of the likelihood of late epilepsy rests on accurate information about the nature of the injury and early complications. Thus injuries complicated by early epilepsy, by intracranial hæmatoma or by depressed fracture have more than 25% incidence of late epilepsy. Depressed fracture has long been considered a potent

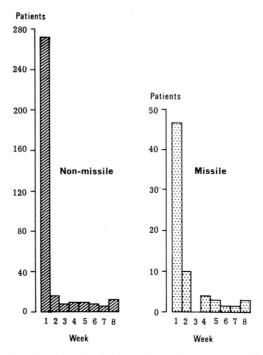

TIME of FIRST FIT
(within 8 weeks of injury)

Two series of patients developing epilepsy during the first 8 weeks after injury, showing the week during which the first fit occurred. The predominance of the first week is obvious.

FIG. 58 Early epilepsy

cause of epilepsy but closer examination has revealed that the risk varies greatly (from 5–80%) according to various factors, and an accurate estimate of the risks depends on having information about these influences (fig. 59). The risk of late epilepsy after depressed fracture is much higher when there has been 24 hours PTA; penetration of the dura and early epilepsy also add to the risk. However, these complicating factors are relatively uncommon and 70% of depressed fractures are in the categories carrying less than 20% risk of late epilepsy and 40% have less than 5% chance of developing this complication. It would seem wise to recommend anti-convulsants for 18 months or 2 years to all patients with 24 hours PTA and a depressed fracture, and also to those who have suffered both early epilepsy and dural tearing even though the PTA has been less than 24 hours. The EEG has proved of little value in predicting epilepsy. About half the patients

LATE EPILEPSY AFTER COMPOUND DEPRESSED FRACTURE

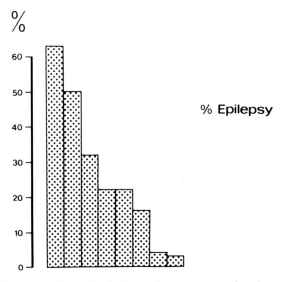

(a) Incidence of epilepsy in relation to the occurrence of prolonged PTA (> 24 hours), early epilepsy and dural penetration.

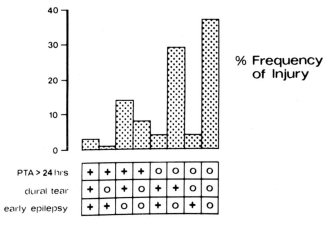

(b) Frequency of various combinations of predisposing factors in a series of 400 non-missile fractures: note inverse relationship to epilepsy incidence, i.e. types of injury most strongly diposed to develop epilepsy are the least common.

FIG. 59 Late epilepsy after depressed fracture

(Predisposing factors for (b) also apply to (a))

with established post-traumatic epilepsy have a normal record, whilst an abnormal record is not uncommon in head injured patients who have never had a fit.

Treatment
Immediate management

When a fit occurs soon after injury (or after an elective surgical opinion) it is important to resist the urge to give immediate large doses of drugs, which by depressing consciousness will make serial observations difficult to rely upon. If status develops it is of course vital to control the seizures; but often these early fits are focal, not associated with loss of consciousness and in themselves constitute no immediate threat. Epanutin (250–500 mg.) or valium (diazepam) (10 mg.) can be given intramuscularly, and a regular dose then given orally.

Status Epilepticus

This is potentially fatal and the possibility of this serious development must be entertained whenever a series of fits occurs over a few hours. Epilepsy is liable to take this form when it develops within a week of operation, when the underlying brain damage is frontal and when the patient is known to have had status on some previous occasion. The term is applied to a series of generalised convulsions without recovery of consciousness between attacks. It must be distinguished from continuing local fits without impairment of consciousness—epilepsia partialis continuans (p. 36).

The ill effects of status are cumulative. Eventually a vicious circle is set up wich it may be impossible to break, and the sooner it is stopped the better the chance of recovery without permanent brain damage. The venous congestion and hypoxia associated with respiratory arrest at the height of each successive seizure cause repeated episodes of cerebral anoxia and swelling, eventually leading to irreversible brain damage which may be fatal. The brains of fatal cases, particularly those of children, show a characteristic pattern of neuronal necrosis; this is most severe in the basal ganglia, the cerebellar cortex (Purkinje cells), the third layer of the cerebral cortex and the medial temporal lobe structures (hippocampus, Ammon's horn and amygdala). Medial temporal lobe sclerosis is frequently found in adults with temporal lobe epilepsy, many have suffered one or more bouts of status in childhood which may have caused the temporal lobe damage. Some children who survive status are left blind and others severely mentally retarded.

Clearly status must be controlled as quickly as possible and treatment must not only stop the seizures but also ensure that maintenance of adequate cerebral oxygenation, by establishing a clear airway and by counteracting the effects which anticonvulsant drugs may have on respiration or blood pressure. As anticonvulsants may have to be given in doses which produce coma, in order to control seizures, the services of an anæsthetist or the facilities of an intensive care unit should be enrolled as a soon as possible, together with laboratory monitoring to check $PaCO_2$, PaO_2 and metabolic acidosis.

Valium (diazepam) has been identified as perhaps the drug of first choice. An intravenous injection of 10 mg. coupled with an intramuscular injection of 10 mg. will often suffice; if fits either fail to respond or soon recur an intravenous drip should be set up with a Y tube so that either valium or glucose saline can be given (50–100 mg. in 500 ml.); up to 40 mg. per hours is safe but hypotension should be watched for if other drugs have already been given to control the fits.

Paraldehyde is certainly effective and has a wide margin of safety; its drawback is the irritant nature of the intramuscular injection which must be deeply placed (5 ml. repeated in 30 minutes if necessary). Although an intravenous drip can be used, cases requiring this are probably better treated with valium.

Phenobarbitone (180 mg.) is probably worth giving once (intramuscularly) but is less effective in arresting established epilepsy than in its prevention. Repeated large doses are certainly contra-indicated for they are cumulative, and may lead to barbiturate intoxication with respiratory depression.

Epanutin (phenytoin sodium: dilantin) is sometimes effective in doses of 250–500 mg. given intravenously or intramuscularly, repeated once after half an hour and then six hourly.

Thiopentone (pentothal) is the most reliable drug but as it may induce hypotension or laryngeal spasm it should not be used until safer drugs have proved ineffective, and an anæsthetist is available. After an initial dose of 25–100 mg. intravenously a drip with a Y tube allows the dose to be titrated to the needs of the individual case (100 mg. in 500 ml.).

Resistant cases of status are rare if really aggressive treatment is applied promptly, and care is taken to maintain adequate oxygenation by keeping the airway clear by position, suction and, if necessary endotracheal intubation. If epilepsy does persist it may require the ultimate deterrent of curarisation and controlled respiration. Tracheostomy is probably always a wise precaution before doing this, because the patient will already have had some hours of respiratory difficulty together with the trauma of mouth gags, suction and a bitten tongue, and he is likely to require assisted respiration for sometime. A cuffed rubber tracheostomy tube is required for positive pressure respiration. Although convulsive movements will obviously cease as soon as the patient is curarised, full doage of epanutin should be continued; paraldehyde and phenobarbitone are best withdrawn so that spontaneous respiration will be readily re-established when the decision is made to allow it. This is probably worth trying after 12 hours. Once the vicious circle is broken by this method there is often no tendency for fits to recur but it may take longer than this; EEG may indicate when it is safe to discontinue curarisation. If a case is resistant to conventional treatment, nothing short of the full regime of controlled respiration should be considered; giving small doses of pentothal without intubation is most unwise.

Prophylaxis

Epanutin (dilantin) (50–100 mg. three times a day) may be given in the early post-operative period without risk of depressing the conscious level and interfering with routine observations; later phenobarbitone (30 mg. twice or three times a day) is added to the epanutin. The importance of regular dosage must be impressed on the patient, for there is a risk of precipitating status if drugs are suddenly withdrawn; the fear of drug addiction which often leads to misgivings must be dispelled, and the rationale of prophylactic treatment should be explained to forestall the tendency of some patients to take their anticonvulsants only when they "feel a bit low" or "are having an off day". In patients who have never had seizures it should be possible to do this without discussing the possibility of epilepsy in concrete terms. They will readily accept the need for regular medication to "help the brain settle down", especially if they have just successfully weathered a major craniotomy; it would be quite wrong, as well as unnecessary, to threaten a patient with the possibility of epilepsy when he may never develop it. It is an easier matter to convince those who have already suffered some attacks and who are anxious to prevent a recurrence, even so some patients and their doctors are curiously resistant to the idea of the long; term treatment, which should be regarded as a small price to pay for freedom from fits. The efficiency of anticonvulsants is shown by the frequency with which patients have their first fit in years the day after they stop their tablets, perhaps because they went on holiday and left them behind, or went into hospital and failed to impress on the resident the importance of continuing their drugs.

But treatment is not always successful. If frequent seizures persist the dosage may be increased. Drowsiness usually limits phenobarbitone to 30 mg. four times a day in patients who are at work, whilst toxicity to epanutin is liable to develop on 100 mg. t.d.s. This takes the form of hyperplasia of the gums and gingivitis, and later ataxia and nystagmus which may be wrongly regarded as signs of tumour recurrence. If a patient's seizures tend to recur regularly at certain times of day, or in women in relation to the menses, the timing of medication should be adjusted accordingly. If fits still persist, another drug must be tried, mysoline 250 mg. t.d.s. being the next best. It should not be given with phenobarbitone, as the cumulative toxicity often causes drowsiness and mental peculiarities, as may mysoline itself if abruptly introduced in full dosage; it should replace phenobarbitone gradually, substituting only one tablet at a time. Other drugs are introduced from time to time, and refractory cases should certainly be given the opportunity of trying them. It seems wise to persist with prophylactic anticonvulsants for 18 months to 2 years; and it would appear unwise to look to the EEG for guidance about the likelihood of epilepsy developing or the wisdom of stopping treatment—common sense and clinical judgement are more reliable.

Epilepsy can spoil an otherwise good recovery after head injury (or any supratentorial surgical procedure), and the social implications of even a single fit are such that anticonvulsants should be considered in patients in whom the likelihood of epilepsy is high. After head injury this will include all patients who have had an early fit, or an acute intracranial hæmatoma, and certain patients with depressed fracture (fig. 59). How long to continue treatment depends on many factors including the temperament and social situation of the patient and the degree of risk. As half the patients who will suffer epilepsy begin to do so within a year of injury it could be reasonable to suggest 18 months to 2 years as the usual period of treatment, but to keep it up for longer in high risk cases.

New drugs appear from time to time and it is possible here to mention only those in most common use at the time of writing. Every patient is a law unto himself, in regard to the pattern of seizures, the reaction to drugs and in the effect of drugs on seizures frequency. There is nothing for it but trial and error, in respect of choice of drug and of dosage. What is of great importance is regular and continuous medication; the availability of tests for drug levels reveals what many doctors already suspected—that not all drugs prescribed are taken, and that patients do not always tell the truth. Epilepsy which is considered drug resistant is more likely to be due to inadequate treatment.

Fat embolism

Cerebral symptoms due to fat embolism may mistakenly lead to suspicion of an intracranial hæmatoma or other complication. Sometimes the accompanying features suggest the correct diagnosis, or it may be made only retrospectively when burr holes have excluded cerebral compression.

Pulmonary fat embolism is an almost invariable finding in autopsies after fracture of a marrow bone; only a few have systemic emboli, concentrated in the brain and the renal glomeruli. Because of the large reserves of function in the lungs, and the enormous capillary bed, pulmonary fat embolism is harmless and cannot account for the chest symptoms which are characteristic of systemic embolism. These are probably secondary to **cerebral embolism**, as pulmonary œdema is known to develop following primary or secondary hypothalamic or brain stem lesions of various kinds.

Cerebral symptoms are the most common, consisting of drowsiness, confusion, epilepsy and cerebral irritation. *Pulmonary symptoms* come on at the same time, suddenly, usually during the first 24 hours. Dyspnœa with tachypnœa, tachycardia and pyrexia tend to suggest broncho-pneumonia. The *petechial rash* is a later development on the second or third day, and appears over the base of the neck, front of the shoulders and upper chest.

Diagnosis is certain when the rash is recognised. Fat in the sputum is of no significance for it indicates only the common pulmonary embolism. Fat droplets in the urine are important, though they may be found only in catheter specimens emptying the whole bladder, as the fat floats and remains with any residual urine. Rarely intravascular fat may be seen in the optic fundus. Needle biopsy of the kidney is diagnostic if glomerular emboli are found, but this drastic method should be used only in obscure cases.

Carotico-cavernous fistula (aneurysm)

This may follow relatively trivial blunt head injuries and is commonest in middle-aged women. Whether these patients already have an aneurysmal or arteriosclerotic weakness of the carotid artery in the cavernous sinus cannot be determined, but as a quarter of the patients develop a fistula spontaneously, without any remembered trauma, this is probably a factor in some cases.

It is usually a few days after the injury when the patient suddenly becomes aware of a noise in the head, a continuous to-and-fro murmur synchronous with the pulse. The clinician can readily hear it with a stethoscope placed over the eyeball, and usually from a much wider area in the frontal region; the bruit may be reduced or even abolished by compression of the carotid artery in the neck. Pain may accompany the onset of the bruit and proptosis develops after a delay which can vary from hours to months. This may be quite mild or so severe as to lead to corneal ulceration, because the lids cannot close over the protruded globe; it usually affects the ipsilateral eye only, but, because of variations in the pattern of the ophthalmic veins which drain into the cavernous sinus, both eyes may be affected or occasionally only the contralateral one. The protruding eye may pulsate and there is usually marked chemosis and congestion of conjunctival vessels; the œdematous conjunctival sacs may hang down over the cheek in severe cases. Eye movements may be restricted mechanically or because of ophthalmoplegia, giving rise to diplopia. The fundus may show hæmorrhages and congested, pulsating veins, but it can remain normal.

Carotid angiography shows the escape of contrast from the carotid siphon into the cavernous sinus and its draining veins; (fig. 60) there may be poor filling of the intracranial branches if the fistula is a large one. The other causes of severe exophthalmos, cavernous sinus thrombosis, endocrine exophthalmos and carotid aneurysm do not produce a bruit or this angiographic appearance.

The course is variable. Spontaneous cures do occur, and seem sometimes to be precipitated by angiography—the bruit abruptly stops and the proptosis subsequently subsides. In other cases although the bruit persists the proptosis is not severe, equilibrium is reached and no treatment is called for. However, the bruit may be so loud and so annoying to the patient that he demands relief; or the proptosis is so severe that something has to be done either because of the unsightly appearance of the eye or the threat to vision.

Common or internal carotid ligation in the neck is the traditional first line of attack. If the bruit persists the aneurysm is then "trapped", by applying an occluding clip to the carotid immediately above the cavernous sinus; these two procedures can be carried out simultaneously as the initial treatment. These often prove ineffective and it is becoming more usual now to try to acclude the fistula itself. Various methods are possible—"posting" muscle emboli up the carotid from the neck in the hope that one will plug the communication; or using fine balloon cathers passed up the carotid artery; or direct electrothrombosis. The ophthalmic artery, as well as the fistula, is arising from the segment of the carotid which lies between the two occlusions but it normally receives sufficient collateral circulation through the orbit from branches of the external carotid artery to maintain an adequate supply to the optic nerve and retina.

Repair of skull defects (Cranioplasty)

Different materials are available. The most reliable, both for acceptance by the tissues and for a satisfactory cosmetic result, is the patient's own *bone flap* if this has been preserved (p. 100). Metal plates (of *tantalum*) need most careful working both before and during operation to achieve a satisfactory contour; they require screws for fixation, which may work loose; and they are radio-opaque, which makes for difficulties if any late complications call for radiological studies. If the plate slips, or is at all inexact or has a sharp edge, it may ulcerate through the skin and has then to be removed.

Plastic materials (such as *acrylic*) are more satisfactory. These can now be moulded in one stage, at operation; they can be worked into shape whilst they set rapidly in the bone defect. They are radiotranslucent, require no screws and excite no tissue reaction.

Attempts at cranioplasty should not be made if there has been local infection until the wound has been completely healed and free of inflammation for 6 or 12 months. Young children should not have a defect repaired until after the age of 5 years because of skull growth. Small defects covered by thick scalp do not need to be repaired as there is very little risk of damage to the underlying brain; sometimes patients are worried about such defects, and it may then be reasonable to offer to close them. But no promise should be made that symptoms such as

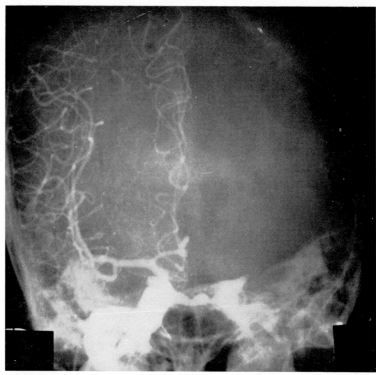

(a) Contrast has escaped from carotid artery to fill cavernous sinus on both sides.

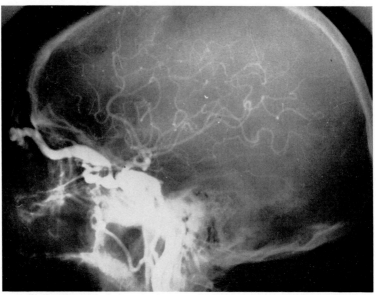

(b) Large ophthalmic vein draining cavernous sinus has filled whilst contrast is still in intracranial arteries and in the external carotid branches in the neck.

Fig. 60 Carotico-cavernous fistula

headache or other post-traumatic symptoms will resolve after cranioplasty, as patients sometimes hope they will.

FURTHER READING

Caldicott, W. J. H., North, J. B. and Simpson, D. A. (1973). Traumatic cerebro-
spinal fluid fistulas in children. *Journal of Neurosurgery*, **38**, 1–9.
Galbraith, S. (1976). Misdiagnosis and delayed diagnosis in traumatic intracranial
hæmatoma. *British Medical Journal*, **1**, 1438–1439.
Gallagher, J. P. and Browder, E. J. (1968). Extradural hæmatoma. *Journal of
Neurosurgery*, **29**, 1–12.
Jamieson, K. G. and Yelland, J. D. (1968). Extradural hæmatoma. *Journal of
Neurosurgery*, **29**, 13–23.
Jamieson, K. G. and Yelland, J. D. N. (1973). Surgical repair of the anterior fossa
because of rhinorrhœe, aerocele or meningitis. *Journal of Neurosurgery*, **39**,
328–331.
Jennett, B. (1975). Epilepsy after non-missile head injuries. Heinemann, London.
Jennett, B. (1976). Some medicolegal aspects of the management of acute head
injuries. *British Medical Journal*, **1**, 1385–1385.
Leech, P. J. (1974). CSF leakage, dural fistulæ and meningitis after basal skull
fractures. *Injury*, **6**, 141–149.
McKissock, W., Richardson, A. and Bloom, W. H. (1969). Subdural hæmatoma—
a review of 389 cases. *Lancet*, **i**, 1365–1370.
Rietz, K. A. (1958). One stage method of cranioplasty with acrylic plastic. *Journal
of Neurosurgery*, **15**, 176–182.
Robe, E. F., Flynn, R. E. and Dodge, P. R. (1968). Subudural collections of fluid
in infants and children. *Neurology* (Minneapolis) **18**, 559–570.
Sevitt, S. (1960). The significance and classification of fat embolism. *Lancet*, **ii**,
825–828.
Stern, W. E., Brown, W. J. and Alksne, J. F. (1967). The surgical challenge of
carotid-cavernous fistula: the critical role of intracranial circulatory dynamics.
Journal of Neurosurgery, **27**, 298–308.
Sumner, D. (1964). Post-traumatic anosmia. *Brain*, **87**, 107–120.
Till, K. (1968). Subdural hæmatoma and effusion in infancy. *British Medical Journal*,
3, 400–402.

IV: Spinal Lesions

CHAPTER 15

Spinal Compression

General features
  Clinical
  Investigation
  Causes of spinal compression

Spinal tumour

Vascular spinal conditions

Infective lesions

Spinal injuries

General features

Spinal compression, whatever its cause, demands surgical relief. Even when the cord has been distorted and compressed for years function may return to a surprising degree if the compression is relieved.

Many conditions can bring about spinal compression but, as with brain compression, the resulting clinical state is similar whether it is due to tumour or abscess or some other pathological process. It is important to recognise spinal compression itself rather than to try to diagnose the underlying pathology, the nature of which may be revealed only at operation. Unfortunately many of the features of compression are also produced by several of the much more common intrinsic diseases of the spinal cord such as disseminated sclerosis, motor neurone disease, and subacute combined degeneration. Because compression is readily relieved in many cases physicians are rightly anxious not to overlook it by accepting a diagnosis which condemns a patient to progressive paralysis without hope of cure.

CLINICAL

Spinal compression causes a tranverse spinal lesion, affecting to some extent all cord functions (motor, sensory and autonomic) *below that level* (fig. 61). In addition involvement of roots *at the level* of compression gives rise to pain and loss of function in a radicular distribution (fig. 62).

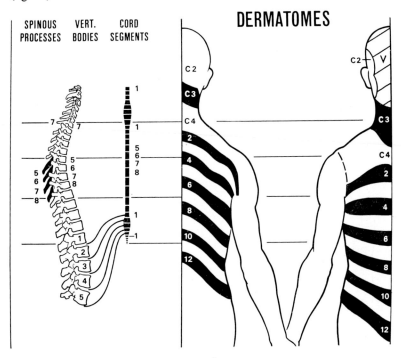

SPINOUS PROCESSES	VERT. BODIES	CORD SEGMENTS

DERMATOMES

Lower thoracic dermatomes are very steep, with T_{12} running from the last rib behind to symphysis pubis in front. Spinal *cord segments* do not correspond with *vertebral bodies*, and *spinous processes* correspond with neither; *dermatomes* are different again.

Fig. 61 Segmental innervation of trunk

Cord lesions produce spastic weakness with increased tendon reflexes and an extensor plantar response, because the upper motor neurone is affected. When there is a partial lesion, sensory loss from cord damage is dissociated, different modalities being affected in varying degrees because of the disposition of the long tracts in the cord. Compression on one side of the cord will affect the uncrossed pyramidal tract and posterior columns, giving spastic weakness and loss of vibration and joint position sense on the same side as the compression; involvement of the crossed spinothalamic tract causes loss of pain and temperature sense on the opposite side. Hemisection to the cord such as this is not to be expected in a pure form; it is sometimes termed the Brown–Sequard syndrome (fig. 76).

Root lesions tend to affect motor and sensory functions to the same degree, and all sensory modalities are equally involved. Motor weakness

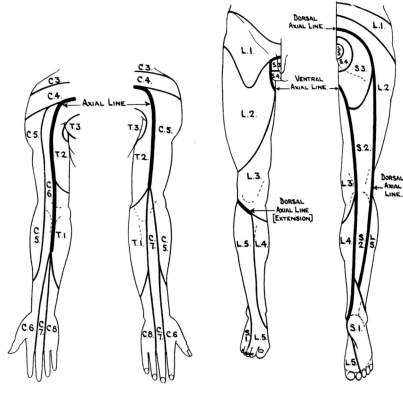

(a) Upper limit monopolises segments C5–T1, leaving C4 and T2 adjoining on the trunk. Axial lines mark where non-consecutive segments meet in the limbs.

(b) Lower limb monopolises segments L3–S2, leaving L2 adjoining S2 and S3 on the buttock.

(*From M.R.C.*)

FIG. 62 Root Dermatomes

is flaccid with loss or depression of tendon reflexes, a lower motor neurone lesion. If one root only is affected there may be severe radicular pain, but very little weakness or sensory loss may be detected because of the overlap between adjacent territories.

Cervical compression shows most clearly the combination of radicular and cord signs, because failure of function of the roots at this level is immediately evident to the patient in the muscles of the arm and hand. The level of the sensory loss due to cord involvement is commonly several segments lower than expected, and sacral sensation is often spared although the lesion appears to be otherwise complete.

Thoracic compression presents as a cord lesion with a clear-cut sensory level in the expected situation; radicular involvement is limited to girdle pain.

Lumbar lesions are predominantly radicular because the cord ends about the level L1/2, below which only the roots of the cauda equina are affected. Flaccid paraplegia with absent reflexes is associated with radicular sensory loss and an atonic bladder. High lumbar lesions may affect also the upper motor neurones of the sacral segments in the conus medullaris, making for a mixed clinical syndrome with absent tendon reflexes and the plantar responses (if still active) extensor.

Intermittent claudication of the cauda equina consists of paræsthesiæ, numbness or weakness developing consistently after a certain amount of exercise; there may also be some calf pain. In most instances a compressing lesion is found which may be a central disc protrusion or a congenital or acquired narrowing of the bony canal; the mechanism is uncertain but may be related to dilatation of intraspinal vessels or to increase in CSF pressure beyond the obstruction.

INVESTIGATION

Lumbar puncture can yield invaluable information which may verify a suspicion of spinal compression, or at least point to the need for further tests. Whilst its universal availability commends it, the results can be misleading if care is not taken with technique.

Careful manometry will reveal a block if it is complete. Compression of the jugular veins produces no rise in the resting pressure, providing the needle is below the level of the block. However, if the neck is roughly handled, and the patient reacts by straining or drawing the knees tight up against the abdomen, a spurious rise may occur due to abcominal venous distension being transferred to the intraspinal venous plexus. Partial blocks are more difficult to demonstrate with certainty, but a slow rise and an even slower return of the pressure to the previous resting level are suspicous. But the subarachnoid space may be almost completely obliterated before manometry is affected; compression is not excluded by normal manometry.

CSF stagnates below a block, the protein level rises and the fluid becomes xanthochromic. Only a few drops of syrupy yellow fluid, which coagulates on exposure to air in the test-tube, may be obtained on puncture; the pressure is sometimes too low to measure. Protein levels up to 5 G. (5,000 mg.) per 100 ml. occur; a high protein level with xanthochromia but no cells (the Froin syndrome) is the result of mechanical block and not of any particular condition.

A dry tap may occur if the needle enters a tumour which is filling the lumbar sac. This may also happen with cisternal puncture, when there is a tumour at the foramen magnum.

Plain X-rays of the spine frequently show evidence of the underlying condition, such as tumour or tuberculosis, but they do not directly reveal spinal compression per se.

Myelography alone will demonstrate a spinal block, showing exactly its level and how complete it is.

MYELOGRAPHY

Technique

Myodil (pantopaque) is normally employed, a viscous iodine-containing oil which is heavier than CSF. After intrathecal injection of contrast the patient is placed on a tilting table, and the oil run up and down the spine whilst the radiologist carries out continuous screening to observe irregularities of flow and any temporary block. Films are taken to be examined in detail later but are often less informative than the direct observation of the oil moving on the television screen.

Contrast can be injected either by lumbar or cisternal puncture, according to where the lesion is expected to be and what information is required. Lumbar and high cervical tumours may obliterate the subarachnoid space locally and the contrast must then be injected at the opposite end of the spine.

The level of a total block may be adequately demonstrated with 3 ml., but full examination calls for at least 5 or 6 ml. If more is used the dye should be removed at the end of the examination, using fluoroscopic control, and some surgeons insist on this no matter how little has been injected because of possible arachnoiditis. This can be time-consuming and painful and once it is done the opportunity of re-screening the myodil to resolve doubtful appearances is lost. To reduce the amount of contrast used, yet have an adequate volume of radio-opaque material, 3 ml. of myodil may be mixed before injection with an equal volume of the patient's CSF; the resulting emulsion is evenly and densely opaque. Water-soluble media are rapidly and completely absorbed but they cause so much pain that a spinal anæsthetic has to be given; air is being increasingly used but it demands careful technique and a high standard of radiography.

If myelography seems likely to be necessary lumbar puncture should be postponed and the CSF taken off in the X-ray department used for analysis; previous puncture often leaves an extradural or subdural pocket of CSF into which the myodil can be injected in error. No information is gained, and if myodil is later successfully introduced into the subarachnoid space a filling defect, or even a block, may be found opposite the previous faulty injection. Lumbar puncture is, however, often an essential part of the initial investigation and only when it has been done may the need for myelography be apparent; in such circumstances the myelogram is best postponed for a week or ten days after the puncture.

Complications

Transient **meningism** with pyrexia and a mild cellular reaction in the CSF is common, and may last 24–48 hours. For this reason patients should always remain in hospital for a few days after myelography. When a more serious reaction occurs it may be due to imperfect technique or the development of mild infection. Low pressure **headache** occasionally develops and is treated by bed and rest and high fluid intake. Aggravation of **CNS signs** occurs rarely, probably due to a critically poised tumour changing position after CSF is removed. This is likely to occur only when signs of cord compression are already very obvious, and is therefore not a contra-indication to lumbar puncture in the doubtful case for which it is such an essential investigation.

Late arachnoiditis is believed to occur only rarely, but it is the fear of this which has led to the search for alternative contrast media and to the practice of removing oil at the end of myelography. There have been reports of a dense plastic inflammatory reaction emmeshing small globules of oil and dividing the subarachnoid space into a number of loculi. The vast majority of patients suffer no ill effects from myelography, and why a few should is not clear; the risk of arachnoiditis

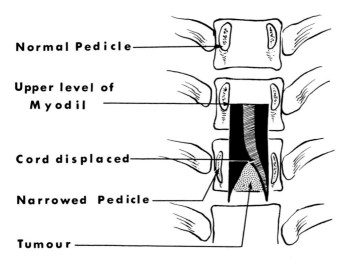

Block of subarachnoid space with lateral displacement of the cord "shadow", an area of diminished density of myodil.

FIG. 63 Myelogram of intradural tumour

may be increased by the occurrence of hæmorrhage when dye is injected, and if bloody CSF is obtained it is probably wise to postpone myelography for a few days, unless the situation is an urgent one.

Information

A block in the subarachnoid space may be discovered, and the level of the obstruction can be marked for the surgeon. This requires care if it is not to mislead. The block should be in the centre of the field so that X-rays are incident at right angles; a metal marker is strapped on and a film taken to check the level. The skin is then marked with a dye such as Bonney's blue or gentian violet (not scratched, because of the risk of sepsis); the skin must not be stretched unnaturally during marking or the mark may no longer be at the correct level when the patient is on the operating table.

The **outline of the cord** itself can be recognised as an area of diminished density, and its displacement to one or other side points to the site of an intradural compression (fig. 63). It may also be possible to deduce whether the mass is situated inside or outside the dura, and also its relation to the spinal cord (p. 274).

Spinal tumours

This term includes all tumours encroaching on the bony spinal canal, and these account for most instances of spinal compression.

CAUSES OF SPINAL COMPRESSION

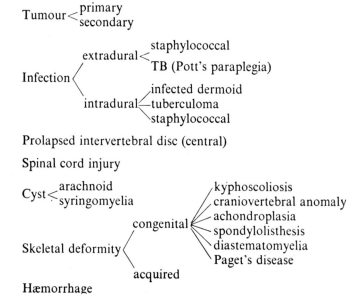

PATHOLOGY

Tumours are classified according to their relationship to the dura and the cord (medulla) (fig. 64), and by histological types. Certain tumours favour particular situations and the following cross-classification results:

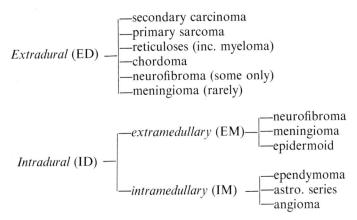

Extradural (ED) —
- secondary carcinoma
- primary sarcoma
- reticuloses (inc. myeloma)
- chordoma
- neurofibroma (some only)
- meningioma (rarely)

Intradural (ID) —
- *extramedullary* (EM)—
  - neurofibroma
  - meningioma
  - epidermoid
- *intramedullary* (IM) —
  - ependymoma
  - astro. series
  - angioma

Malignant extradural tumours are the commonest spinal neoplasms encountered by the surgeon. They can arise either in the vertebræ, where they cause pathological fracture and collapse, or in the extradural tissue between theca and bone. The dura is seldom invaded even though tumour has completely encircled it like a cuff. Hæmatogenous spread of carcinoma is common, from bronchus, breast or prostate. Myeloma forms a destructive vertebral lesion, but other reticuloses and sarcoma commonly affect soft tissue without bony involvement. Sometimes the spinal canal is directly invaded by a neighbouring tumour in the lung, chest wall or retroperitoneal tissues. Later X-rays may show vertebral collapse, the AP view erosion of a single pedicle (fig. 68).

Neurofibroma is the commonest tumour making up rather less than a third of all tumours. Any spinal level may be affected and most tumours are intradural; combined extradural and intradural forms occur in the cervical region, and thoracic neurofibromas are sometimes wholly extradural. Arising in relation to a nerve root, they form either a lozenge-shaped intraspinal mass or a dumbell tumour growing through an intervertebral foramen, partly intra- and partly extraspinal (fig. 64). The intraspinal part may be extradural or intradural or both; the extraspinal may present as a lump in the neck or a shadow in the posterior mediastinum which is discovered when the chest is X-rayed for some other reason. If there is evidence of neurofibromatosis (café au lait skin marks or cutaneous polyps) the possibility of multiple tumours must be considered, some of which may be on cranial nerves. Radiological bone change is common, either pedicular erosion or expansion of an intervertebral foramen (figs. 65, 66).

Meningiomas are rather less common, and are almost confined to the thoracic spine and to middle-aged women. Rarely they occur at the foramen magnum where they lie anteriorly. An oval mass is formed which is adherent to the inner surface of the dura, but separates readily from the cord although it may have deeply indented it and displaced it to one side of the spinal canal. Bone change is unusual (fig. 67) but calcification in the tumour is occasionally recognised radiologically.

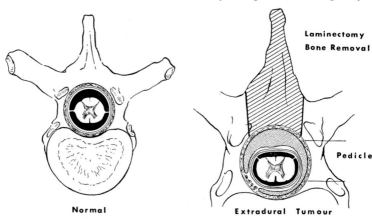

Normal   Extradural Tumour

(a) Normal—cord suspended by dentate ligaments within the subarachnoid space (black), outside which is extradural space.

(b) Extradural tumour (stippled), surrounding dural sac like a cuff.

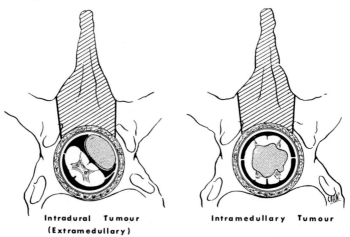

Intradural Tumour   Intramedullary Tumour
(Extramedullary)

(c) Intradural (extramedullary) tumour, displacing the cord.

(d) Intramedullary tumour, expanding the cord.

(*After Reid.*)

Fig. 64 Anatomical types of spinal tumour

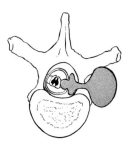

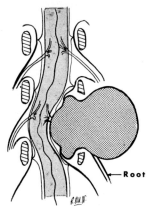

(*a*) Intraspinal part may be partly intradural.

(*b*) Tumour originates on a root and escapes by enlarging bony foramen of exit, eroding pedicles.

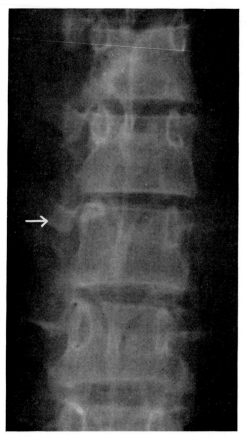

(*c*) Lower part of one pedicle eroded by neurofibroma in foramen.

(*After Eden.*)

FIG. 65 Thoracic dumbell tumour

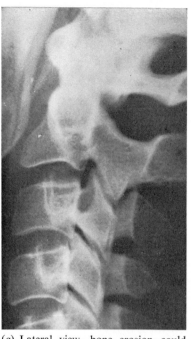 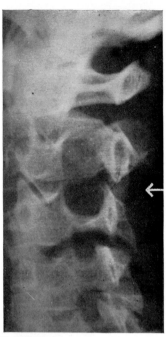

(a) Lateral view—bone erosion could be overlooked as foramina are largely hidden.

(b) Oblique view—smoothly enlarged C2–3 foramen.

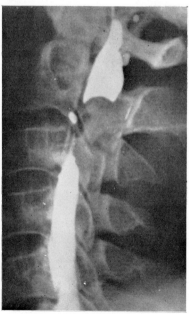

(c) Filling defect in myodil column at appropriate level.

FIG. 66 Cervical dumbell tumour

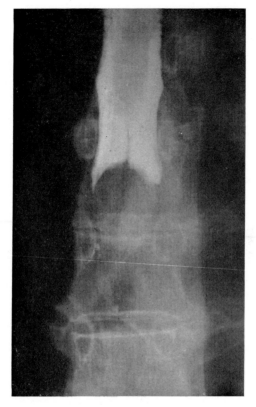

FIG. 67 Meningioma

Complete myelographic block with no pedicular erosion.

Gliomas form tumours within the cord itself in 80% cases. About half of these are ependymomas, the remainder astrocytomas of varying grades of malignancy. The whole cord is swollen, and the bony spinal canal is expanded with narrowing of the pedicles over several segments. Glioma is the only common intradural tumour, but angiomas also occur in this situation (p. 284). Most of the other 20% of gliomas occur in the lumbosacral canal, arising from the filum terminale below the end of the cord. They displace the roots and cause scolloping of the posterior aspect of the vertebral bodies. Almost all are ependymomas, and are sometimes termed "giant tumours of the cauda equina". Sometimes an intracranial ependymoma or medulloblastoma seeds into the spinal subarachnoid space, and multiple deposits are found.

Epidermoids also occur in the lumbosacral canal; many appear to be the result of implanted skin tissue from the use of a lumbar puncture

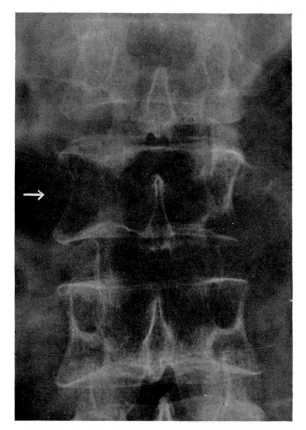

FIG. 68 Metastasis

Missing pedicle due to destructive deposit.

needle without a stilette. Most have developed in children previously treated for tuberculous meningitis, who have had many punctures for which serum needles may have been used because small needles with stilettes were not available.

Dermoids occur as intradural tumours, which may also be intra-medullary; they are truly congenital tumours containing hair and sebaceous material, and may be connected with the skin by a sinus and thereby liable to infection.

Lipomas are also probably dermoids of a kind, because fat is not normally found within the theca; these are usually combined intra-medullary and extramedullary tumours by the time they come to operation, and it is hard to determine in which situation the growth began.

CLINICAL

Tumour compression may be acute or chronic, producing two quite distinct syndromes.

Acute compression most often results from malignant extradural tumours, paraplegia developing over hours or days, perhaps after a week or so of backache or root pain. If sudden vertebral collapse occurs, such as may happen with a carcinomatous deposit or myeloma, the onset of cord compression is associated with the most agonising pain. Spinal tenderness and local kyphosis may be found. This clinical syndrome of rapidly developing flaccid paraplegia can also be produced by extradural staphylococcal abscess or by massive central protrusion of a disc. As all three conditions demand urgent surgery it is not vital to distinguish between them.

There are other causes of a sudden transverse lesion which do not call for operation. The commonest are acute demyelinating and vascular occlusions in the cord, but all are included in the term "transverse myelitis" which is no more than a label for rapidly developing paraplegia without evidence of compression. Although some mild prodromal root irritation does sometimes occur with these conditions pain is usually much less common than with compression. If there is any evidence to suggest compression the spine should be explored.

Chronic compression is the mode of onset for the common intradural tumour, and presents an entirely different clinical appearance.

There is no limit to the length of time over which a spinal tumour may give rise to symptoms, nor is there any combination of neurological signs which a tumour may not bring about. *Pain* is the earliest feature as a rule; this may be either backache due to bone erosion or disturbance of spinal mechanics or root pain. This is an acute lancinating pain, referred along the length of a root, which in the thoracic region is described as girdle pain; movement, or raising intrathecal pressure by coughing or sneezing, may precipitate a spasm. Spinal tumour pain is often worse at night, the patient walking the floor in an attempt to gain relief, in contrast to pain due to prolapsed disc which is almost always improved by bed rest.

Eventually most patients develop *weakness, wasting, spasticity or sensory and sphincter disorders*. But pain may persist for many years before CNS signs appear, in particular with lumbosacral tumours. The spinal canal is so capacious here that giant tumours can develop with bone erosion before the roots of the cauda equina are embarrassed. However, *disorders of spinal movement* are usually produced, and these closely resemble those due to prolapsed disc—scoliosis, muscle spasm and restricted straight-leg raising. Tumours at the foramen magnum form another puzzling group, because the last cranial nerves may be involved so that an intracranial tumour is suspected. Pain and sensory loss are restricted to a narrow collar distribution, whilst motor symptoms may involve any combination of the four limbs. Both plain X-rays

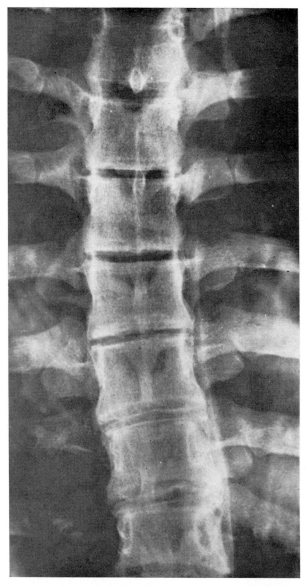

(a) Pedicles eroded over many segments; normal pedicles can be seen in the uppermost vertebrae, and in the two lowermost vertebrae the pedicles are visilble but thinner on their medial aspects.

FIG. 69 Intramedullary tumour

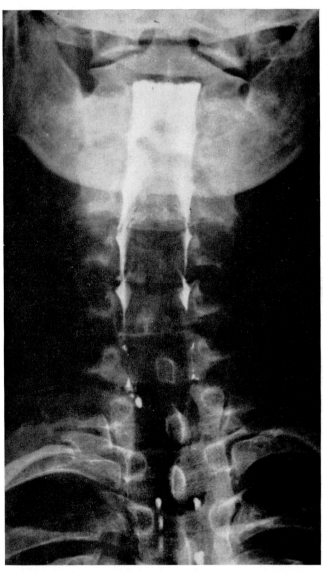

(b) Myelogram (different case)—widening of spinal subarachnoid space; contrast trickles around the edge of the central tumour filling root pockets like rose thorns.

FIG. 69 (continued)

and myelograms are difficult to interpret in this region but diagnosis is important because most tumours are meningiomas and can be removed.

When a spinal tumour is suspected, confirmation can frequently be obtained from two simple procedures. **Lumbar puncture** may show a manometric block, but even without this the CSF protein level is almost always abnormally high. **Plain X-rays** show some vertebral abnormality in about half the patients with spinal tumour. Lateral views may show altered bone density or collapse, AP views abnormalities of the pedicles, and oblique views the intervertebral foraminæ (figs. 65, 66, 68, 69).

Myelography may not be needed for the diagnosis of a spinal tumour, but is the only way of determining its size and situation which may help in planning the operative approach. *Extradural* masses produce an abrupt cut-off, and the displacement of the theca away from the bone may be observed in lateral projections. *Intradural* extramedullary tumours may cause a curved margin (fig. 67); they may displace the cord to one side, and produce asymmetrical tails of contrast (fig. 63). *Intramedullary* tumours cause the shadow of the cord itself to be widened and the root pockets may be expanded (fig. 69), but allowance must be made for the normal lumbar and cervical enlargements. Irregular curly filling defects denote vessels and are suggestive of an angioma, but are sometimes seen at the poles of a meningioma or neurofibroma.

Spinal tumour is a rarity compared with the many common conditions which it can simulate during its clinical evolution. Lumbar backache and sciatica will suggest **prolapsed disc**, but when due to tumour these symptoms seldom settle with rest. Backache alone may lead to suspicion of **ankylosing spondylitis** especially if muscle spasm leads to a frozen spine. The seeming anomaly of pain presumed of skeletal origin, which fails to respond to rest, sometimes leads to the suspicion that the patient's complaints have a **psychosomatic** explanation, and not infrequently the psychiatrist sees the patient before the surgeon does. **Visceral** disease may be simulated by lower thoracic radicular pain, so much so that the abdomen is opened. When retention of urine appears before other signs CNS primary **genito-urinary disease** may be suspected, whereas if motor signs predominate intrinsic disease of the cord such as **disseminated (multiple) sclerosis** or **motor neurone disease** may be considered.

Few spinal tumours will be overlooked if at least a lumbar puncture and good X-rays of the spine are done on all patients who have persistent backache or root pain, which does not respond as expected to adequate rest. With so uncommon a condition giving rise to such prosaic symptoms, many patients will necessarily be investigated with negative results, but this is justified by the high likelihood of successful removal if a tumour is found.

TREATMENT

Laminectomy should be performed whenever a spinal tumour is diagnosed unless it is an unquestionably malignant one in a patient already dying of cancer. The more rapidly paraplegia has developed the greater the urgency for decompression of the cord by operation. **Meningiomas and neurofibromas** can be removed completely in most instances; but the extraspinal part of a neurofibroma may require a second operation by a different approach. Sometimes this part of the tumour is doing little harm and can be left, although sarcomatous change is always a possibility.

If a tumour is found at operation to be **intramedullary** little can be done. Manipulation within the cord almost always disturbs disastrously whatever function remains; there is much less leeway than in the brain where quite large amounts of nervous tissue can be sacrificed to improve access. Sometimes such a tumour is cystic; if so, improvement may follow release of the fluid contents through a small incision strictly in the posterior median raphe of the cord. This may also help cases of syringomyelia. In both conditions recurrence is usual and is seldom effectively delayed by attempting to encourage continuous drainage of the cyst into the subarachnoid space by leaving a small tube in place. Occasionally an intramedullary tumour comes to the surface of the cord and appears to have a plane of cleavage from normal nervous tissue; it can sometimes be encouraged to extrude itself slowly, and therefore relatively safely, by a two-stage procedure. At the first operation the posterior median raphe is split, down to the surface of the tumour, and the wound closed leaving the dura open; several weeks later the tumour may be found to have largely delivered itself from the cord and can be removed. It has been suggested that when paraplegia is total the thoraco-lumbar cord containing an intramedullary tumour might be removed completely in the hope of relieving local pain and preventing upward spread of the tumour.

Ependymomas, alone of gliomas, have a fairly good outlook. They are radiosensitive so that even incompletely removed tumours can be controlled for a time. Many occur in the lumbosacral canal where a total, but piecemeal, removal is often possible by teasing tumour away from the roots of the cauda equina.

Malignant extradural tumours cannot be extirpated completely, but laminectomy and removal of as much growth as possible, without opening the dura, may relieve root pain and backache satisfactorily. Some of the *primary extradural tumours* respond well to radiation post-operatively, and reticulosarcoma in particular may not recur for 10 years or more. When recurrence is long delayed there is always the possibility that the new symptoms are due to radiation effects on the cord. This diagnosis must also be thought of whenever a patient who has had radiation for other conditions in the neighbourhood of the cord begins to suffer from any kind of myelpoathy; those at risk include case of carcinoma larynx or œsophagus and ankylosing spondylitis. *Secondary carcinoma* has a poor outlook, with three quarters of patients dead within six months of operation; prognosis is particularly poor when the primary is in the bronchus and the onset of paraplegia has been rapid, whilst the 5% or so who survive more than a year are mostly from breast or prostate. Unfortunately the presence of primary carcinoma is not recognised before operation in 40–50% of patients, and urgent surgery must be carried out lest the compression be due to one of the more favourable primary (though malignant) tumours; even when histology of the spinal mass is available the site of the primary may remain a mystery, but most such cases prove to have small bronchial tumours.

Recovery of function after the removal of a benign extramedullary tumour can be dramatic, and patients who were bedridden may walk again in weeks. More often the final stages of improvement are slow, and active rehabilitation is vital if the most is to be made of the benefits of operation in patients already severely paralysed. Recovery of neurological function may continue for many months, and, in the case of regenerating cauda equina lesions, for as long as two years; both patient and physiotherapist may need to be reminded of this when morale flags.

Initially careful nursing is needed (p. 288) but the patient may get out of bed as soon as the sutures are removed, provided there is not gross vertebral body destruction. Even the most extensive laminectomy does not affect the weight-bearing components of the spine, and no special support or care is called for. Splints, toe-raising springs and calipers may be needed as temporary measures together with sticks or tripods.

Vascular lesions of the cord

Angiomas are better regarded as congenital malformations than as tumours. Cord function is probably more often affected by deprivation of blood supply, aggravated by episodes of hæmorrhage and thrombosis, than by compression. Occurring below the mid-thoracic level these irregular collections of abnormal vessels lie partly on the surface and partly within the cord, and so are not amenable to total excision. Only one or two largish veins may be seen on the posterior surface of the cord at laminectomy, but it will usually be obvious that the vessels disappear into the cord itself.

Clinically there may be a steadily progressive neurological deficit, but more often the course is episodic and remitting, simulating disseminated sclerosis. Moreover both conditions may be aggravated by pregnancy. Some relapses may be recognised as hæmorrhagic, either because of symptoms of spinal subarachnoid hæmorrhage, or because bloody or xanthochromic fluid is obtained on lumbar puncture. Myelography may show tortuous filling defects due to large vessels, which may also be demonstrated by intraspinous vertebral venography; water-soluble contrast (urographin) is injected into the marrow of the spinous process at the level of the lesion and fills the veins of the spinal canal in retrograde fashion. Teasing away part of the tumour may afford some relief and the operating microscope makes this a safer and more precise procedure.

Hæmorrhage compressing the cord is a rare event. Extradural, subdural or intramedullary (hæmatomylia) occur, as complications of trauma, angioma, or hæmophilia.

Thrombosis of the anterior spinal artery is an occasional cause of "transverse myelitis", usually causing an incomplete transverse lesion affecting motor more than sensory function. Many cases previously regarded as primarily vascular may have been due to cervical spondylosis producing myelopathy (p. 304).

Epidural spinal abscess

This commonly takes the form of an **acute** infection at the thoraco-lumbar junction, and is one of the causes of rapidly developing paraplegia.

Following a distant infection, usually a staphylococcal skin lesion such as a boil, a small focus of vertebral osteomyelitis develops and extradural pus accumulates. Bone changes can seldom be detected on X-ray; the diagnosis rests on a history of backache and root pain associated with pyrexia and malaise, followed after a few days by spreading numbness and later weakness of the legs. The spine is tender locally, and there may be muscle spasm and scoliosis; a band of hyperæsthesia is often found at the level of the compression. The white blood cell count is raised and also the sedimentation rate. Lumbar puncture and myelography can safely be carried out below the lesion, but a high puncture with a low lesion can result in the needle entering the abscess and draining pus, or even passing through the cavity carrying infection into the theca.

Cord function is threatened both by compression and spreading thrombosis. To be successful surgical drainage must be carried out before vascular changes have brought about total paraplegia. Urgent laminectomy is required; as much pus as possible is removed, but the dura is not opened. Two or three small rubber catheters with multiple holes are left in the extradural space, and through these dilute penicillin (3 ml. of 5,000 units/ml.) is irrigated every six hours for 48 hours. Maximal doses of systemic antibiotics are given on the presumption that the organisms are staphylococci, pending a bacteriological report. Provided surgery is expeditious the outlook is good.

Occasionally a **chronic** staphylococcal spinal abscess develops a cold abscess, with gross vertebral destruction and a paravertebral shadow. It is likely to be confused with tuberculous infection, but is most commonly found in the cervical region, and is confined to a single body. Rarely, an intradural abscess is found, either as a solitary lesion or due to infection of a dermoid, and this too is usually a chronic staphylococcal condition.

Pott's paraplegia

Spinal tuberculosis is still an occasional cause of cord compression. Initially infection is bony, an osteomyelitis affecting two or more adjacent vertebral bodies (rarely laminæ) and destroying the intervening discs. Collapse and kyphosis develop, and a paravertebral abscess collects on one or both sides. Cord compression *early* in the illness is usually due to the abscess, but when occurring *late* in the healing or quiescent phase is due to bone deformity. At either time it may be ascribed to sequestrated bone or disc, or to accumulations of granulation tissue or caseous material, and there is always the possibility of infective thrombosis.

Cord involvement complicates about 30% of cases of thoracic tuberculosis, the part of the spine most often affected. All degrees of compression occur, from altered reflexes to total paraplegia. Before antituberculous chemotherapy was available only about 50% of patients with Pott's paraplegia recovered sufficiently to walk usefully, and 25% died. Operation did little to help, both because it was often complicated by meningitis or by chronic wound sinuses, and because laminectomy (the only procedure performed) failed to deal with the compressing material which was situated anterior to the cord.

Chemotherapy has improved the control and shortened the duration of spinal tuberculosis; but cord complications still develop, sometimes as the presenting feature in hitherto undiagnosed and untreated cases. Surgery can now be performed *safely* even in the active phase, under cover of antituberculous drugs, and an *effective* operation has been devised for relieving cord compression, namely **antero-lateral decompression**. It should be performed without delay whenever paraplegia is progressive, or already of marked degree. If the signs of cord involvement are limited to reflex or sensory changes the patient may be observed for a time, whilst full doses of antituberculous drugs are given and the spine immobilised. Operation is done if there is any evidence of progression. If plain X-rays show a large paravertebral abscess, this should be drained by the limited operation of costotransversectomy, even if there is no evidence of cord involvement, in the hope of preventing paraplegia. Except for this, X-rays, lumbar puncture and myelography are of little help in deciding on the need for operation, or in planning the approach—which should always be centred on the clinical kyphos.

Antero-lateral decompression begins with the removal of the posterior four inches of at least three ribs on one side. This usually releases the paravertebral pus, and the intercostal nerves can then be identified. They enable the theca to be recognised, and the pedicles can then be nibbled away, leaving the laminæ, posterior intervertebral joints and the opposite pedicle intact in order to maintain the stability of the spine. The diseased tissue anterior to the theca can then be evacuated without the need to risk damaging the cord by retraction. Post-operative improvement is often noticed within 48 hours, almost always within a week.

Spinal injuries

These are largely the concern of orthopædic surgeons, and no detailed account will be given of the mechanics of injury or X-ray appearances.

The vast majority of closed spinal injuries leave the cord and roots quite unscathed. Most of those which are associated with CNS involvement have a fracture-dislocation in the cervical region, or at the thoraco-lumbar junction, the result of flexion strains. Some cervical injuries follow hyperextension and may then be associated with a head injury (a frontal blow causing the hyperextension). A relatively trivial injury of this kind, without a fracture, may produce profound paralysis if the patient already suffers from cervical spondylosis (p. 302).

CLINICAL

Both the spinal cord and the roots at the level of the injury are usually damaged. There may be a transient loss of function from concussion of the cord. Recovery from this may begin within 6 hours, and should be readily detected within 48 hours. When there is a complete lesion immediately after injury it is therefore impossible for some time to predict the chances of recovery, but if there is any evidence of conduction of impulses past the area of injury a considerable degree of recovery can confidently be expected. If on the other hand no function at all has returned by 48 hours it can safely be assumed that the lesion is a complete and permanent one, provided it is the cord itself which is involved.

With thoraco-lumbar injuries, however, it is the roots of the cauda equina which are damaged. It is vital to distinguish between root and cord lesions, because even though there is no sign of returning root activity some weeks after injury, recovery can still occur by a process of regeneration similar to that observed after peripheral nerve injuries. No such regeneration is possible in the spinal cord. When a mixed lesion of cauda equina and conus medullaris occurs, the root damage may give a false idea of the level of the lesion.

X-rays are unhelpful. Especially with hyperextension injuries there may be no apparent bony damage, even though the patient is totally paraplegic. But careful inspection may reveal small avulsion fractures of the spinous process, or of the antero-inferior margin of the body, which indicate that there has been hyperflexion or hyperextension although the spine now has a normal alignment.

Occasionally, in a patient with an incomplete lesion, the signs increase during the first few hours or days. This may be due to further damage to cord, or more often roots, by an unstable fracture, or by extrusion of intervertebral disc tissue. More rarely it may be due to pressure from a spicule of bone encroaching on the spinal canal or even to intramedullary hæmorrhage (hæmatomyelia). When a progressive spinal lesion is suspected it is important to determine, by lumbar puncture manometry and myelography, whether there is a spinal block, as laminectomy may then be indicated.

TREATMENT

In principle this closely resembles the management of head injuries in that little or nothing can be done to restore damage already done, and efforts are therefore directed to the prevention of complications and to providing the best conditions for natural recovery. Again, as with head injuries, the success of treatment depends more on skilled nursing than on operative surgery, which is seldom called for.

Active nursing of the paraplegic patient is the same whether the primary pathology is trauma, tumour or infection. It assumes particular importance after spinal injuries, because the problem presents itself suddenly in any hospital in the country where accidents are accepted. Failure to institute proper nursing care promptly can have disastrous effects; it can take months to heal sores or cure urinary tract infections which became established in the first week after injury. Yet no special skills are needed, only the conviction that active care is required, and that none of these complications need develop.

The skin

Pressure sores are quite simply the result of pressure on vulnerable areas of skin, where bone closely underlines it. The paraplegic patient has lost both the sensory urge and the motor power to shift position. But in addition to this, in the acute phase of spinal injury the skin is exceptionally liable to pressure damage, because of autonomic disturbance, and the patient needs to be turned every two hours, day and night. Lateral, prone and supine positions should all be assumed, in turn; divided mattresses allow the pressure points (anterior superior iliac spine, trochanters or sacrum) to be left free of pressure between two parts of the mattress.

The spine

This demand for regular turning must be met with the minimum risk of further damage to the spinal cord and roots at the level of the fracture.

Until the stability of the fracture has been assessed, which should be done as soon as possible, the spine must be handled with great care.

The danger of inflicting additional damage is greatest in the cervical region. A **temporary collar**, either of leather or improvised out of cardboard or newspaper, will prevent sudden flexion or extension. During turning in bed, positioning for X-rays, or transferring the patient from his bed to a trolley, firm traction should be exerted manually.

If the injury proves to be of the hyperextension type a collar will suffice as definitive treatment, because this is a stable fracture. Flexion injuries are best treated with **continuous skull traction**, even when this is not required to achieve initial reduction. Skull calipers are the safest way of maintaining traction, and are easily put in under local anæsthesia; the patient need not be moved from his bed or trolley for this minor procedure. The points are placed symmetrically above the external auditory meati; a small nick is made in the skin with a tenotome and the outer table drilled with a guarded bit. About 5 lb. traction is enough to keep the neck in a safe, neutral position, but much greater weights may be needed to reduce a difficult fracture-dislocation. Using a variety of pulley-holders the patient can assume almost any position in bed, and nursing procedures are both easier and safer once calipers are in position. Muscle spasm rapidly subsides and the patient is soon much more comfortable.

Thoraco-lumbar fracture-dislocations are usually relatively stable, and, if the patient is moved with care, and nursed in slight hyper-extension with a pillow in the small of the back, most remain reduced. When there is instability, and particularly if the lesion is incomplete and can therefore be made worse, **internal fixation** with plates and screws may be advisable so that regular turning can be continued.

The bladder

At first the bladder is without tone, and when it is full there is over-flow incontinence. After a few weeks, if the lesion is above the mid-thoracic segments, an **automatic bladder** is established, because a reflex arc is left intact between the bladder and the isolated lower part of the spinal cord. Active voiding occurs in response to stimuli such as distension by a sufficient volume of urine, or by scratching the skin in the region of the genitalia. Some patients learn to use this reflex regularly before distension causes involuntary emptying of the bladder. However, unexpected stimuli are always liable to trigger this mechanism, and few patients can rely on keeping dry without wearing a urinal of some kind. Lower lesions involving the sacral segments or roots leave the bladder permanently **atonic**, and some form of drainage has to be established; if overflow incontinence is allowed to persist infection invariably develops in the stagnant bladder.

No special care is required in the first 24 hours, but if the bladder cannot be emptied naturally at the end of this period something must be done. **Urethral catheterisation** is currently the method of choice, and this demands meticulous surgical technique if infection is to be avoided. Either a small Foley catheter or a plastic Gibbon type is used; drainage is intermittent, by releasing the clamp every four hours, in order to distend the bladder regularly in a natural manner. It is wise to prescribe a systemic antibiotic for the first two weeks; daily washouts of the bladder with 1:5,000 chlorhexidene should be continued as long as a catheter remains in the bladder. The catheter is changed weekly, or sooner if it becomes blocked. If urethritis develops it may respond to local irrigation; a Foley catheter should be removed and a small Gibbon type passed twice a day until the inflammation has settled.

When there are no facilities for aseptic catheterisation, it may be safest to temporise with **manual expression**; in women a bimanual technique achieves fairly complete emptying of the bladder. **Closed suprapubic drainage**, using a small catheter introduced by a stab method (Riches) is good emergency treatment, especially if there is a perineal injury making it impossible to establish urethral drainage. **Open suprapubic drainage** is now seldom employed. Even with suction the bladder is rarely completely emptied and it is impossible to prevent infection; because it is never distended the bladder may contract and it is then difficult to close the fistula and establish an automatic bladder.

The later management of the bladder cannot be discussed in detail. In principle it consists of maintaining adequate bladder drainage so as to prevent dilatation of the upper urinary tract, and of recognising and treating infections. These are easily overlooked in a paraplegic patient who cannot complain of dysuria or frequency; the common signs are headache, pyrexia and an increase in spasticity and flexor spasms. If drainage is unsatisfactory, the risk of recurrent infection is higher; a residual urine of less than 50 ml. should be the aim of treatment.

The limbs

From the start all joints in the paralysed limbs should be put through their full range of movements daily. As tone returns and spasticity develops, physiotherapy becomes vital in preventing contractures. Carefully padded splints, best made of plaster for the individual patient, may be required to prevent deformities developing. Flexor spasms, usually the most troublesome, are reduced in the prone position, and the patient should learn to sleep on his face; this will also tend to overcome the tendency to fixed hip flexion. At the same time the unaffected muscles of the shoulder girdles (in thoraco-lumbar lesions) are developed by active exercises against increasing resistance so that the patient will be able to hoist himself about with his arms when he becomes mobile again.

Spasticity is sometimes so severe that an attempt has to be made to achieve a balance of reflex activity by cutting tendons, muscles or peripheral nerves. Intrathecal injections of phenol or alcohol are less selective than peripheral operations, but are suitable for some patients with complete spinal lesions which cannot be aggravated by these injections.

General condition

In the early weeks after injury patients frequently develop a negative nitrogen balance and become anæmic. If bed sores and urinary infections are allowed to develop they may aggravate these metabolic disorders, which in turn hinder the control of infection and the healing of sores. Frequent blood transfusions are most helpful, even when the anæmia is not severe and the plasma proteins not unduly low.

Final rehabilitation

The paraplegic (except those with high cervical lesions) now has a reasonable expectation of leaving hospital within six months, and leading an independent life. This aim is most likely to be realised by rehabilitation in a special unit where there are no concessions to invalidism, and where the patient can be rigorously trained in the discipline necessary to avoid pressure sores and urinary infections, complications which remain threats even after he leaves hospital. A wheel-chair life may call for special arrangements at home and at work, but with determination these adjustments can be made, provided the patient is willing and well-advised.

FURTHER READING

Bloom, H. J. G., Ellis, H. and Jennett, W. B. (1955). The early diagnosis of spinal tumours. *British Medical Journal*, **1**, 10–16.

Brice, J. and McKissock, W. (1965). Surgical treatment of malignant extradural spinal tumours. *British Medical Journal*, **2**, 1341–1344.

Editorial (1968). Pott's paraplegia. *British Medical Journal*, **1**, 638.

Editorial (1969). Neurogenic intermittent claudication. *British Medical Journal*, **1**, 662.

Gautier-Smith, P. C. (1967). Clinical aspects of spinal neurofibromas. *Brain*, **90**, 359–394.

Guttman, L. (1976). Spinal cord injuries. 2nd Edition. Blackwell, Oxford.

Greenwood, J. (1963). Intramedullary tumours of spinal cord. *Journal of Neurosurgery*, **20**, 665–668.

Nathan, P. W. (1965). Chemical rhizotomy for relief of spasticity in ambulant patients. *British Medical Journal*, **2**, 1096–1100.

Newman, M. J. D. (1959). Racemose angioma of the spinal cord. *Quarterly Journal of Medicine*, **28**, 97–109.

Ommaya, A. K., Di Chiro, G. and Doppman, J. (1969). Ligation of arterial supply in the treatment of spinal cord arteriovenous malformation. *Journal of Neurosurgery*, **30**, 679–691.

Shaw, N. E. and Thomas, T. G. (1963). Surgical treatment of chronic infective lesions of the spine. *British Medical Journal*, **1**, 162–164.

Smith, R. (1965). An evaluation of surgical treatment for spinal cord compression due to metastatic carcinoma. *Journal of Neurology, Neurosurgery and Psychiatry*, **28**, 152–158.

CHAPTER 16

Prolapsed Intervertebral Disc

Introduction

Lumbar spine

Cervical spine
Acute disc prolapse
Cervical spondylosis

Thoracic spine

Degeneration and trauma combine to produce disc lesions, the two factors operating in varying proportions in different parts of the spine, and from one individual to another. Degeneration is a normal ageing process, the large fluid nucleus pulposus of childhood undergoing progressive dehydration and shrinkage throughout life. Trauma, in the form of a single major incident or of repeated minor stresses (sometimes occupational), may directly precipitate prolapse or it may accentuate degenerative changes which predispose to prolapse in the future.

The highly mobile cervical spine is more prone to degenerative changes, and most disc protrusions in this region occur at or past middle age. In the lumbar region trauma is more often predominant, and young persons in physically stressful occupations (such as miners or nurses) are common sufferers. A disc protrusion may be *lateral*, compressing a single nerve root, or *central* causing pressure on the spinal cord or, in the lumbar region, the cauda equina (fig. 70).

Lumbar spine

PATHOGENESIS

Almost all protrusions are at one of the lower two spaces; L5/S1 is affected twice as often as L4/5, but both discs are affected in about 10% of patients. Most lesions are lateral and affect either the L5 or the SI nerve root; but the few central protrusions that occur are important because they can produce paraplegia with sphincter involvement.

Often the onset is undramatic, sometimes following unaccustomed activity such as digging the garden or playing games after a long interval. No immediate ill effect is felt, but the patient wakes next morning with severe backache and may be unable to get out of bed at all. After several days in bed the pain usually subsides, often without there having been any sciatica; further attacks follow similar strains, perhaps with years of freedom between episodes. Usually after one or more incidents of backache alone the pain begins to spread into the buttock and down the leg, but this can occur in the first attack.

A single sudden injury or strain is the obvious cause in some cases. As the incident recurs, often when lifting a heavy weight, the patient is struck by severe pain in the back with or without sciatica. He may be unable to get up off the ground or be able only to hobble away bent double. A few cases develop during pregnancy, and may recur only in subsequent pregnancies; physiological laxity of ligaments may be a factor in these cases, and the protrusions are often central rather than lateral.

Some patients are unable to recall any unusual strain before their first attack, which may have been dismissed as mild lumbago. Even patients who do claim some obvious cause for their condition may remember attacks of mild lumbago years before, and it is likely that these were due to the early stages of their disc disease.

For so common a disease we are surprisingly ignorant of the ætiology, but clearly trauma is seldom the sole factor, even in the lumbar region. Operative findings are often difficult to relate to clinical manifestations; the removal of a small protrusion may afford dramatic relief from severe symptoms, whilst operation during an acute episode of pain may reveal a totally sequestrated fragment of disc so adherent to its surroundings that it must have been extruded months previously. Radiculitis is probably an important factor, and the nerve root is sometimes seen to be inflamed at operation during an acute attack. Resolution of symptoms with conservative treatment is more likely to be due to subsidence of this inflammation, or to the root changing position in relation to the disc, than to the protrusion reducing itself. Swelling of protruded disc material by the absorption of water may account for root compression developing some time after the incident which produced the initial prolapse, and subsequent desiccation could account for spontaneous improvement in symptoms without treatment.

CLINICAL SYNDROMES

Two components can be recognised in most instances, the spinal and the radicular, but either may occur alone.

Spinal pain probably results from the torn annulus fibrosus in the acute stage, but when the condition becomes chronic secondary factors such as arthritis of the interarticular joints may contribute. The mechanics of the spine are disturbed, giving rise to characteristic signs—

loss of lumbar lordosis (rare in any other condition), scoliosis and acute spasm of the erector spinæ. This may result in a completely "frozen" spine, attempts at toe-touching producing movement only at the hip joint whilst the lumbar spine remains rigid.

Radicular pain from the lower two disc spaces is reported as sciatica, and may spread only as far as the buttock or radiate to the calf and ankle. The rare upper disc protrusions cause anterior crural pain, affecting the front of the thigh. Root pain is aggravated by movement, by strains such as coughing and sneezing which increase intrathecal pressure, and by straight-leg raising. The sciatic nerve may be tender to palpation in the buttock. Paræsthesiæ may be complained of in the affected dermatomes around the foot, and are often precipitated by the same factors as aggravate the pain.

Objective evidence of root compression may be found, but even with severe sciatica there may be no neurological signs. Sensory loss is usually limited to diminished appreciation of pin-prick in part of the L5 or S1 dermatome, according to the root affected (fig. 62). Weakness of the extensor hallucis longus and wasting of extensor digitorum brevis (which normally forms a bulge on the dorsum of the foot) are frequent with L5 root lesions; occasionally severe foot drop develops and persists after the pain has subsided. Reduction or complete absence of the ankle jerk usually indicates compression of S1 root. However, neither this, nor the distribution of motor and sensory signs and symptoms, can be relied on to localise the level of the protrusion; there are variations in the distribution of the roots forming the lumbosacral plexus, whilst a disc at the upper level (L4/5) can compress both the lower roots at the same time (fig. 70a), moreover both discs may be prolapsed.

About 2% of operated lumbar disc protrusions are **central** in situation (fig. 70(*b*)) and cause compression of the cauda equina. This serious development can occur in the very first attack, but more often there is a story of recurrent sciatica which often involves *both* legs, either in turn or at the same time. Both ankle jerks may be absent. When there is evidence of bilateral root involvement operation should be recommended lest the next attack be complicated by sphincter paralysis and bilateral foot drop. Sometimes paraplegia comes on insidiously without a great deal of pain, or the patient may wake up after manipulation under anæsthesia to find the pain gone but the legs paralysed.

INVESTIGATION

The diagnosis of a disc lesion is made on the history and clinical examination; investigations are undertaken to exclude other conditions rather than to confirm a prolapse. **Plain X-rays** show narrowing of the disc space in less than half the patients with proved disc lesions. Scoliosis, too limited to be obvious clinically, may be recognised and loss of lumbar lordosis confirmed. Evidence of a spinal tumour, ankylosing

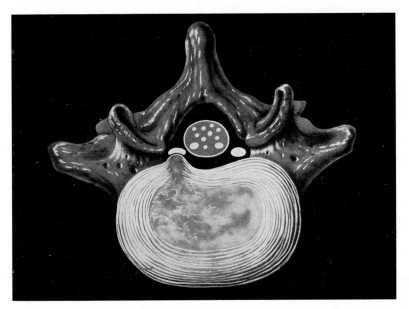

(a) *Lateral* lesions affect one, or at most two, roots causing unilateral symptoms.

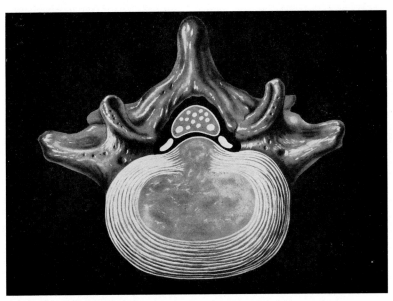

(b) *Central* lesions may compress emerging roots (extradurally) on both sides, but can also affect all the roots of the cauda equina (intradurally) at that level.

FIG. 70 Lumbar disc prolapse

spondylitis or vertebral tuberculosis may be found and explain the pain.

Lumbar puncture will usually show normal dynamics but the protein may be increased up to 100 mg/100 ml; a central protrusion may produce a spinal block with yellow proteinaceous fluid if the needle is inserted below it, but even above the disc the fluid may be similar. Clearly the discovery of a high protein will not distinguish between disc and tumour, but in such circumstances this is not vital because both call for exploration.

Myelography is not a very reliable method for detecting disc lesions and false findings, both positive and negative, occur in even the most skilled hands. It is less likely to miss a lesion at L4/5 than at the lower space, where the canal is wider. It is therefore doubtful whether the decision to operate should be based on myelographic findings; the clinical history and findings are more important. These do not reliably indicate the level of the protrusion—but as the myelogram is not wholly reliable, and as some patients have lesions at both spaces, it is probably best to deal with this problem by making it a rule always to inspect both spaces at operation. Oil myelography may be needed if a high disc lesion, or a spinal tumour is suspected.

Water-soluble media are becoming available for the demonstration of the lower spaces, and being less dense they are able to show more detail. They can (at present) be used only for the lower lumbar spine because if contrast comes in contact with the conus medullaris painful muscle spasms occur (controllable by Diazepam). For this reason the patient must sit up for about six hours after injection; less irritant media are under development.

CONSERVATIVE TREATMENT

The majority of episodes diagnosed as disc protrusions settle in time without operative treatment. Complete **bed-rest**, lying flat with only one pillow, accelerates resolution as well as affording immediate relief of pain in most cases. A hard mattress is better than a soft one, and this may be achieved with fracture boards or by putting the mattress on the floor. An unyielding mattress limits spinal flexion, which is painful, and it is much easier to turn over on a flat surface than in a hollow. A severe attack requires at least a fortnight strictly in bed, followed by gradual mobilisation. Continuous **skin traction** applied to the legs (7 lb. on each side with the foot elevated 12 in.) may give relief from acute pain when bed-rest alone has proved ineffective.

If pain recurs as soon as the patient gets up but is not very severe a **plaster jacket** may give some degree of rest to the spine without the necessity of returning to bed. A steel reinforced long **spinal support** has the advantage that as improvement sets in it can be put off for gradually increasing periods and is still available should a recurrence develop.

These devices do not so much support the spine as prevent excessive movement which might aggravate the root lesion.

Manipulation is practised much more widely than many doctors imagine. Numerous patients find someone willing to give them local treatment of this kind when they feel they are receiving insufficient sympathy or attention from their ordinary medical attendants. Chronic recurring disc pain is very demoralising, and it is small comfort to be assured that it is a common condition, that it will settle in time, and that it is unlikely to result in serious disability. Many patients report dramatic cures from manipulation and in skilled hands and with proper precautions it has a limited place in treatment. But when manipulations have to be repeated they tend to be of less value each time. It is unlikely that a prolapsed disc is ever restored to its rightful place; more likely a loose fragment is slipped away from the root or secondary non-articular adhesions are broken down. Excessive flexion, especially under anæsthesia, is dangerous, and no manipulation should be considered if a central lesion is suspected; patients have been made paraplegic by manipulation in these circumstances.

OPERATION

Surgery is necessary only when conservative measures fail, and, except when there is cauda equina compression, should not be offered to a patient who has not given bed rest a serious trial. Many patients diagnosed as having a disc lesion enjoy long remissions or suffer only one attack. The **indications** for surgery are:

1. **Recurrent episodes** of pain, especially when sciatica predominates over backache.

2. **An unrelieved acute attack** of sciatica, even when it is the first episode. A few patients, most of whom prove to have extruded a massive fragment of disc, continue to experience excruciating pain even in bed and on traction; on one should under-estimate the severity of this pain which can reduce the toughest stoic to tears. In such instances early operation is indicated even if there are no neurological signs.

3. **Progressive CNS involvement**, either extending sensory loss or rapidly worsening paralysis of the dorsiflexors. The place of surgery is disputed when the patient presents with an established foot-drop of some weeks duration but is quite free of pain. Some surgeons believe that little good comes from exploration in such circumstances, but it is probably wise to operate because recovery can occur by regeneration in a motor nerve root and continuing compression is likely to hinder this.

4. **Suspected central protrusion**, as indicated by bilateral sciatica or bilateral radicular signs, even though limited to absent ankle jerks or sensory loss. Once paraplegia is established recovery is extremely slow and usually incomplete, and operation in these cases should be urged whether or not pain is severe.

5. **Doubt about the diagnosis** may justify exploration. If a spinal

tumour is suspected, either clinically or because of equivocal myelographic findings, there may be no alternative.

Technique

Neurosurgeons usually perform this operation in the prone position, in which case the hips should be supported so that the abdomen is free of the table; this greatly reduces congestion in the extradural veins and makes for an easier exposure. Alternatively the lateral position may be used, or the patient may crouch on the table over bent knees and hips with the object of opening up the interlaminar spaces.

Although loosely referred to as laminectomy, such a complete exposure is usually reserved for large central protrusions. For the usual lateral lesions the muscles need be stripped from the spinous processes on the affected side only. The margins of the laminæ above and below the space are nibbled away, and the ligamentum flavum removed to expose the root and the disc beyond it. The posterior longitudinal ligament is usually intact over the disc, and must be incised before disc material can be removed, but sometimes it has already ruptured and disc fragments are found free in the spinal canal; they may then migrate some distance from the level of the disc from which they sequestrated.

It is not enough to remove only the sequestrated fragment because more may prolapse later; the disc space should be emptied as far as possible, using a scraping instrument until bone is felt above and below. Because lesions are found at both the lower two lumbar spaces in 10% of cases, and even myelography cannot reliably exclude a lesion, it is wise always to explore both spaces even when a lesion is found at the first space exposed. The operation does not weaken the spine as no weight-bearing structures are removed.

Free movement in bed may be permitted immediately after operation, and the patient can get up in two or three days if he is comfortable in bed. Fairly rapid mobilisation under the supervision of a physiotherapist is valuable. Although many patients are ready to leave hospital by the tenth day, it is unwise to send a patient home until his confidence is fully restored, and this takes longer in some patients than in others. Normal activities should be resumed gradually; a man might return to office work within a month, but heavy work or strenuous games should not be considered until two or three months after operation. After this no restriction is necessary, and there is no reason for wearing any form of support.

Complications

Only infection is at all common, but if wound infection develops it may be slow to resolve, because the blood supply in the midline of the back is rather meagre. Occasionally patients develop severe back pain a week or so after operation, sometimes worse than their original disc pain, and relief comes only by nursing in a plaster bed for a month or so. This condition appears to be related to the development of fusion between the two vertebræ across the operated disc space, perhaps precipitated by low-grade infection. The ultimate results in patients who have this complication are particularly good. Attempts to encourage fusion by inserting bone chips into the empty disc space are seldom successful, but some surgeons carry out posterior spinal fusion in selected cases, usually when back pain is the principal complaint and persists after disc removal.

Results

The outcome of operation for disc removal is very good in about 80% of cases, provided selection has been judicious. As soon as the patient recovers from the anæsthetic, he may remark that his leg or his back feels free again and that the pain has gone. However, the continuation or the re-appearance of sciatica during the first fortnight after operation is common, and is no reason for anxiety. It is probably due to inflammatory changes in the compressed root which may have been temporarily aggravated by retraction at operation. Neurological signs recover variably, and some degree of sensory loss and a depressed ankle jerk may persist indefinitely. Sciatica is more reliably relieved than backache and the patients who rate the success of operation as only "fair" mostly suffer from continuing backache or stiffness; a few patients claim not to be any better after operation and continue to suffer from episodic sciatica but no patient should be worse. Sometimes persisting symptoms are due to a migrated fragment missed at operation or to a second protrusion not discovered at operation. Apart from these obvious causes for failure results are less favourable in patients over 40 years of age, in those with heavy manual occupations and when sciatica has persisted for more than a year before operation. Patients with occupations or leisure activities which inevitably put strain on the back should be strongly advised to seek an alternative job or sport, even though pain has satisfactorily subsided either with conservative measures or after operation. After major cauda equina compression motor recovery continues slowly over 18 months or more; control of the bladder is regained only slowly and often incompletely.

Recurrence

Reappearance of pain, or of a complete disc syndrome, occurs in up to 10% of patients after successful operation, sometimes after several years complete freedom from symptoms. The usual explanations are:

(1) Recurrent protrusion at the operated site.
(2) Protrusion of a previously unaffected disc.
(3) Adhesions between the root and the operated disc.
(4) Arachnoiditis, with associated radiculitis at one or more levels.

Cervical spine

Disc disease in the cervical region seldom takes the form of the protrusion of a single nucleus pulposus. Degenerative changes affecting several discs are more usual, giving rise to the radiological appearance of cervical spondylosis—although this may be accompanied by no signs or symptoms whatever.

Acute disc prolapse

This can occur at any age, and in a spine showing no radiological evidence of spondylosis, although it may be superimposed on this degenerative condition. Often a single incident of trauma is remembered, which was followed at first by only neck stiffness but later by signs of CNS disorder. Acute prolapse is more commonly central than lateral, and causes weakness and spasticity of the legs; but some root pain, muscle wasting and paræsthesiæ in the upper limb may also occur. A relatively acute onset, sometimes days or even weeks after the original trauma, is not uncommon, and may be followed by a period of relative improvement. But the signs may be steadily progressive, strongly suggestive of a spinal tumour; the myelogram may show a complete block and sometimes the kind of fading defect associated with intramedullary tumour. A late sequel is focal spondylosis with disc collapse and osteophytosis confined to one space only.

Operation is urgently required for this condition, and the neck must be handled with extreme caution during induction of anæsthesia and positioning on the table (p. 302). When the dura is opened at laminectomy the backward bulge of the cord is usually obvious. The dura is cut laterally and dissected off the disc which is incised; the central protrusion is milked laterally to the incision into the space where it can safely be picked out in small pieces. This may have to de done from both sides, leaving the dura intact anteriorly in front of the cord. The patient wears a soft collar for a month or so after operation, and the results are usually satisfactory.

Cervical spondylosis

This results from an ageing process. Radiological changes are found in 75% of patients over 50 years of age who have no spontaneous complaints referable to the neck. Because these changes appear earlier in men than in women they are presumed to be related in part to occupational trauma, but seldom is any direct association demonstrated. However, trauma may clearly be the factor precipitating symptoms in a patient already afflicted with spondylosis.

PATHOLOGY

The primary lesion is probably collapse of the disc with annular protrusion around its whole circumference. As ligaments are pulled away from their attachment to the margins of the vertebral bodies, reactive osteophytosis develops, and the ligaments themselves thicken. Together with the low annular protrusion, osteophytes and ligaments reduce the antero-posterior diameter of the spinal canal. Arthritis of the neuro-central joints, which abut on the foraminæ from C3 to C7, leads to further bony proliferation, which encroaches on the intervertebral foraminæ already narrowed by disc protrusion and osteophytes. Fibrosis in the dural root sleeves in this situation constricts the root, and tethers both it and the cord during spinal movements. The mobility of the spine itself is also impaired, restricted where disc changes are advanced and excessive at unaffected levels above and below.

Many factors contribute to the production of symptoms and signs when these do appear. The spinal cord, lying tethered in a narrowed spinal canal is liable to suffer additional compression during even normal neck movements. In extension, for example, the ligamenta flava wrinkle and can form a posterior compressing agent. When extremes of move-ment are reached the cord is in great jeopardy, and sudden symptoms may follow excessive flexion or extension due to accidental trauma or to seemingly uneventful endoscopy under anæsthesia (p 304). But compression of the cord or roots is seldom the whole story. Both the anterior spinal artery and the radicular arteries in the foraminæ are in vulnerable situations, and the site of cord damage found pathologic-ally corresponds closely to that resulting from thrombosis of the anterior spinal artery. Indeed it now seems likely that many patients formerly regarded as suffering from primary vascular occlusions in the spinal cord were in fact spondylotics.

RADIOLOGICAL SIGNS

1. **Narrowing of the disc space**, affecting one space only in 40%, two spaces in 40%, and more than two in the rest. In rather more than a third, C5/6 is affected, and in rather less than a third C6/7 or C4/5; less often C3/4 is involved and C7/T1 only rarely.

2. **Change in the normal curve**, commonly a loss of the natural lordosis; this may be restricted to two adjacent vertebræ, and limited mobility between them is best demonstrated by comparing films taken in flexion and extension.

3. **Osteophytes** are more obvious anteriorly but posterior overgrowth is more important; foraminal narrowing is seen only in oblique views.

4. **Myelographic indentations** of the anterior dura do not always conform to the levels of maximum disc collapse and osteophytosis. Posterior indentations due to ligamenta flava are rarely seen, probably because films are not often taken in extension. A complete block is unusual, but when it occurs may indicate acute disc prolapse.

CLINICAL SYNDROMES

Advanced radiological changes can occur without any clinical accom-paniments; but a number of asymptomatic patients, in whom spondyl-osis is a chance finding, prove on careful examination to have evidence of mild cord compression (spasticity, increased reflexes, or sensory changes). When there are florid symptoms and signs they do not always correspond to the level of maximum radiological change. Even when both radicular and cord involvement occur one or other is usually predominant.

In consequence two main syndromes are recognised.

Brachial neuropathy

Pain is the principal complaint, dull and aching in the neck and shoulder with shooting pain down the arm to the elbow or wrist. Although only one root is affected the pain spreads beyond the dermatome distribution, probably because it develops also within muscles supplied by that root. Pain may also arise from the disc itself.

Muscle spasm and tenderness may give rise to secondary spread of pain, especially to the occipital region where it is complained of as headache.

Paræsthesiæ are frequently experienced in the arm and the tip of the thumb (C6 root from C5/6 lesion) or the middle finger (C7 from C6/7 lesion). Sensory loss, weakness, wasting and reflex changes are usually slight.

These complaints may appear relatively suddenly, sometimes precipitated by trauma; or they can develop insidiously; repeated attacks of acute pain occur in some patients. Very often the pain is related to movement and position, and there is not a clear distinction between the syndromes of lateral disc lesion, spondylosis, brachial neuritis and the various anatomical types of thoracic outlet syndrome (scalenus anticus, costoclavicular and cervical rib compressions). Whilst occasional pure cases of these are recognised, it seems likely that in the majority a combination of factors contrive to produce a similar type of disorder. Some believe that whatever the level of the initial lesion there is liable to be a secondary spread, to higher and lower branches of the brachial plexus, of interstitial changes in the nerve trunks, limiting their elasticity and making them susceptible to damage during normal movements. The relief of a syndrome by surgical attack at one level does not necessarily prove that this was the site of the original pathological lesion. An example is found in cases of carpal tunnel compression associated with pain in the upper arm and shoulder which is relieved by operation at the wrist.

TREATMENT OF BRACHIAL NEUROPATHY

Providing rest for the affected part is the basis of all methods. Aggravating movements must be avoided, whatever these are in the individual case. The arm may be supported from the unaffected shoulder with a **sling,** and this together with analgesics, injections of procaine into tender spots and local heat and shortwave diathermy may be sufficient to give relief. Active physiotherapy is contraindicated apart from shoulder girdle strengthening exercises.

More effective immobilisation is provided by a **collar.** Whilst a plastic model is being made to the patient's measurements, a simple substitute of sorbo rubber and cardboard is well worth wearing and considerable relief follows in a few days. Some surgeons prefer a light Minerva **plaster of paris cast** which incorporates the head, neck and shoulders, and this may have to be used if a collar is not giving good relief. A collar is preferable because its use can be discontinued gradually, it can be kept to wear again if a recurrence threatens, and it is not so socially embarrassing as a plaster cast. Patients can often be induced to return to work whilst still wearing a collar, and this is advantageous because immobilisation should be continued for three or four weeks after pain has subsided; relapse often follows premature return to normal free movement.

Skull traction, using ice-tong calipers and 5–6 lb. weight (p. 289), is reserved for those who fail to respond to simpler methods. Manual traction in various directions is first tried until the right one is found. Traction often relieves acute pain rapidly, and can be replaced by a collar after 2 or 3 weeks. Manipulation may be of value in skilled hands, and always provided there is no evidence of cord compression.

Many **operations** have been devised, mostly directed at relieving pressure on the affected root. These include simple decompression of the foraminæ, removal of discs and osteophytes, and fusion of the spine at the affected level by bone grafts placed from the front. Few surgeons remain enthusiastic about these operations for long, and fortunately conservative measures, with proper application and persistence are at least equally effective.

Cervical myelopathy

Insidious development of **spasticity in the legs** is the most frequent mode of onset, noticed first either as slowness or clumsiness in walking. **Weakness** is less striking than increased tone and exaggerated deep reflexes. Rather more than two-thirds have some **sensory loss,** but in only half of these is there a definite sensory level, and then it is often upper thoracic rather than cervical; in the rest the deficit is radicular in pattern or, occasionally, a suspended area of loss over the thorax such as accompanies syringomyelia. About a third complain of **neck pain and stiffness**, and a similar number have **clumsy hands** with wasting, and occasionally fasciculation, of the small muscles of the hand and paræsthesiæ are also common.

Sudden aggravation of cervical myelopathy, or even the abrupt appearance of spinal cord symptoms for the first time, may follow **trauma.** Hyperextension injuries insufficient to cause fracture or dislocation are particularly liable to precipitate a transverse spinal lesion in a patient with cervical spondylosis, even when this has hitherto been asymptomatic. Tripping and falling on the head (with resulting frontal abrasions) is a common mechanism, but another is hyperextension during surgical procedures such as tonsillectomy, bronchoscopy or œsophagoscopy; even the manipulations required to pass an endotracheal tube by an anæsthetist can jeopardise the cord especially when all protective muscle spasm has been abolished by relaxant drugs.

Sometimes a person with spondylosis develops paraplegia over a period of minutes without any obvious trauma; either normal neck movements have been sufficient to cause further damage in a situation already critical; or a vascular occlusion or acute disc protrusion has occurred. Before accepting spinal cord symptoms as due to spondylosis, it is vital to exclude other treatable conditions such as spinal cord tumour, sub-acute combined degeneration and neurosyphilis; also to distinguish primary degenerations such as motor neurone disease and disseminated sclerosis which have a less favourable prognosis than spondylotic myelopathy and are not helped by operation. Considering the frequency with which radiological changes occur there is a danger of attributing to spondylosis any cervical cord disorder first appearing in middle age.

TREATMENT OF MYELOPATHY

Because the natural history of this condition is imperfectly understood, it is difficult to assess the need for treatment, let alone its effectiveness. Asymptomatic and mild cases occur with severe radiological changes, and many probably remain in this stage unless trauma precipitates a crisis. Even then recovery from acute paraplegia is often quite rapid without any special measures being taken, but it is wise to fit a collar to limit neck movements. **Immobilisation** seldom improves myelopathy of the chronic type, but may relieve neck and arm pain if these are prominent.

The question of **surgery** arises when an acute incident is associated with a spinal block or fails to improve rapidly. In chronic cases operation is often urged when there is severe and progressive disability, if there is doubt about the diagnosis, or if the myelogram shows a marked indentation at one disc level.

Operation may be confined to providing a wide posterior decompression by *laminectomy*, opening the dura and cutting dentate ligaments at several levels. This deals with the antero-posterior narrowing of the spinal canal, removes the possibility of ligamenta flava impinging on the cord from behind, and may allow the cord to ride away from the anterior irregularities of discs and osteophytes. Some patients are improved for a time but are liable to relapse within a couple of years.

The hazards and practical difficulties of removing the bony bars and ridges anterior to the cord, perhaps at several levels, are formidable. Simple decompression owes its popularity to this. But some surgeons believe that only if these are adequately dealt with will worthwhile relief be obtained, and certainly the best results are in those cases in which a large anterior indentation is seen, both on the myelogram and at operation, and is removed. Such cases merge with acute disc protrusions which give the best operative results of all. The difficulty is that the already damaged cord will not tolerate retraction, and the offending bony mass must be approached from the lateral aspect and this can be a tedious and difficult process. A period in a collar is advisable after operation, followed by a spell of active rehabilitation.

A different approach is *anterior interbody fusion* (Cloward's operation). A peg of bone from the patient, from the human bone bank or from the selection of prepared animal bones which are available, replaces a core of tissue of the same size consisting of parts of the opposing vertebral bodies and the intervening degenerated disc. This may be done at two or three levels if necessary.

Thoracic spine

Only two or three disc lesions in a thousand are thoracic, and all these occur below the fifth thoracic vertebra. Most patients are between 40 and 50, and a number recall an injury before the onset of symptoms. Radicular pain is abdominal in distribution and is readily mistaken for visceral disease. Spinal cord compression can develop without any pain at all, and may then resemble primary degenerative disease of the cord. Paraplegia may develop rapidly over a few days or increase gradually over many months, or even years. An anterior lesion is produced, akin to anterior spinal artery thrombosis, with spastic weakness of the legs and spinothalamic rather than posterior column sensory loss.

Radiological evidence of degeneration in the thoracic spine takes the form of calcification in the disc spaces, not narrowing or osteophytic lipping. Calcified discs are an occasional incidental finding in the middle aged, and when a clinical disc syndrome does develop this may not correspond to one of the calcified interspaces. Myelography does not often demonstrate a complete block, but the lesion can usually be localised by its filling defect much more reliably than from the clinical level of disc calcification.

Operation is difficult because the thoracic spinal canal is naturally narrow and largely filled by the spinal cord. The disc lesion is central and anterior to the cord, which is even less tolerant to retraction when already stretched over a hump than in the cervical region. A careful attack from the side is necessary, and it has even been suggested that an antero-lateral decompression (p. 296) makes the best approach. The disc is usually partly calcified and must be nibbled and worn away gradually. Some patients already severely paraplegic fail to improve after operation, probably because there are secondary vascular changes in the anterior spinal artery distribution which the removal of the disc does nothing to reverse.

FURTHER READING

Armstrong, J. R. (1965). Lumbar disc lesions. 3rd edition. Livingstone, Edinburgh.

Brain, R. and Wilkinson, M. (1967). *Cervical spondylosis and other disorders of the cervical spine.* Heinemann, London.

Chrispin, A. R. and Lees, F. (1963). The spinal canal and cervical spondylosis. *Journal of Neurology, Neurosurgery and Psychiatry*, **26**, 166–170.

Cloward, R. (1958). The anterior approach for the removal of ruptured cervical discs. *Journal of Neurosurgery*, **15**, 602–617.

Epstein, J. A. and Lavine, L. S. (1964). Herniated lumbar intervertebral discs in teenage children. *Journal of Neurosurgery*, **21**, 1070–1075.

Fisher, R. G (1965). Protrusions of thoracic disc. *Journal of Neurosurgery*, **22**, 591–593.

Jennett, W. B. (1958). A study of 25 cases of compression of the cauda equina by prolapsed intervertebral discs. *Journal of Neurology, Neurosurgery and Psychiatry*, **19**, 109–116.

Lees, F. and Turner, J. W. A. (1963). Natural history and prognosis of cervical spondylosis. *British Medical Journal*, **2**, 1607–1610.

Le Vay, D. (1967). A survey of surgical management of lumbar disc prolapse in the United Kingdom and Eire. *Lancet*, **i**, 1211–1213.

Marshall, W. J. S. and Schorstein, J. (1968). Factors affectng the results of surgery for prolapsed lumbar intervertebral disc. *Scottish Medical Journal*, **13**, 38–42.

Naylor, A. (1951). Brachial neuritis with particular reference to lesions of the cervical intervertebral discs. *Annals of the Royal College of Surgeons of England*, **13**, 158–187.

O'Connell, J. E. A. (1950). The indications for and results of the excision of lumbar intervertebral disc protusions: a review of 500 cases. *Annals of the Royal College of Surgeons of England*, **6**, 403–412.

Pearce, J. and Moll, J. M. H. (1967). Conservative treatment and natural history of acute lumbar disc lesions. *Journal of Neurology, Neurosurgery and Psychiatry*, **30**, 13–17.

Stern, W. E. and Crandall, P. H. (1959). Inflammatory intervertebral disc diseases as a complication of the operative treatment of lumbar herniations. *Journal of Neurosurgery*, **26**, 261–276.

Symon, L. and Lavender, P. (1967). The surgical treatment of cervical spondylotic myelopathy. *Neurology* (Minneapolis), **17**, 117–126.

Verbiest, H. and Paz Y. Geuse, H. D. (1966). Anterolateral surgery for cervical spondylosis and cases of myelopathy or nerve root compression. *Journal of Neurosurgery*, **25**, 611–622.

V: Congenital Conditions

CHAPTER 17

Hydrocephalus and other Cranial Abnormalities

Infantile hydrocephalus

Juvenile and adult hydrocephalus
  aqueduct stricture
  low-pressure hydrocephalus

Craniostenosis

Infantile hydrocephalus

PATHOLOGY

Non-communicating (obstructive) hydrocephalus is due to a block within the ventricular system which prevents the escape of CSF into the subarachnoid space. The block is normally at one of the narrows: foramen of Monro, aqueduct of Sylvius or the foraminæ of exit from the fourth ventricle (figs. 3).

In **communicating** hydrocephalus the ventricles and the subarachnoid space are in communication; the cause is still most often an *obstruction* but placed more distally, in the basal cisterns. Although CSF can escape into the cisterna magna and the lumbar theca it cannot reach the supratentorial subarachnoid space, over the surface of the cerebral hemispheres, where absorption normally takes place. Occasional cases of communicating hydrocephalus are due to *overproduction of CSF*, such as when there is a papilloma of the choroid plexus. Very occasionally it may develop due to obstruction in the superior longitudinal sinus (and *reduced absorption of CSF*).

Communicating and non-communicating forms of hydrocephalus are about equally common in infancy; sometimes secondary block develops, converting one form into the other. It is seldom easy, even at post-mortem examination, to determine with certainty the primary cause of hydrocephalus. The commonest factors appear to be **birth trauma** and **meningitis**, each of which excites a meningeal reaction with subsequent adhesions at several sites. The commonest site is the cisterna ambiens, the narrow space between the midbrain and the tentorial edge (figs. 9, 25); the arachnoid villi elated to the superior longitudinal sinus may also be involved in adhesions. Congenital **malformations** are found in about a quarter, most commonly a narrowed aqueduct, atresia of the exit foramina of the fourth ventricle, or an Arnold–Chiari malformation. This last is almost always found when hydrocephalus is associated with spina bifida (see p. 330).

Occasional cases of infantile hydrocephalus are due to **tumour**. In almost a quarter **no obvious cause** can be found, but as both birth trauma and neonatal infections are readily overlooked it is quite likely that these account for most of the remaining cases.

CLINICAL

In the first six months of life raised pressure produces an enlarging head and bulging fontanelle rather than headaches and papillœdema. The parents may have noticed the **big head** since birth, or it may only have been obvious recently. The head circumference can be compared with a chart showing the normal limits (fig. 71). The **rate of growth** can be assessed by repeating the measurement in two or three weeks, if the circumference is not already very abnormal. Doubt may arise in families who tend to have big heads, but the top of the head is then usually rather flat, and the face is large in proportion to the skull vault rather than dwarfed by it as in hydrocephalus.

A **bulging fontanelle** is a more reliable sign of raised pressure if the head is not very big, but it must be felt while the child is quiet. Dehydration due to vomiting or poor feeding, not uncommon in hydrocephalus, may cause the fontanelle to feel soft in spite of expanding ventricles.

Less constant features are epilepsy of some kind, major convulsions being less common than minor twitchings, or sudden head sagging, or eye rolling; mental retardation evidenced by slowness in passing the normal milestones; blindness with pale optic discs; and spasticity of one or more limbs. Many of these signs are probably due to underlying brain damage (e.g. birth trauma or congenital malformation) rather than to the effects of the dilated ventricles.

INVESTIGATIONS

Plain X-rays may show separation of the sutures. If there is a blocked aqueduct the posterior fossa may be small because the cisterna magna has never developed. Craniovertebral or other bony anomalies may suggest the possibility of a malformation of the brain.

EMI scanning is the safest way to confirm the diagnosis of hydrocephalus, and because it can be repeated the progress of these conditions can be followed. From the distribution of the dilatation the site of the block may be deduced, and a tumour may be shown. It will not, however, give the detailed information which ventriculography will.

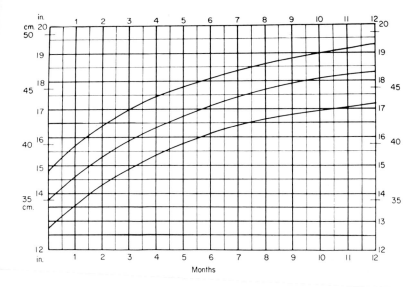

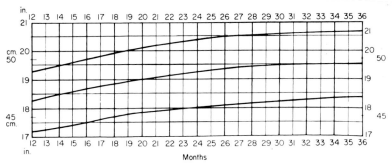

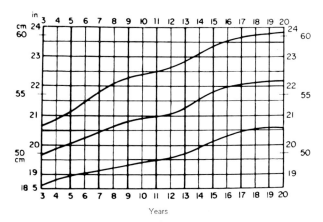

FIG. 71 Normal head circumference in infancy

Chart shows *upper limit* of normal for 90% of average infants;
average values are ½ in. less.

Ventriculography (fig. 24) will often be needed in order to make as accurate a diagnosis as possible, and in particular to localise the level of the block and exclude a tumour. The replacement of large volumes of CSF with air is dangerous because it may precipitate brain shifts or hæmorrhage. However, a "bubble" of 10–20 ml. of air injected with a sharp needle through the fontanelle into the lateral ventricles is safer and can be equally informative if the child is successively positioned to move the air into the various likely sites for pathology. It is probably wise to tap the subdural space immediately before needling the ventricle, in order to exclude a subdural hæmatoma or effusion which are common causes of an enlarging head after trauma or meningitis.

Isotope ventriculography or cisternography makes it possible to study the circulation of the CSF and is a much more effective technique than the use of dyes (p. 69).

NATURAL HISTORY

The natural outcome of hydrocephalus is uncertain, but recent studies suggest that only 25% of those diagnosed within the first three months of life will attain adult life. Two-thirds of the **deaths** are in the first 18 months, and more than half are ascribed to hydrocephalus itself without an obvious complication. Meningitis and chest infection are frequently recognised as the cause of death, but these infants readily succumb to intercurrent infection of all kinds.

If a child lives for one or two years, his chances of surviving without treatment rise to about 50%, although he may remain handicapped. The survivors include those whose hydrocephalus has undergone natural **"arrest"** which most often occurs between nine months and two years of age. The head never gets smaller, but resumes growth when the normal head–body ratio is restored by development of the rest of the body.

About a third of cases which arrest naturally or are controlled by treatment have normal intelligence, and a third have no physical abnormality; but less than a fifth are free of both mental and physical handicap. Physical disabilities include blindness and spasticity, and the latter may be severe enough to render a child bedridden. Severe mental and physical handicaps tend to be associated, but neither appears to be related to the duration of head enlargement, to the thickness of cortex, or to head size except when this is extreme. Hydrocephalus with spina bifida rarely survives without disability. It seems likely that continuing disabilities are more often related to underlying brain damage than solely to ventricular dilatation.

TREATMENT

Progressive hydrocephalus demands treatment unless brain damage or malformation is obviously so severe as to make useful survival unlikely. Even though some cases do become arrested this may not occur before irreparable damage has been done. If the head is still actively enlarging operation should not be postponed in the hope of a spontaneous cure.

Three different types of operation are available, but some patients require more than one procedure before the hydrocephalus is controlled.

1. Direct attack on the block

Obstruction at the foramen magnum due to Arnold–Chiari malformation may be relieved by *posterior fossa decompression*. If the outlets from the fourth ventricle are blocked, but the subarachnoid space is patent, relief may follow *opening the ventricle*. Both these procedures are more successful in mild cases in older children; in infancy the posterior fossa is difficult to explore—large venous sinuses in the dura make access difficult and the cisterna magna is often very small.

2. Short-circuits (by-passing the block)

These attempt to re-establish the circulation of CSF by providing a by-pass around the block, the level of which must be known before the

OPERATIONS for HYDROCEPHALUS

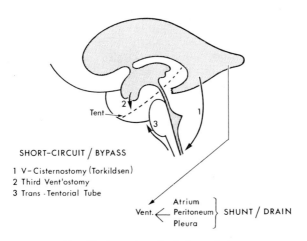

SHORT-CIRCUIT / BYPASS

1 V–Cisternostomy (Torkildsen)
2 Third Vent'ostomy
3 Trans-Tentorial Tube

Vent. ⟨ Atrium
Peritoneum ⟩ SHUNT / DRAIN
Pleura

FIG. 72 Operations for hydrocephalus

appropriate procedure can be done (fig. 72). The most consistently successful is *Torkildsen's operation* (ventriculo-cisternostomy) in which one or both lateral ventricles are put in communication with the cisterna magna (p. 315). Because of the frequency of blockage in the basal cisterns this is less effective for infantile hydrocephalus than it is for pure aqueduct blockage in older children and adults. An attempt may be made to bypass this blockage in the basal cistern by a *transtentorial tube* passed from the lateral ventricle through the cisterna ambiens into the cisterna chiasmaticus. *Third ventriculostomy* consists of making a hole in the lamina terminalis to allow CSF to escape from the ventricle into the chiasmatic cistern, but it seldom drains effectively for long.

3. Shunts (drains)

CSF can be diverted to other body cavities from which it is absorbed. Shunts from the lumbar theca are effective only for communicating hydrocephalus and are now rarely used. But all types can be treated by ventricular shunts, which are also effective when there are multiple obstructions in the CSF pathways (fig. 72). The simplest to perform is ventriculo-peritoneal drainage, with the lower end of the tube placed above the liver to minimise omental adhesions. An occipital burr hole enables the tube to be placed in the lateral ventricle, and it is then led subcutaneously down the neck and trunk, making subcutaneous incisions where needed. If it works, this type of operation is probably the best. It is applicable to all types of hydrocephalus, simple and safe to perform and to adjust if necessary when blockage occurs. A flushing device can be placed in the burr hole to help keep the system clear and a valve may be put in the system to prevent too rapid drainage, but in most cases this can be controlled by posture in the post-operative period.

The introduction of a unidirectional valve, capable of functioning indefinitely when embedded in the tissues, has made possible the drainage of CSF into the vascular system. *Ventriculo-caval* shunt (syn. v.-jugular, v.-atrial) is now a widely practised operation. A one-way valve is essential to prevent reflux of blood and it is placed subcutaneously behind the right ear, and connected by fine plastic tubing to the lateral ventricle above and, via the internal jugular vein, to the superior vena cava below; some surgeons prefer the tip to be in the atrium, but in any event the position is checked by an X-ray on the operating table. Valves opening at different pressures are available, but a low pressure one is needed for babies whose skulls offer less resistance than the high pressure valves which therefore fail to work.

Complications

In about 10% there is some complication other than simple blockage, the most important being infection; this is particularly serious if the shunt is to the vascular system. Ulceration of the skin over the valve may occur or organisms of low virulence colonise the valve itself, causing chronic bacteræmia. The result is persistent pyrexia, progressive anæmia, splenomegaly and positive blood cultures with sterile CSF. Antibiotics are powerless to control this and the valve must be removed. Infection is much less common if no valve is used.

How long these various shunts continue to function is uncertain, because even if they cease to drain on account of blockage of the tube, or growth of the child, hydrocephalus does not necessarily recur. Other channels may have opened up by this time, or the "active" phase of the hydrocephalus may have passed. In either event a temporary diversion of CSF may effect a permanent cure. On the other hand some children develop raised pressure again after many years, indicating that they require continued drainage. Revision operations are often quite effective and can usually be limited to replacement of the lower tubing but if the jugular vein thromboses the shunt must be transferred to the other side or an alternative diversion (e.g. peritoneal) used. Occasionally the valve resistance increases with time and replacement is then needed.

Most obstructive hydrocephalus after infancy is secondary to a tumour in the posterior fossa, midbrain or third ventricle. However, some are due to primary aqueduct blocks which failed to produce a markedly enlarged head in infancy, perhaps because they were incomplete.

JUVENILE AND ADULT HYDROCEPHALUS

aqueduct stenosis (iter stricture)

PATHOLOGY

Stenosis consists of simple narrowing of the iter without any other surrounding abnormality or any associated developmental defect. **Gliosis,** said by some to be the commonest type when hydrocephalus develops late, consists of a narrow iter surrounded by dense gliotic proliferation in the periaqueductal grey matter. Neurofibromatosis is a frequent accompaniment. **Forking** of the aqueduct is more often found in infancy, associated with Arnold–Chiari malformation. A relatively large dorsal channel and several tiny ventral ones do not together comprise a sufficient cross-section to deal adequately with the CSF flow.

When hydrocephalus develops slowly over the years many secondary changes are found within the cranium. Constant pulsatile pressure of the convolutions of the brain against the bone of the skull erodes the inner table, causing irregular recesses filled by small herniæ of brain. In places the skull sometimes gives way completely; if this is over one of the paranasal air sinuses and the dura is breached, "spontaneous" (i.e. non-traumatic) CSF rhinorrhœa develops. Diverticula of the ventricle may push out into the subarachnoid space, especially from the region of the trigone of the lateral ventricle into the cisterns in the pineal region. If a diverticulum ruptures, the tension of the hydrocephalus is relieved, and this self-cure may account for the long survival of some patients with advanced dilatation. Such a diverticulum can act as a local "tumour" and compress the midbrain, producing local signs and displacement on ventriculography.

CLINICAL

Most patients are first seen in late childhood and are rather plump, with a somewhat large head; a mild degree of infantilism may be observed, probably the result of pressure from the dilated third ventricle on the suprasellar region. Some present with headache, vomiting and signs of raised pressure. These may have been precipitated by a recent mild head injury or one of the infectious diseases of childhood, which have disturbed the delicate equilibrium so far maintained. Sometimes this condition is discovered by chance when the fundi are examined or the skull X-rayed for some other reason.

Chronic papilloedema with commencing atrophy is usually found on examination. Midbrain compression frequently results in loss of upward gaze of the eyes, and the pupils react sluggishly to light. A mild tremor is common and may suggest a cerebellar lesion; a number of these patients are investigated in the expectation of finding a posterior fossa tumour.

X-ray of skull may show the beaten silver appearance (digital markings) of the vault together with other signs of long-standing raised pressure—the sutures are widened and the pituitary fossa enlarged with erosion of the dorsum sellæ (fig. 73). A shallow posterior fossa, as judged by the position of the grooves for the transverse sinus and the low-lying torcula, is also characteristic.

EMI scanning may provide enough information, but **positive contrast ventriculography** will usually be necessary; this is better than using air which may disturb existing internal herniations and precipitate an acute crisis, or the patient may go into a slow decline and die in spite of surgical relief of the pressure. Contrast must be given time to trickle through a narrowed aqueduct, hours for the maximum information to be obtained.

TREATMENT

Torkildsen's ventriculo-cisternostomy was designed for treating this condition and since its introduction the outlook for these patients has become favourable. Unless there is doubt about the diagnosis, a full posterior fossa exploration is not necessary, and the cisterna magna can be exposed through a limited midline incision. The arch of the atlas is taken off, and the posterior rim of the foramen magnum nibbled away. An occipital burr hole is made and a catheter passed through it into the lateral ventricle; the outer end is led subcutaneously to the midline exposure, and the end placed in the cisterna magna, or the subarachnoid space of the cervical spine (fig. 72). The tube may not drain immediately, but lumbar punctures for a few days may encourage it to start. There may be a cellular reaction for the first week. Many patients have now had these tubes in place for 15 years, and those seen at post-mortem usually look as clean as the day they were put in, with no ventricular reaction. The ventricular shunts introduced for infantile hydrocephalus can also be used in adults and should not require revision due to growth; they are simpler to perform than Torkildsen's operations.

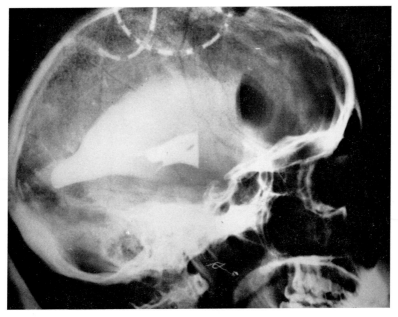

FIG. 73 Conray ventriculogram in case of aqueduct stenosis—note large lateral ventricles and block in aqueduct.

Normal pressure hydrocephalus

Certain patients with presenile dementia associated with marked disorder of gait, and often incontinence, have been shown to have enlarged ventricles associated with relatively little cortical atrophy. Because some of these patients improve markedly after ventricular shunting operations it has been suggested their neurological dysfunction may be due to a pressure effect on the brain from the increased internal surface of the ventricles. ICP monitoring indicates that pressure is normal, or subject to only minor peaks (usually at night). Isotope encephalography suggests that the hydrocephalus may be due to failure of normal processing of absorptive CSF to the supratentorial subarachnoid space; tests show isotope still in the ventricles at a time when it should have disappeared. Artificial CSF infusions have demonstrated reduced absorptive capacity. No investigations so far devised can reliably predict which patients will benefit from shunting operations; it is probably only about a third that do so and many of these have a history of a preceding event, such as subarachnoid hæmorrhage, head injury or meningitis which might have blocked absorptive capacity.

Craniostenosis

Premature fusion of one or more of the cranial sutures causes deformity of the skull which is usually evident within the first year of life. The most striking abnormality follows fusion of the coronal sutures, the forehead being very high—brachiocephaly or turricephaly; in this and in oxycephaly (all sutures affected) the anterior fossa floor is short and steep, there are often digital markings on the skull X-ray and proptosis results from the shallow orbits. Other abnormalities (syndactyly, cleft palate, facial deformity and mental defect) are common. The question is whether any symptoms are in fact due to raised pressure, or the orbital deformity. Fusion of the sagittal suture alone is much more common, and causes an elongated narrow head (scaphocephaly); other abnormalities are unusual and raised pressure rarely develops.

Operations are designed to make artificial sutures, but some manœuvre is needed to prevent fusion after operation. Either some inert material is interposed (plastic sheeting or tin foil), or else the dura is painted with Zenker-acetic solutions to destroy its osteogenic function. Under the age of 10 months or so, the sutures are restored by double saw-cuts, or nibbling; but after this scalp flaps must be turned and free bone plates formed by cutting all round areas of vault bone. If proptosis is marked, with optic nerve changes, then orbital decompression may be required in addition. To be effective surgery should be performed in the first 3–6 months of life.

FURTHER READING

Anderson, F. M. and Geiger, L. (1965). Craniosynostosis: a survey of 204 cases. *Journal of Neurosurgery*, **22**, 229–240.

Appenzeller, O. and Salmon, J. H. (1967). Treatment of parenchymatous degeneration of the brain by ventriculo-atrial shunting of the cerebrospinal fluid. *Journal of Neurosurgery*, **26**, 478–482.

Cohen, S. J. and Callaghan, R. P. (1961). A syndrome due to bacterial colonisation of Spitz-Holter valves. *British Medical Journal*, **2**, 677–680.

Editorial (1969). Treatment of hydrocephalus. *Lancet*, **i**, 191–192.

Forrest, D. M. and Cooper, D. G. W. (1968). Complications of ventriculoatrial shunts. A review of 455 cases. *Journal of Neurosurgery*, **29**, 506–512.

Fox, J. L., McCullough, D. C. and Green, R. C. (1973). Effect of cerebrospinal fluid shunts on intracranial pressure and on cerebrospinal fluid dynamics. 2. A new technique of pressure measurements: results and concepts. 3. A concept of hydrocephalus. *Journal of Neurology, Neurosurgery and Psychiatry*, **36**, 302–312.

Laurence, K. M. and Coates, S. (1962). The natural history of hydrocephalus. *Archives of Disease in Childhood*, **37**, 345–362.

Laurence, K. M. (1969). Neurological and intellectual sequelae of hydrocephalus. *Archives of Neurology*, **20**, 73–81.

Nag, T. K. and Falconer, M. A. (1966). Non-tumral stenosis of the aqueduct in adults. *British Medical Journal*, **4**, 1168–1170.

Ojemann, R. G. (1969). Further experience with normal pressure hydrocephalus. *Journal of Neurosurgery*, **31**, 279–294.

Paine, K. W. E. and McKissock, W. (1955). Aqueduct stenosis. *Journal of Neurosurgery*, **12**, 127–145.

Raimondi, A. J., Samuelson, G., Yarzagaray, L. and Norton, T. (1969). Atresia of the Foramina of Luschka and Magendie: The Dandy Walker Cyst. *Journal of Neurosurgery*, **31**, 202–216.

Russell, D. S. (1949). Observations on the pathology of hydrocephalus. *H.M.S.O. Spec. Ser. Med. Res. Coun. No. 265*. London.

CHAPTER 18

Congenital Spinal Abnormalities

Spinal dysraphism
  spina bifida cystica
  spina bifida occulta

Neural anomalies
  cerebellar ectopia
  syringomyelia

Vertebral anomalies
  craniovertebral anomalies
  spondylolisthesis

Anomalies of development in the spine most commonly derive from failure of fusion of the neural tube and adjacent cutaneous, muscular and osseous structures; these are embraced by the term "spinal dysraphism" which includes defects which may affect neural tissues only indirectly, such as lumbosacral lipomas. Clearly different are anomalies which primarily affect the neural tube and need not be associated with any bony abnormality, although in practice such an association is very common (e.g. cerebellar ectopia with lumbosacral spina bifida). Separate again are anomalies primarily of the vertebræ which may affect the neural contents of the canal only after many years as a result of the deformity produced.

SPINAL DYSRAPHISM

Spina bifida cystica (aperta)

  This major abnormality occurs once in 300 live births but the possibility of detection in utero at an early enough stage to justify abortion promises to reduce its incidence. It affects the lumbosacral region in 80% of cases. Simple **meningocele** accounts for only 5% and consists of a herniation of the subarachnoid spaces only, without any nervous tissue. Survival without disability is the rule, and hydrocephalus seldom develops; when it does it usually undergoes natural arrest. The swelling may already be covered with skin at birth, but if not the membrane soon epithelialises and thickens to form a firm covering. Excision is simple and free from risk.

Myelomeningocele is much more serious, consisting of abnormal spinal cord and roots exposed by a skin defect. Some degree of paralysis of the legs and bladder is common, and in severe cases the anal sphincter is lax. Three quarters develop hydrocephalus, usually due to associated cerebellar ectopia (see below), and this makes for a less favourable prognosis; indeed hydrocephalus and infection were largely responsible for the 90% mortality which was usual in the first year of life until the last decade. Since the introduction of effective operations for hydrocephalus, the availability of antibiotics, and the practice of early closure of the skin defect, over 50% of those who survive the first 24 hours now reach school age. Even with the spinal lesion healed and the hydrocephalus controlled some persisting handicap is usual, but the frequency and severity of this varies considerably in different series: the combination of urinary incontinence, some degree of paraplegia (perhaps with talipes or congenital dislocation of the hip), and possibly mental retardation, presents formidable social and educational problems, as well as the need for continuing medical supervision by a team of experts. Because of this there is now increasing acceptance of the view that surgical closure should be carried out only on these babies with a restricted lesion, good sphincter tone, reasonable limb movements and in whom there are no other associated congenital anomalies. For the best results in those chosen for surgery the skin closure should be done in the first 24–48 hours, in order to prevent infection and scabbing of the exposed neural tube. A decision must therefore be reached quickly, which is best done by a team of surgeons and pædiatricans, having decided on criteria beforehand, and then applying these in individual cases as they occur.

Operation in the first 48 hours causes very little upset and can be done under local or general anæsthesia. Elaborate flaps of skin, fascia or muscle are unwise. The head is kept low for a few days to minimise the risk of CSF leakage, and care is taken to avoid fæcal contamination of the wound. The head circumference is regularly checked for evidence of hydrocephalus; orthopædic and urological assessment and follow-up are arranged.

Spina bifida occulta

A bony defect in the lamina of the first sacral vertebra is frequently seen on X-ray, and is of no significance. When a more extensive laminar defect is found, often with widening of the inter-pedicular distances, one of a number of other lesions may be discovered which can lead to progressive neurological deficit in the lower limbs. The clinical syndrome is similar for all lesions, consisting of disordered gait and a deformed foot (usually cavovarus); these are progressive and may be associated with an obvious neurological deficit or a neurogenic bladder disorder.

Myelography shows either a low conus medullaris (below body of L3), or a mass (lipoma or dermoid), or spinal cord deformity (diastemato-myelia). The latter consists of duplication of the spinal cord over a few segments, sometimes with separate dural tubes, separated by an intervening bony spur which can stretch neural structures. Intra-spinal lipoma may be connected with a subcutaneous lipoma over the sacrum, whilst patients with any of these lesions may have a tuft of long hairs or a sinus over the lumbosacral region. Although the disability caused by these lesions may be only slowly progressive there is a good case for exploration in order to prevent further damage by ascent of a tethered cord with the growth of the child, or by growth of a mass (lipoma or dermoid) which impinges on the roots and cord.

NEURAL ANOMALIES

Cerebellar ectopia or encephalo-cranial disproportion is an invariable finding when meningo-myelocele is associated with hydrocephalus. The most obvious abnormality is elongation of the cerebellar vermis which may reach the lower cervical vertebræ; it is bound by vascular adhesions to the herniated medulla, and the lower cranial nerves and upper cervical nerve roots have to travel upwards to their exit foraminæ. This component of the abnormality, which leads to obstruction of CSF flow, is sometimes termed the Arold–Chiari malformation. In fact the cerebral hemispheres are usually enlarged and the tentorium low, resulting in a small posterior fossa with crowding of structures through the foramen magnum. A third of brains with this abnormality also have aqueduct stenosis, and hydromyelia is also common (see below, syringomyelia). Milder degrees of ectopia may be symptomless and may occur without any abnormality in the spinal column.

Syringomyelia is applied to the syndrome of central cord dysfunction associated with a cystic cavitation; the cyst fluid has often the composition of normal CSF and it is now believed that the condition is in fact hydromyelia. Dilatation of the central canal is believed to result from CSF being forced into this situation by a valvular action due to a hind-brain anomaly. Certainly in many patients with syringomyelia, who are subjected to posterior fossa exploration, cerebellar ectopia is found.

The clinical features consist of gradually developing wasting of the small muscles of the hand and loss of spinothalamic sensation (pain and temperature). This may lead to inadvertent burns, and to trophic joint changes. Spasticity of the legs may develop, and if the medulla is involved nystagmus and bulbar palsy. Progress may be very gradual, but sudden or steady worsening can occur. Radiation is now held to be of limited value, as is laminectomy and aspiration of the cyst; tubes or other devices to maintain drainage have only a temporary effect. But posterior fossa exploration and freeing of adhesions around the cerebellar ectopia may have a more lasting effect.

VERTEBRAL ANOMALIES

Craniovertebral anomalies. Development defects of the bony spine are particularly common in the cervical region. The consequences for the cord are largely similar to those associated with cervical spondylosis, which may indeed develop due to the abnormalities of intervertebral movement. Chronic myelopathy, and the liability to profound paralysis following minor trauma, are shared by both conditions.

Basilar impression is the commonest anomaly, consisting of invagination of part of the rim of the foramen magnum into the skull so that it is higher than the occipital squama immediately lateral to it. Basilar impression is often associated with other anomalies, and it may also develop, as an acquired rather than congenital disease, secondary to Paget's disease, rickets or other diseases causing softening of bone.

Fusion of adjacent cervical vertebræ is commonest at the C2/3 interspace, but the atlas is often occipitalised in addition. This anomaly is particularly likely to be followed by spondylosis at joints below the fusion, and to be associated with a short neck recognisable clinically, (the Klippel–Feil syndrome). *Myelograms* may show a complete or partial block at the foramen magnum; the subarachnoid space is distorted by the rim of the foramen magnum, an abnormally high odontoid process, secondary dural bands and arachnoid adhesions, or abnormally low tonsils: any of these may block the outlet from the fourth ventricle with consequent hydrocephalus.

All degrees of *clinical abnormality* are encountered from the incidental radiological finding of vertebral fusion to paraplegia. Certain signs are probably due to associated maldevelopment within the nervous system (vertical nystagmus, mirror movements in the limbs, and loss of postural sense in the arms and legs) but a chronic myelopathy can develop with basilar impression. A spastic quadriparesis is the most obvious feature, but cerebellar ataxia, dysarthria and lateral nystagmus also occur, and there may be hydrocephalus with papillœdema in addition. The removal of bone in the course of a posterior fossa decompression, and division of the dural bands which are usually found, release the pressure on the structures at the foramen magnum and may be enough to re-establish circulation of the CSF without a short-circuit operation.

Spondylolisthesis is a defect in development of the vertebral pars interarticularis of usually L4 or 5. As a result of the bony disconnection between the laminæ and the body, the body may gradually be displaced forwards, so that there is a step between it and the body below. It is doubtful whether this ever causes nerve root pressure, although it may produce backache; however, a disc lesion is liable to develop, and that may cause a root lesion in the usual way. Whether such a disc lesion should be treated in the usual way, or the removal of the disc should be followed by an interbody fusion, is a matter of controversy.

FURTHER READING

Applyby, A., Foster, J. B., Hankinson, J. and Hudgson, P. (1968). The diagnosis and management of the Chiari anomalies in adult life. *Brain*, **91**, 131–140.

Bharucha, E. P. and Dastur, H. M. (1964) Craniovertebral anomalies. A report on 40 cases. *Brain*, **87**, 469–480.

Brocklehurst, G., Gleave, J. R. W. and Lewin, W. (1967). Early closure of myelo-meningocele with special reference to leg movement. *British Medical Journal*, **1**, 666–669.

Dale, A. J. D. (1969). Diastematomyelia. *Archives of Neurology*, **20**, 309–317.

Doran, P. A. and Guthkelch, A. N. (1961). Studies in spina bifida cystica. *Journal of Neurology, Neurosurgery and Psychiatry*, **24**, 431–345.

Gardner, W. J. (1965). Hydrodynamic mechanism of syringomyelia: its relationship to myelocele. *Journal of Neurology, Neurosurgery and Psychiatry*, **28**, 247–259.

James, M. C. C. (1967). Results of treatment of progressive lesions in spina bifida occulta five to ten years after laminectomy. *Lancet*, **ii**, 1277–1279.

Lassman, L. P. and James, M. C. C. (1967). Lumbosacral lipomas: critical survey of 26 cases submitted to laminectomy. *Journal of Neurology, Neurosurgery and Psychiatry*, **30**, 174–181.

Mawdsley, T., Rickham, P. P. and Roberts, J. R. (1967). Longterm results of early operation of open myelomeningoceles and encephaloceles. *British Medical Journal*, **1**, 663–666.

Sharrard, W. J. W. (1963). A controlled trial of immediate and delayed closure of spina bifida cystica. *Archives of Disease in Childhood*, **38**, 18–22.

Spillane, J. D., Pallis, C. and Jones, A. M. (1957). Developmental abnormalities in the region of the foramen magnum. *Brain*, **80**, 11–48.

VI: Lesion Making in the Nervous System

CHAPTER 19

Principles and Applications of Lesion-making

Modification of the function of some part of the nervous system by the planned destruction of certain structures in the brain, spinal cord or nerves now forms an important part of neurosurgery. Certain structures may readily be exposed and dealt with under direct vision but many of the targets are deeply situated and can be reached only by needles or probes directed from outside. However the target is reached, several methods of lesion-making are available.

Lesion making

Mechanical lesions are usually employed when direct exposure of the target is possible, e.g. section of spinal or trigeminal roots, excision of the temporal lobe or frontal leucotomy. For closed stereotaxic techniques a probe has been developed with an extrudable wire loop to effect a mechanical lesion. The shape and size of the lesion made by this probe can be determined to some extent by the degree of extrusion of the wire loop and the amount of rotation applied to the probe.

    Chemical lesions have been used for many years, notably alcohol injections into the trigeminal ganglion, and a range of intrathecal injections has been developed for the treatment of pain.

    Thermal and cryogenic lesions are now most commonly used, at least for stereotaxic lesion making. Both present problems which derive from the uneven susceptibility of brain tissue to destruction which is partly due to varying physical properties of the grey and white matter. An advantage of these lesions is the degree of control possible; with a thermistor in the probe tip the temperature can be monitored and if only a limited deviation from normal temperature is allowed (up to 40°C or down to 0°C) a temporary lesion may be produced and its effects observed. This is more readily achieved with cryogenic lesions; hemiparesis produced at a temperature of 0°C may recover completely within 10–15 minutes of restoring normal temperature. Even as a

333

permanent lesion is being made at a lower temperature a zone of reversible inactivation will precede the enlarging permanent lesion and if undesired side-effects arise the lesion may be halted at that stage. Heat lesions are usually made by passing a radio-frequency current of megacycle frequency through a fine monopolar electrode bared for the last few millimetres of its shaft; cold lesions are produced by circulating liquid nitrogen through a probe. The size of the lesion in either case is determined by the size of the probe and by the extent of the temperature change and its duration; after one minute the lesion probably does not increase much in size. The shape of a thermal lesion can be varied to some extent by varying the amount of proble which is left uninsulated but the basic shape is ovoid.

Internal radiation with a beta emitter has been extensively used for hypophysectomy, using yttrium 90.

External radiation with conventional X-rays is of limited value because it is not possible to focus down to a volume much less than 5 cm^3; it is therefore useful only for tumours and cannot be employed for anatomical lesion-making. With a proton beam, generated by a cyclotron, a very precise lesion can be made; no energy is imparted to the tissue through which the beam passes, but at a certain distance all the energy is given up (the Bragg peak effect). This is an attractive method which requires no probe to be passed into the brain or even a burr hole (if radiological reference points are outlined by air-encephalography); its limitation is the availability of a powerful cyclotron and of suitable medical facilities adjacent to it.

Ultrasound has proved disappointing so far, because although an external source is used the energy is too low to penetrate the skull and a craniotomy is required.

No doubt technical ingenuity will result in new methods which will answer more completely the surgeon's demand for a tool which will produce a tailor-made lesion in the depths of the brain, without the need to penetrate or damage the overlying structures. Induction heating of a metal seed implanted in the target area by passing a radio-frequency current through an external coil shows some promise, but electrolytic lesions, seem disappointing.

Stereotaxic Surgery

A whole new dimension of surgery was opened up by stereotaxic techniques whereby a surgical probe can be directed to any desired target site within the nervous system without the prohibitive risks which direct exposure would involve or the inaccuracies associated with free-hand introduction. Stereotaxic surgery is now used for the relief of symptoms due to a wide variety of conditions including Parkinsonism and other movement disorders, intractable pain, acromegaly, mental abnormalities and epilepsy; there is every reason to believe that in time it may find even wider application. Success depends on accurate delineation of the appropriate target area beforehand, and on the attainment of sufficient precision in reaching the target in the operating theatre; the latter is achieved with the help of radiological and physiological monitoring which can be likened to the coarse and fine adjustment in this technique.

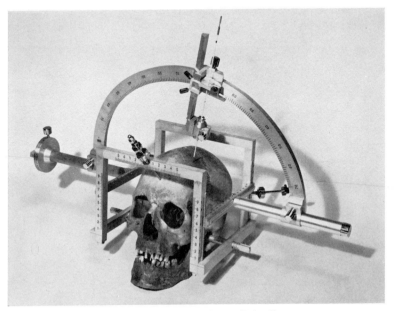

FIG. 74 Stereotaxic frame (Leksell)

Frame is fixed to skull by three pins (right posterior one is obscured); electrode carried on arc with electrode against skull where burr hole would normally have been made. Ear bars are in position, but would normally be removed as soon as pins inserted in skull.

Stereotaxic operations on the brain require three main manœuvres:

1. Fixing to the skull a rigid frame carrying an adjustable probe-holder, designed to guide the probe through a burr hole to the target (fig. 74).

2. Outlining intermediate reference points within the ventricular system by contrast radiology. The relationship of these reference points to the target is shown in a brain atlas, and is transposed to the patient's skull film on which both the ventricles and the scale on the frame are displayed (fig. 75).

3. Adjusting the probe-holder on the basis of these measurements and then guiding the probe to the target area.

4. Verifying the probe position by physiological monitoring by observing the effect of electrical stimulation or of a temporary lesion

on brain function, or by making electrical recordings from the tip of the probe. Since it is function that is to be modified by the operation it is the functional rather than the anatomical localisation which is important; however accurate the instruments, individual anatomical variations will always limit the accuracy of placement and verification is therefore essential. This monitoring may indicate the need for further adjustment before a permanent lesion is made.

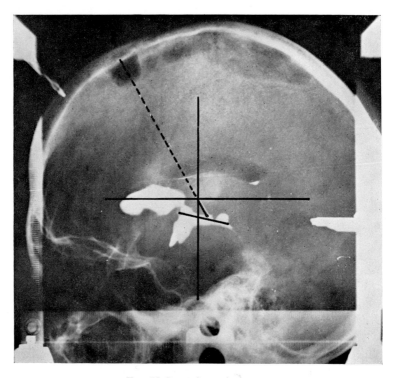

FIG. 75 Lateral ventriculogram

Lateral myodil ventriculogram with frame in place. The short solid line indicates the inter-commissural line, and the intersection of the longer lines marks the central point of the instrument, the distance from this point to the target determines the offset required to reach that target.

Local anæsthesia is usually employed because physiological verification is then much easier, and be detected in time to prevent their being permanent untoward side-effects of the lesion in relieving symptoms can be directly observed may the efficacy. In children and in patients with mental disorders or very violent involuntary movements there may be no alternative to general anæsthesia, but neuroleptanalgesia (p. 101) is making this less often necessary than previously.

Stereotaxic frames

Innumerable instruments have been developed in recent years as successive surgeons have tried to improve on existing machinery by modification or by completely new designs. One problem which demands solution is the magnification produced by X-rays taken at conventional tube film distances; two main methods have been introduced to overcome this, one being to impose a fixed tube-film distance such that the same magnification, which is calculable, will occur on all films; the other is to employ tele-radiology, which involves placing the X-ray tube a sufficient distance (usually > 4 metres) from the head so that the rays will be for practical purposes parallel and therefore non-distorting. Most of the stereotaxic frames are developments of the Horsley-Clarke instrument which was designed for animal work and patented in anticipation of human use in 1912.

FURTHER READING

Brodkey, J. S., Miyazaki, Y., Ervin, F. R. and Mark, V. H. (1964). Reversible heat lesions with radiofrequency current. *J. Neurosurg.*, **21**, 49–53.
Editorial. (1965). Prospects in radiosurgery. *Lancet*, **i**, 1373–4.
Kalyanaraman, S. and Gillingham, F. J. (1964). Stereotaxic biopsy. *J. Neurosurg.*, **21**, 854–858.
Rand, R. W., Rinfret, A. P. and Von Leden, H. (1968). *Cryosurgery*. Springfield: C. Thomas.

Movement disorders

Surgery for dyskinesias began with treating Parkinsonism but since the introduction of L-dopa surgery is more often used for certain cases of torsion dystonia, hemiballismus, choreo-athetosis and spasmodic torticollis (now widely regarded as a restricted from of torsion dystonia). It is still used for Parkinsonism when drugs are either ineffective, too toxic, or are not available. A similar lesion is made by most surgeons for all these conditions, in the ventro-lateral nucleus of the thalamus; sometimes an additional or alternative lesion is made in the globus pallidus which is believed by some to be more effective in relieving rigidity or spasticity, whilst the thalamic lesion relieves tremor (fig. 76). In this rapidly expanding field views are liable to change as experience accumulates and new sites for lesions are continually being explored. The size as well as the site of the lesion may be important in determining the outcome; as a principle, the smallest lesion which is effective is usually made, because the unknown factor in every case is the amount of damage already suffered by the brain as the result of the primary disease process. If this is appreciable the additional therapeutic lesion may cause new deficits in motor control, higher sensory function or in subtle features such as motor initiative or sensory awareness. As a result a patient whose tremor or rigidity is relieved may fail to use his improved limb or may have added disabilities related to the motor function of the body as a whole.

The sole objective of surgery for movement disorders is to improve the overall motor function of the patient: not necessarily to eliminate the last remnant of abnormal movement, which in any event often worries the relatives more than the patient, but rather to increase the ease with which the hand or leg can be used: not necessarily to eliminate the dystonia in severe athetosis but to prevent the wild excursions of the limbs and trunk which tend to throw the patient off balance. Much good can be achieved by aiming for a less than perfect elimination of all signs and symptoms in order to avoid any increase in functional impairment in other ways.

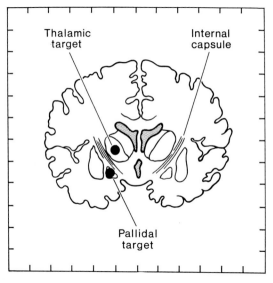

FIG. 76 Basal ganglia targets

Epilepsy

Epilepsy is a presenting feature of many intracranial conditions treated by surgery but in the present context operations specifically designed to relieve epilepsy are considered. These are mostly directed to the removal of areas of abnormally functioning brain, usually scars left by previous brain damage resulting from external violence, ischæmia or infection. The rationale is that the pathological meningocerebral scar is more epileptogenic than the scar which develops subsequent to planned surgery; however, epilepsy returns after some years in over 50% of patients operated on, presumably due to the eventual redevelopment of scar tissue or the resumption of epileptic activity in parts of the brain not removed.

The success of such surgery depends on the identification of that part of the brain which is functioning abnormally. This is less easy then might appear, because secondary epilepsy activity may be induced in areas adjacent, or even remote from the primary lesion. How much benefit may accrue in such circumstances from removal of the primarily abnormal part of brain is debatable The variability of results of surgery for epilepsy may depend in part on the extent to which brain remote from the original lesion has had its epileptogenic threshold permanently lowered by the lesion. Identification of the site of origin of the seizures depends mainly on observations of seizure pattern (p. 27) and of serial EEG recordings. These two may be combined in the technique of activation, in which a seizure is deliberately induced (usually chemically) during an EEG recording; this enables accurate observation both of the evolution of the seizure and of the localisation of the electrical activity accompanying it. If a patient is already suffering very frequent seizures activation will of course be unnecessary. Investigation must also be directed to discovering an underlying lesion such as a tumour and will include angiography and ventriculography; the latter may also show local dilatation of part of the ventricular system due to atrophy related to previous brain damage. Slowly growing gliomas and vascular abnormalities which do not act as space-occupying lesions frequently cause epilepsy; they may escape detection by contrast radiology and be discovered only in the course of surgery for epilepsy, directed at removing a supposed area of scarring.

Three main types of resection are undertaken for epilepsy, each directed at the removal of pathological tissue.

(1) **Temporal lobectomy.** This is the most commonly practised operation for epilepsy. Temporal lobe epilepsy is by far the commonest form of focal epilepsy, now that the wide range of phenomena to which it can give rise has been recognised (p. 27). All attacks are characterised by some alteration in consciousness, however transitory, and many are associated with behavioural abnormalities. The latter may come to dominate the clinical picture, in the form of personality disorders and outbursts of aggression; these may result in the patient's admission to a mental hospital or his coming into conflict with the Law. Whether the episodes of aggressive behaviour are really epileptic equivalents is very doubtful, but the question is often posed in an attempt to plead diminished responsibility for actions committed during them. These factors often make it difficult to reach a decision about operations; reducing the frequency of the epileptic attacks may or may not improve the behavioural component of the patient's disability, although it is often claimed that a difficult personality may be less of a social problem if there is not the added feature of frequent fits. The surgeon must be certain that undoubted fits are occurring with sufficient frequency to

justify operation (say more than one a month) and that anti-convulsant drugs have not only been prescribed but have been taken regularly in sufficient dosage and for long enough to derive maximum benefit.

The electoral criteria for operation are even more difficult to state in clear terms, but a marked predominance of abnormal activity in one temporal lobe is essential; such a predominance should be based on serial recordings including sleep records and the use of sphenoidal electrodes. These are placed in the naso-pharynx and percutaneously (through the infra-orbital region) so as to lie over the anterior and inferior aspects of the temporal lobe. In certain centres depth electrodes have been implanted in the medial temporal lobe structures but they are not strictly necessary.

Operation on the dominant temporal lobe can result in some risk of dysphasia and if there is any doubt in an individual as to which side of the brain is dominant this should be determined by the intracarotid amytal test. A graded injection into the carotid artery, which is punctured percutaneously as for angiography, will cause temporary hemiparesis without consciousness being so far depressed as to make speech testing impossible; the patient is tested for various aspects of language function during recovery.

The operation consists of the removal of the anterior 6 or 7 cms. of the temporal lobe; the most important structures to remove are the medial and deeply placed ones, the uncus, hippocampus and amygdala. In about 75% of operations some pathological abnormality is found in the removed temporal lobe, even though pre-operative radiology has been negative. This may take the form of very low-grade glioma or of an angioma or other vascular malformation which may have partly calcified; in some an active glioma is discovered. The commonest lesion, however, is an atrophic one consisting of sclerosis and loss of neurones in the region of the hippocampus, uncus and Ammon's horn.

The frequency of this medial sclerosis of the temporal lobe naturally raises the question of ætiology. One hypothesis is that this is a sequel of birth trauma, which has caused tentorial herniation and subsequent scarring. A more widely accepted explanation is that medial sclerosis results from one or more bouts of status epilepticus in early childhood. Certainly children who have died from uncontrolled status consistently have neuronal necrosis in these structures which is believed to be ischæmic in origin. Moreover many patients with temporal lobe epilepsy give a history of status epilepticus in childhood.

(2) **Hemispherectomy** can be of benefit to children contracting severe hemiplegia in the first two years of life and who are subject to insistent epilepsy. Such children usually appear retarded in addition to suffering from hemiplegia and epilepsy. Although the operation removes all of the cortex of one cerebral hemisphere, leaving the basal ganglia intact, crude movement and sensation is usually preserved in the contralateral limbs and may indeed improve after operation so that walking is quite

possible. Relieved of the burden of frequent fits the patient may improve greatly in behaviour and apparently in intellectual performance; attendance at a special school and some degree of social integration become possible.

(3) **Local cortical excisions** are seldom called for but the scar left by a penetrating brain wound or an abscess may occasionally be worth resecting. It is in such cases that electrocorticography can be of most help to the surgeon in indicating the exact location and extent of abnormally functioning cortex. The surgeon may test the activity in the remaining brain after the initial excision. It may also help him to avoid excising functionally vital areas such as the motor strip which can be identified by stimulation. When such electrical exploration of the cortex is called for at operation the anæsthesia must be such as not to interfere with the cortical activity. Local anæsthesia is the most reliable and has stood the test of time, but the neuroleptanalgesic drugs form a very useful supplement. Indeed they may be used together with gas and oxygen unless the patient's verbal co-operation is required but care must be taken that the inducing dose of barbiturate is kept to a minimum.

(4) **Stereotaxic lesions** in the upper brain stem are under active investigation for the control of epilepsy. It is to be hoped that a site can be found where a lesion may prevent a local epileptic discharge from becoming sufficiently widespread to cause a major clinical fit.

FURTHER READING

Falconer, M. A. and Taylor, D. C. (1968). Surgical treatment of drug resistant epilepsy due to mesial temporal sclerosis. *Arch. Neurol.*, **19**, 353–361.
Rasmussen, T. (1963). Surgical therapy of frontal lobe epilepsy. *Epilepsia*, **4**, 181–198.
Turner, E. (1963). A new approach to unilateral and bilateral lobotomies for psycho-motor epilepsy. *J. Neurol. Neurosurg. Psychiat.*, **26**, 285–299.

Psycho-surgery

It is 100 years since a survivor of severe frontal lobe damage was observed to have alteration of his personality, becoming uninhibited and emotionally unrestrained. Only in 1933 did Moniz propose a surgical assault on the frontal lobe as a means of treating patients with mental illness. The original procedure, standard leucotomy, cut most fibres to and from the frontal poles and produced marked personality change and intellectual damage as byproducts of its beneficial effects in diminishing tension and aggression. Because of this, and because recently introduced drugs have made it possible to produce reversible control of behaviour, this original operation is now rarely performed. However, more restrictive procedures have been devised, which are beneficial without producing permanent adverse effects on the personality. These are directed at various parts of the limbic system, of which the fronto-thalamic fibres cut in the standard leucotomy are also a part; they include orbital undercutting, limited fronto-thalamic lesions, cingulectomy and amygdalotomy. Most mental conditions originally treated surgically (schizophrenia and depressive psychosis) are now more satisfactorily controlled by drugs, and the indications for these new procedures are limited. Patients suffering from obsessional neuroses or chronic endogenous depression with agitation, who show marked tension, are most likely to be benefited, providing there has been a reasonably stable pre-morbid personality.

Operation calls for only a few days in a surgical unit and the operation can be carried out through a burr hole which needs only a very limited shaving of the head. The effect is seldom immediate and the patient should always return to the care of a psychiatrist, who should continue both drugs and supportive therapy, at least for a time. Organic complications of leucotomy are rare, but post-operative hæmorrhage may occur and epilepsy occasionally develops even after many months.

FURTHER READING

Brown, M. H. and Lighthill, J. A. (1968). Selective anterior cingulotomy: a psychosurgical evaluation. *J. Neurosurg.*, **29**, 513–519.
Editorial (1966). Surgery for mental illness. *Brit. med. J.*, **1**, 310–311.
Knight, G. (1964). The orbital cortex as an objective in the surgical treatment of mental illness. The results of 450 cases of open operation and the development of the stereotactic approach. *Brit. J. Surg.*, **51**, 114–124.
Knight, G. (1969). Bifrontal stereotactic tractotomy: an atraumatic operation of value in the treatment of intractable psychoneurosis. *Brit. J. Psychiat.*, **115**, 257–266.
Lewin, W. (1961). Observations on selective leucotomy. *J. Neurol. Neurosurg Psychiat.*, **24**, 37–44.
Sargant, W. (1962). The present indications for leucotomy. *Lancet*, **i**, 1197–1198.

APPLICATIONS OF LESION MAKING

Pain relief *see* Chapter 20 (p. 343)
Hypophysectomy *see* Chapter 9 (p. 154)

Surgical Relief of Pain

Nature of pain

Personality and pain

Anatomy of pain

Treatment of pain from inoperable cancer

Neuralgia
> trigeminal neuralgia
> glossopharyngeal neuralgia
> atypical facial pain
> traumatic neuralgias

Neurosurgeons are called upon to relieve pain by making lesions in the nervous system when radical treatment of the cause of the pain is impossible. The patients form two main groups:

(1) Those with pain caused by inoperable cancer, uncontrollable ischæmia or some other form of intractable tissue destruction.

(2) Those with pain caused by some disorder of the nervous system itself—neuralgia.

It was at one time the neuralgias which predominantly concerned the neurosurgeons, but with the increasing availability of neurosurgical services more of the former group are being treated.

NATURE OF PAIN

Pain is a complex sensory experience; in most instances it is useful and everyone must experience pain in infancy in order to learn to avoid the circumstances which provoke it. To be without the sensation of pain is a severe and often fatal handicap in children born with congenital insensitivity to tissue damage. As with other sensory experiences there is no single brain centre for pain, although operations on the sensory system appear to modify the sensation. Only the patient can describe his sensation of pain, and only he can say whether it is

343

better or worse and he alone can be the final arbiter for the assessment of operations designed to relieve his pain.

PERSONALITY AND PAIN

Both the experience of pain and the patient's reaction to it may be modified by various psychological factors which include the patient's normal personality and the attitude of those around him. The significance of the pain for the patient may determine the amount of anxiety it causes, whilst basic personality traits may affect the way in which the patient's pain is communicated to those near him, whether the discomfort and anxiety is apparently exaggerated or suppressed. Whilst pain is normally a warning reaction to noxious stimuli it may also form an expression of distress, a cry for help, a form of communication. These complex factors warrant serious attention when major procedures are proposed for the relief of pain which is considered overwhelming, because adjustments in certain factors forming the psychological background may make the situation much more tolerable and the need for surgery may then be less pressing. This is particularly the case with pain from advanced cancer, and to a lesser extent with the traumatic neuralgias.

ANATOMY OF PAIN

The sensory nervous system transmits coded information about the effects produced by the environment, and several nerve fibres are employed in the transmission of information from even the smallest and most localised stimulus. The nerve action potentials or impulses are the basic units which make up the codes, which depend on the patterns of impulses produced. Impulses are distributed in *space* amongst the different neurones from the region of the stimulus, and distributed in *time* by their frequency and their rate of conduction. Different neurones conduct at different rates proportional to their thickness. The result of this system is a temporo-spatial pattern of impulses transmitted to the brain from each stimulus in the periphery. The interpretation of the patterns depends upon the *learning* of their significance, not upon keeping fibres from different parts of the body minutely parcelled within the brain. Enough information is present in the impulse patterns for the brain to *learn* both what they signify and where they come from.

For example, an electrical stimulus from an electrode in the thalamus of a conscious patient may make him complain of a tingling sensation in the hand. Changing the electrical character of the stimulus, without altering the position of the electrode, can result in a different distribution of the sensation produced. The impulse pattern has been changed and the brain changes the interpretation.

The same nerve fibres which serve pain also serve temperature sensation. They are mostly small diameter fibres and form a network throughout the body. In the skin, where they operate in combination with larger nerve fibres connected to hair follicles and touch corpuscles, the power of discrimination is high. In other tissues, where the network is less dense, it is less discriminating.

There are no specific nerve endings or nerve fibres for pain. The sensation of pain depends upon the stimulus of tissue damage. If there is a thermal flow in the same tissue, this new stimulus will produce a different pattern of impulses in the same nerves, and the sensation of a change in temperature results.

Operations for pain do not demand that all the nerve fibres from the painful area should be cut and all sensation from the area abolished. The aim is to produce a *qualitative* change in impulse pattern which eliminates most of the pain by raising the threshold, but affects only slightly the other sensations of touch and joint position. Such a qualitative change in sensation can most readily be brought about by a *quantitative* reduction in the number of sensory fibres from the area.

TREATMENT OF PAIN FROM INOPERABLE CANCER

Not all cancer is painful, even in the terminal stages. But sometimes when growths invade the bones of the spine or face, or extend into the sacral or brachial plexus, or into the posterior root ganglia, pain can surpass all other symptoms by its severity, its persistence and its devastating effect on morale. But care must be taken to confirm that it is in fact pain which is the real cause of distress, and that it is not being used as a distress signal, due to inability to cope with other aspects of progressive disease.

Drugs will not adequately relieve severe and relentless pain for more than a few days. Even cocktails of gin and opium in heroic doses cannot compete for long with the unremitting or spasmodic pain of nerve root invasion. Watched closely, many patients will be seen to forego their euphoric mixtures because they no longer relieve the pain nor make them euphoric. They dislike the be-fuddlement and nausea of continuous medication and long to have a clear head. Yet skilfully used in a sympathetic environment some of the newer analgesics (e.g. pentazocine) may prove effective; the phenothiazine group of drugs (e.g. largactil) may reduce the emotional response to pain, although not altering the threshold to pain sensation.

Operative relief. A short expectancy of life is not necessarily an adequate criterion for withholding a neurosurgical operation for the relief of pain. With only a month to live the pain from an operation wound may be more bearable than that due to invasion, and the morale of everyone will be higher if the patient dies free from distressing pain and from the feeling that every one has given up.

But the patient's sufferings must not be added to; nothing adds more to the suffering than a useless operation. There are many risks and difficulties in the surgery of ill and dying patients, but there is no room for complacency over results. The appropriate procedure must be carefully selected and planned. It must be consistent with the patient's strength, and aim at permanent relief of pain for the rest of the patient's life. In few other instances in surgery is there such a premium on experience and judgement.

Pain can be relieved by intervening in the *sensory nervous system* or, in certain cases by intervening in the *hormonal control* of cancer.

SITES OF OPERATIVE INTERVENTION
IN THE NERVOUS SYSTEM

(1) Posterior nerve roots.
   Posterior rhizotomy in the spinal canal, or in the posterior fossa.
   Partial block of posterior roots by intrathecal injection.
(2) Spinal cord.
   Antero-lateral cordotomy.
   Anterior commisurotomy.
(3) Brain stem.
(4) Thalamus.

Posterior nerve roots

Posterior rhizotomy implies section of the whole posterior root and this abolishes all sensation. In the trunk, three or four roots need to be cut before any one dermatome is anæsthetic because of the overlap of skin fibres. Complete anæsthesia is no disadvantage in the chest wall or in the neck, but complete anæsthesia of one side of the face from trigeminal rhizotomy leaves an irritating numbness which many patients dislike intensely. Posterior rhizotomy of the nerves which contribute to the major limb plexuses will relieve pain only at the expense of motor function. The action of muscles depends on intact afferent as well as efferent fibres and a *totally* de-afferented limb is largely useless.

Thoracic pain from tumour invasion, root infiltration or even from other causes such as the stripping of the parietal pleura by aneurysmal dilatation of the left auricle, is most readily treated by rhizotomy. Unfortunately the pain from post-herpetic neuralgia, or the hypersensitivity and distressing pain occasionally persisting in thoracotomy wounds, is not always relieved. These pains continue to be felt in the anæsthetic area.

Shoulder and arm pain from brachial plexus invasion often defies other methods of surgical relief and some sacrifice of usefulness may have to be accepted in the arm and hand to ensure relief of pain.

Facial and head pain is sometimes best treated by extensive unilateral rhizotomy which includes not only the posterior root of the fifth but also the ninth nerve, the upper fibres of the tenth nerve and the upper three cervical posterior roots. This involves a major procedure through the posterior fossa but it can be almost guaranteed to relieve pain and prevent recurrence of pain from continued growth. Cutting the sensory root of the trigeminal nerve leaves the cornea insensitive and constant care must be taken to protect it from unnoticed damage. Injection to the Gasserian ganglion (p. 352) may give temporary relief but most tumours soon spread beyond the trigeminal area and pain recurs.

Partial block posterior roots by intrathecal chemicals was introduced in 1956 using phenol, and subsequently hypertonic saline was found to be effective. Dilute phenol (2% or 5% in lipid solutions, myodil or glycerine) when injected into the spinal canal produces a *quantitative* reduction in the fibres of the nerve roots with which it comes in contact. This in turn produces a *qualitative* change in the function of the nerves. There is a very slight decrease in the power and tone of the muscles supplied by the anterior roots, for it is impossible to keep the phenol strictly in contact with only the posterior nerve roots. Most useful of all is the *considerable rise in the threshold to pain*.

But the ease with which this small procedure can be *attempted* bears little relation to the skill needed for its *safe* performance. The phenol does not discriminate in its action on nervous tissue and as much care must be spent in keeping the phenol away from the cord, the conus and the lower sacral nerves (supplying the sphincters), as in guiding it to the roots selected for partial block. Incontinence is too high a price to pay for relief, and the sphincteric nerves lie too close to the upper sacral roots to make the method safe for low leg or perineal pain. If disease or surgery has destroyed the sphincters it can be used for low pain but otherwise it is best kept for pain in the distribution of the lumbar roots.

Phenol in lipid solution is heavier than CSF and the patient must be carefully positioned with the selected root pockets dependent in every plane. 0·2 ml. is first injected at the selected level and a subjective feeling of warmth in part of the underlying leg will indicate that the phenol is acting on the nerve root supplying that part. The injection must be stopped if the warmth is felt in the foot, perineum or buttock, or worse still in the opposite (uppermost) leg.

When hypertonic saline (7%) is used the patient lies with a head-up tilt. The affected side should be dependent, and the patient's head be raised above the level of the lumbar puncture. General anæsthesia is required, and 20–30 ml. are rapidly injected at room temperature.

The spinal cord

The spinal cord is not merely a cable carrying fibres upwards and downwards for the brain; it is part of the central nervous system and shares with it a multiplicity of collateral connections—many of the nerve fibres which enter synapse within the cord and contribute to the extensive integration of activity present at all spinal levels. A large number of the small diameter fibres believed to carry pain sensation enter the cord from the sensory roots' cross to the opposite side within

three to four segments of entering to form the spino-thalamic tracts
(fig. 77).

Antero-lateral cordotomy divides these smaller fibres in the antero-
lateral quadrant and raises the threshold to pain on the opposite side.
It is a safer and more reliable method than intrathecal phenol for pain
in the lower leg or pelvis. The two levels of choice for the operation
are at T2 and between C1 and C2. The T2 level is high enough for low
pains (the level of relative analgesia always tends to drop in the post-
operative period, often by several segments) but avoids any damage to

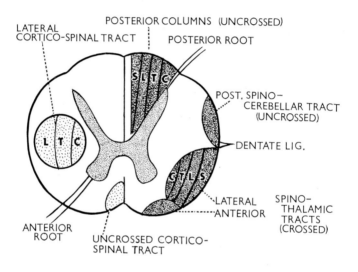

c = cervical, t = thoracic, l = lumbar, s = sacral.

Fig. 77 Spinal cord tracts, descending on left and ascending on right

the cervical enlargement. The high cervical level is necessary for all
high thoracic, arm and shoulder pain; it is a more difficult and more
dangerous procedure.

Bilateral cordotomy may be necessary for bilateral pain. It can
sometimes be judged that pain on the other side will be manageable
with drugs once it is the only pain left. At other times bilateral cordotomy is clearly going to be needed and the value of pain relief must be
weighed against the increased risks of the bilateral operation.

As many as two-thirds of the patients will have bladder difficulty,
after bilateral cord incision, and in half of these it will be permanent.

One-fifth will have noticeable loss of power in the legs. To try to minimise these dangers the two cordotomies should be performed at different levels, either at opposite ends of the exposure or at two operations, one at T1, the other at C1. Bilateral cordotomy is rarely justified for non-fatal conditions.

Percutaneous cordotomy has now replaced the open operation; it avoids a major procedure under general anaesthesia, and the lesion can be accurately titrated because the patient is fully awake and co-operative. A needle is introduced into the cord under radiographic control, usually by a lateral approach between C1 and C2 vertebræ. The site can be verified by observing the effects of electrical stimulation, andt hermal lesion is then made.

Anterior commisurotomy. The thin fibres which enter the cord from the posterior roots and cross over to the opposite side are the only group of fibres that do cross in any number. They may be cut by splitting the cord down the midline, and this may relieve pain on both sides in the segmental area corresponding to the incision.

The brain stem has been a disappointing site for surgery. After selective tractotomy either the pain relief is too incomplete and too brief, or sensory loss and ataxia are too extensive and too profound to make this a reliable method.

The thalamus can only be operated upon stereotaxically but little reliance can be placed on these operations for pain at the present time. Small lesions in the posterior thalamus might give poorly localised sensory loss, even to pin prick, but there will not necessarily be any relief of pain. The altered sensation, if it persists, may even make the pain seem worse and give an uncomfortable hypersensitivity to the skin.

On the other hand some small lesions near the midline and in the region of the ventro-postero-medial and para-fascicular nuclei may give considerable relief of pain without any detectable sensory loss. There is a tendency for pain to recur after this operation but it is possible to leave pliable electrodes within the thalamus. After a few months, when the pain recurs, more current can be passed down the electrode, the lesion further increased in size, and the pain relieved for a further period.

Neuralgia

Changes in the sensory system due to trauma, disease or degeneration can alter the conducting mechanism and thereby change the impulse patterns at any level. It appears that "non-painful" impulse patterns may be changed into "painful" impulse patterns en route. This probably plays some part in the genesis of the altered sensation in causalgia, post-herpetic neuralgia, the thalamic syndrome and painful phantom limb. When certain types of neuralgia have been established for some time they become almost impossible to eradicate. It is as though the mechanism for learning has associated pain, and nothing but pain, with the one area for so long that it eventually interprets all stimuli as pain.

Neurosurgical operations aimed at relieving neuralgias may not only be ineffective but may even initiate a new pain or unpleasant sensation which is worse than the old. One misfortune is the appearance of "anæsthesia dolorosa" where severe and continuous pain is felt in a denervated area which is quite insensitive to all external stimulation.

TRIGEMINAL NEURALGIA

Trigeminal neuralgia is the term applied to a particular facial pain which is unique amongst the neuralgias in that the pain can nearly always be completely controlled by treatment. If the same treatment is mistakenly given to patients with other forms of facial pain, they are unlikely to be improved and may be made worse.

The *age of onset* is usually over 50 years, and many patients are in the eighth or ninth decades; but it may start in patients as young as twenty-five. Its occurrence in younger patients arouses the suspicion of an associated disseminated sclerosis.

The main *clinical feature* is the sudden and severe pain that only lasts a moment and then goes, leaving nothing behind—except the fear of its return. Shaving, talking, washing or even a cold wind may disturb the skin of the upper lip and trigger a paroxysm of pain which is so severe that the patient is immobilised in agony. It is initially localised to one division of the trigeminal nerve, usually the second, but with time tends to spread to other divisions and increase in severity. Its course is interrupted by remissions of months or years of complete freedom from pain, and an elderly patient may die of an unrelated cause before it returns. It may become bilateral, either soon after its onset or after years of unilateral pain.

The trigger area may be in the gums or teeth. Some patients are given dental treatment for what is in fact trigeminal neuralgia; others seem to develop trigeminal neuralgia after prolonged and painful treatment for dental disease.

Rarely does the first paroxysm of pain occur in the ophthalmic division, but it may spread to the forehead from the cheek and later appear to start from behind the eye.

Physical signs are few. The patient may present with a scarf around his head, and talk very little and out of the corner of his mouth. Thinness and dehydration from not eating, a dirty face from not washing or shaving, all from fear of precipitating an attack of pain, may be the only signs there are. Sometimes a slight subjective loss to pin prick is found over the one side—when it can be tested for—but the corneal reflexes, which are rarely brisk in old age, are usually equal.

Treatment of Trigeminal Neuralgia

The only permanent and effective cure lies in denervation by cutting the sensory root of the trigeminal nerve. This inevitably makes that side of the face anæsthetic which is subjectively unpleasant and puts the cornea at risk from ulceration. Because many of the patients are elderly, and because there may be spontaneous remissions of pain lasting several years, there is a natural desire to try less radical measures first, and to avoid a major operation if possible. Not only are there now drugs which are adequate for many patients but there are new techniques for producing partial trigeminal nerve destruction through a needle or electrode introduced percutaneously. Open operations on the trigeminal root are therefore much less often used than previously, but may still have a place—particularly in younger patients who may be reluctant to contemplate repeated procedures. Injection methods rarely produce permanent denervation and when there is suspicion of a mass lesion adjacent to the ganglion causes the neuralgia.

Drugs

Tegretol (carbamazepine) has transformed the treatment of trigeminal neuralgia; injections and operations are much less frequently required since its introduction. In doses of 200 mg. tablets up to 4 or 5 times daily it usually controls pain within 24 hours; the dose should be the smallest needed for the relief of pain, because some ataxia and blurring of vision may occur. Indeed most patients now coming to surgery are those who require such a high dosage to control their pain that toxic effects are troublesome; virtually all patients respond with adequate dosage, and the drug may be given as a therapeutic test when the diagnosis is in doubt. Long term treatment with tegretol is not advised, as very occasionally it may cause marrow suppression; after two to three weeks freedom from pain the dosage is reduced to ascertain if a natural remission has occurred, and if it has the drug is discontinued. Analgesic drugs are virtually useless for this sudden type of pain, and should not be used.

Electro-coagulation of the retro-gasserian rootlets or the ganglion of the trigeminal nerve can bring about analgesia in a selected area of the trigeminal distribution and a differential loss of pain sensation with retention of light touch sensation. A lumbar puncture needle is inserted under radiological control through the foramen ovale at the base of the skull, into the retro-gasserian rootlets. The needle enters the cheek just above and lateral to the angle of the mouth and passes upwards and backwards between the maxilla and the vertical ramus of the mandible to the foramen ovale; it is advanced into the intracranial cavity until it lies in the trigeminal cave, which can be identified by the flow of a clear colourless cerebro-spinal fluid from the needle. The stilette is replaced by an electrode through which low voltage electric stimuli can be applied to the trigeminal rootlets. The needle is adjusted in position until the patient experiences sensations (usually paræsthesiæ, occasionally pain) in the area of which he complained of his original pain. A radiofrequency thermal lesion is made until analgesia, without anaesthesia is produced in the appropriate area of the face. This procedure has a high overall success rate and the advantage over previous procedures is that it can usually achieve pain control with much less troublesome anæsthesia of the face, mouth and tongue. If, however, only a partial lesion is made there may be recurrence; the procedure can be repeated.

Alcohol injection of the trigeminal ganglion or root has been a standard method for many years. Improved technique, using radiological control, now enables the roots to be more reliably selected—which should fire more long lasting anaesthesia; because there should be no regeneration after a root lesion. It is much more difficult to selectively save the first division with an alcohol injection, and there is therefore a risk of keratitis.

Injection or avulsion of the infra-orbital or supra-orbital nerves is sometimes of use for localized pain when there is good reason to avoid more radical measures. Injections are likely to last only 6–18 months, avulsions rather longer.

Trigeminal root section remains the most reliable and effective way of permanent denervation. The usual approach is extradurally in the middle fossa, but an alternative is intradurally through the posterior fossa—originally introduced as the best way of excluding (in dealing with) tumours involving the root. The operating microscope has made this procedure more precise, and differential section of only the affected roots can be more reliably undertaken; and the complication of facial palsy has been reduced to a rarity. The dreaded complication of neuroparalytic keratitis is therefore now seldom encountered. Although this is a major operation it is quite well tolerated by the elderly patients, who comprise most victims of this condition.

With the patient sitting up, or lying in the lateral position, a hole of about 5 cm. diameter is nibbled in the temporal bone through a vertical scalp incision above the mid-point of the zygoma. The dura is lifted from the floor of the middle fossa (and protects the temporal lobe); the middle meningeal artery is followed to the foramen spinosum, coagulated and cut. As the dura is stripped up to expose the mandibular division above the foramen ovale, care has to be taken to avoid damaging or pulling the greater superficial petrosal nerve. This little nerve arises from the geniculate ganglion, and a pull transmitted to this ganglion may produce a permanent facial palsy. The paralysed eyelid will then leave the cornea exposed; if the cornea is also made anæsthetic, and if the lacrimal gland stops secreting tears (the greater superficial petrosal nerve supplies secretor motor fibres to the gland) it will be in the greatest possible danger—dry, insensitive and exposed—and will certainly need a tarsorrhaphy to prevent neuroparalytic keratitis.

The nerve is protected at operation by splitting the thickness of the temporal dura. The lower split layer stays attached to bone and covers the nerve, and the upper split layer continues the protection of the temporal lobe.

By incising the dura of Meckel's cave it is possible to see the rootlets entering the ganglion. These are then lifted on a small hook and cut, sparing the ophthalmic rootlets, if desired. The motor root can be identified by its greater thickness and its greater obliquity as it passes medially to the ganglion on its way non-stop to the foramen ovale. It must be spared, especially if there is a chance of neuralgia developing on the other side also.

GLOSSOPHARYNGEAL NEURALGIA

The one feature that most cases of glossopharyngeal neuralgia have in common is pain triggered by swallowing. There are two main sites of the pain, the throat or tongue and the ear. If the pain appears in the one it commonly radiates to the other. The patient usually indicates the site of the pain in the throat by pointing his finger to the tip of the hyoid bone below the angle of the jaw. Long remissions of pain are common; in some patients the pain never becomes unbearable. Rarely it occurs on both sides and very occasionally it is associated with trigeminal neuralgia. When pain on swallowing is severe there is soon a temptation to stop eating and old patients may become alarmingly cachectic. There are no abnormal physical signs. The trigger spot can occasionally be identified on the back of the tongue and the pain briefly relieved by a lignocaine spray. When paroxysmal throat pain on swallowing is associated with transient syncope it certainly incriminates the ninth nerve: the innervation of the carotid sinus in the neck is responsible for the reflex bradycardia and hypotension.

There is little that will relieve glossopharyngeal neuralgia short of sectioning the ninth nerve in the posterior fossa. It is also wise to cut the upper one or two rootlets of the tenth nerve which carry sensory fibres from areas close to those in which the pain arises. It is not uncommon to find some unexpected pathology associated with the lower cranial nerves which undoubtedly bears responsibility for the pain. Glossopharyngeal and vagal neuromas are the commonest findings in what is, however, a rare presentation.

In many cases the diagnosis is difficult because the pain is diffuse and only inconstantly related to swallowing. Not all throat and tongue neuralgias will be relieved by denervation, and the operation can be performed safely only on one side; swallowing is very difficult after bilateral section.

ATYPICAL FACIAL PAIN

Facial pain which does not have the features of trigeminal or glossopharyngeal neuralgia, and does not appear to be associated with any other detectable pathology, presents a problem in diagnosis and often defies treatment.

The initial stage of trigeminal neuralgia may present as an atypical facial pain. The possibility always exists, too, that pain in the face is due to inflammation or neoplasia. It is easy for either, in the early stages, to produce pain and yet avoid detection by even the most rigorous clinical and radiological examinations. Dental malocclusion may cause pain which appropriate mechanical adjustments will relieve.

Except where the pain in the face has remained unchanged for many years, and time enough elapsed for any other pathology to manifest itself, atypical facial pain can only be a provisional diagnosis. Alcohol injections to anæsthetise the painful areas rarely relieve the pain and often appear to add to the overall discomfort.

There are a few special types of pain which can be relieved by special procedures. Some types of ear pain can be relieved by sectioning the nervus intermedius—the sensory part of the facial nerve—and other specific operations on the mid-brain tracts for trigeminal neuralgia and facial pain problems are occasionally employed. The rest of the facial neuralgias which are unassociated with any demonstrable pathology, together with many post-traumatic and post-herpetic neuralgias, may respond to local physical measures such as local freezing of the skin or percussion of the painful areas to try and "tire out" the pain, but they do not often respond to neurosurgical operations. The mechanisms of their production are not fully understood and whilst the patients must always be given sympathy they should not necessarily be given an operation, even if they ask for one.

When all these causes have been excluded there remain many patients with long-standing, aching facial pain which has none of the acute exacerbation or triggering qualities of true neuralgias. The pain may date from a dental extraction, and is commonest in middle-aged women in whom it may be the presenting feature of endogenous depression. Alcohol injections to anæsthetise the painful areas rarely relieve the pain and often appear to add to the overall discomfort.

Traumatic Neuralgia

Causalgia usually follows injury to a small nerve trunk at the wrist or in the hand. Following incomplete repair of the nerve the scar overlying it, or the incompletely re-innervated skin beyond, becomes exquisitely tender and this may render the whole arm useless. Cervical sympathectomy may cure the condition if performed early, but it is not unknown for it to be treated by serial amputations up to the shoulder with the pain persisting in either the phantom or the stump after each operation. Posterior rhizotomy, cordotomy and thalamotomy may result in a severely disabled patient with unrelieved pain who eventually takes his own life in despair.

In *post-herpetic neuralgia* the nervous tissue is damaged by infection. In the *thalamic syndrome* the damage arises usually from ischæmia or hæmorrhage. The minor stroke, which is the usual cause, may give an initial hemiparesis with a profound hemianæsthesia and sensory ataxia. Most of the power eventually returns to the side but there may be some altered posture of the limbs at rest and some athetoid movements. Most of the feeling returns to the side also, but with it a distressing hypersensitivy to the slightest stimulus. The sensation may appear to be one of almost spontaneous pain, although it is usually precipitated by light contact with clothing, or exposure to a light draught of air.

FURTHER READING

Bond, M. R. and Pearson, I. B. (1969). Psychological aspects of pain in women with advanced cancer of the cervix. *Journal of Psychosomatic Research*, **13**, 13–19.

Editorial (1968). Intractable pain. *British Medical Journal*, **3**, 513–514.

Gildenberg, P. L. (1974). Percutaneous cervical cordotomy. *Clinical Neurosurgery*, **21**, 246–256.

Henderson, W. R. (1967). Trigeminal neuralgia: the pain and its treatment. *British Medical Journal*, **1**, 7–15.

Hitchcock, E. (1969). Osmolytic neurolysis for intractable facial pain. *Lancet*, **i**, 434.

Hitchcock, E. R. (1970). Hypothermic-saline subarachnoid irrigation. *Lancet*, **i**, 843.

Killian, J. M. and Fromm, G. H. (1968). Carbamazepine in the treatment of neuralgia. *Archives of Neurology*, **19**, 129–136.

Lipton, S. (1968). Percuataneous electric cordotomy in the relief of intractable pain. *British Medical Journal*, **2**, 210.

Maher, R. (1960). Further experiences with intrathecal and subdural phenol. *Lancet*, **i**, 895–899.

Onofrio, B. M. and Campa, H. K. (1972). Evaluation of rhizotomy. Review of 12 years experience. *Journal of Neurosurgery*, **36**, 751–755.

Richards, R. L. (1967). Causalgia. *Archives of Neurology*, **16**, 339–350.

Savitz, M. H. and Mslis, L. I. (1973). Intractable pain treated with intrathecal isotonic iced saline. *Journal of Neurology, Neurosurgery and Psychiatry*, **36**, 417–420.

White, J. C. and Sweet, W. H. (1955). Pain, its mechanisms and neurological control. Thomas, Springfield.

List of Drugs

British name	*American equivalent*
thiopentone	pentothal
halothane	fluothane
methoxyflurane	penthrane
trichlorethylene	trilene
d-tubocurarine	tubarine
chlorpromazine	thorazine
fentanyl + droperidol	innovar
frusemide	lasix
betamethazone	betnesol
dexamethazone	decadron
epanutin	dilantin
pethidine	demerol

Index

Figures in bold type, e.g. **182** *refer to illustrations*